Polymers for Controlled Drug Delivery

Editor
Peter J. Tarcha, Ph.D.
Abbott Laboratories
North Chicago, Illinois

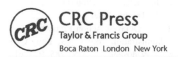

CRC Press
Taylor & Francis Group
Boca Raton London New York

CRC Press is an imprint of the
Taylor & Francis Group, an **informa** business

CRC Press
Taylor & Francis Group
6000 Broken Sound Parkway NW, Suite 300
Boca Raton, FL 33487-2742

© 1991 by Taylor & Francis Group, LLC
CRC Press is an imprint of Taylor & Francis Group, an Informa business

First issued in paperback 2019

No claim to original U.S. Government works

ISBN 13: 978-0-367-45075-5 (pbk)
ISBN 13: 978-0-8493-5652-0 (hbk)

**Visit the Taylor & Francis Web site at
http://www.taylorandfrancis.com**

**and the CRC Press Web site at
http://www.crcpress.com**

Library of Congress Cataloging-in-Publication Data

Polymers for controlled drug delivery/editor, Peter J. Tarcha.
    p. cm.
    Includes bibliographical references.
    Includes index.
    ISBN 0-8493-5652-0
    1. Controlled release preparations. 2. Polymers. 3. Drugs-
-Vehicles. I. Tarcha, Peter J.
    [DNLM: 1. Delayed-Action Preparation—administration & dosage.
2. Drug Administration Routes. 3. Drug Carriers. 4. Polymers—
administration & dosage.   QV 785 P7836]
RS201.C64P67 1990
615'.19—dc20
DLC
for Library of Congress

Library of Congress Card Number 90-2608

To
Angela

PREFACE

Polymer science has advanced to the point where the materials we use every d
been designed for high performance and favorable interaction in their intended enviro
The design and use of polymers for the enhanced delivery of therapeutic agents i:
the newest and most exciting areas in this field. Drug discovery and design has ɪ
us with numerous therapeutic agents exhibiting positive effects, but many have n
close to realizing their fullest potential *in vivo*. This is especially true for those r
from recombinant DNA technology, due to problems in delivering them in active
the desired sites of action. The body has devised elaborate mechanisms to con
production, protection, and delivery of endogenous "drugs" such as hormones, eɪ
antibodies, and mediators of the immune system. Conversely, unwanted endogenous
e.g., tumor cells, have devised ways to evade immunological surveillance. We are be
to understand some of the intricacies of these mechanisms. One of the exciting chä
which remain is the better design of macromolecules that function safely and in conc
the living organism in the delivery of therapeutic agents.

This monograph provides a treatise for the selection of polymer or polymer-based ɪ
vehicles as starting points in the attack on specific drug-delivery problems. Desiɪ
chapter to cover classes of polymers or polymeric vehicles which function by mecɪ
with some commonality, it can serve as a text for the newcomer or as a springbɪ
new ideas for the seasoned drug-delivery scientist.

Experience has taught me that the most innovative solutions are created in resɪ
well-defined problems or goals. In drug delivery, one of these goals must alwayɪ
realization of therapeutic benefit. In order for this to occur, the safety of any systeɪ
consideration must be established. Toxicity, metabolism, and elimination studies are
done in animal models first, so as to predict performance and possible problems in ɪ
Chapter 12 is included to give the drug delivery scientist a feel for what must be unɪ
in this aspect of a drug carrier's evaluation if the system is to have a chance for
trials. Successful completion of animal studies is just the beginning of the process fɪ
delivery system. The U.S. Food and Drug Administration has many stringent aɪ
requirements which must be satisfied to help insure the safety of new drug prodɪ
human use. Chapter 13 reviews this process.

I wish to thank all of the contributors and their institutions for making this moɪ
possible, and sincerely appreciate the support of Abbott Laboratories for my role
project.

Peter J. Tarcha

THE EDITOR

Peter J. Tarcha, Ph.D., is a Section Head at Abbott Laboratories.

Dr. Tarcha graduated with a B.S. in Chemistry and a Ph.D. in Polymer Science from the Institute of Materials Science at the University of Connecticut in 1983. There he specialized in polymer colloid and surface chemistry, and was a presentor at the NATO Advanced Study Institute on Polymer Colloids, Bristol, U.K., 1982.

Since joining Abbott Laboratories in 1983, Dr. Tarcha has been involved in the research and development of polymers, chemically modified surfaces, and spectroscopic methods, applied to health care. In addition, he has led a research group investigating hemoglobin-based resuscitative fluid technologies, and continues to maintain activities in this area. He has published, or has in press, 15 papers and abstracts, and has two patents pending.

CONTRIBUTORS

George A. Agyilirah, Ph.D.
Assistant Professor
College of Pharmacy
University of Minnesota
Minneapolis, Minnesota

Gilbert S. Banker, Ph.D.
Professor and Dean
College of Pharmacy
University of Minnesota
Minneapolis, Minnesota

Saul Borodkin, Ph.D.
Associate Research Fellow
Pharmaceutics R & D
Abbott Laboratories
North Chicago, Illinois

Mitchell B. Friedman, Ph.D.
Head
General Toxicology
Abbott Laboratories
North Chicago, Illinois

Dr. Mou-Ying Fu Lu, Ph.D.
Research Investigator
Control Release Section
Pharmaceutical Products Division
Abbott Laboratories
North Chicago, Illinois

Frederick A. Gustafson, M.S.
Director
HPD Regulatory Affairs
Abbott Laboratories
North Chicago, Illinois

Ann Hsu, Ph.D.
Senior Research Pharmacist
Solid Formulation Development
Abbott Laboratories
North Chicago, Illinois

Richard D. Kiernan
Manager
Department of Drug Regulatory Affairs
Burroughs Wellcome Company
Research Triangle Park, North Carolina

Richard W. Korsmeyer
Pfizer Central Research
Pfizer, Inc.
Groton, Connecticut

Kam W. Leong, Ph.D.
Assistant Professor
Department of Biomedical Engineer
School of Medicine
Johns Hopkins University
Baltimore, Maryland

R. Saul Levinson, Ph.D.
Director
Pharmaceutical Research
R. P. Scherer Corporation
Ann Arbor, Michigan

Kenneth R. Majors, M.S.
Toxicologist/Research Investigator
Department of Toxicology
Abbott Laboratories
North Chicago, Illinois

David W. Newton, Ph.D.
Chairman and Associate Professor
Department of Pharmaceutics
Albany College of Pharmacy
Albany, New York

David A. Pecosky, M.S.
Pharmaceutical Scientist
Pharmaceutical Development
Hospital Products Division
Abbott Laboratories
Abbott Park, Illinois

James C. Price, Ph.D.
Associate Professor
Department of Pharmaceutics
College of Pharmacy
University of Georgia
Athens, Georgia

Steven L. Regen, Ph.D.
Professor
Department of Chemistry
Lehigh University
Bethlehem, Pennsylvania

Joseph R. Robinson, Ph.D.
Professor
School of Pharmacy
University of Wisconsin
Madison, Wisconsin

Irving R. Schmolka, Ph.D.
Private Consultant
Gross Ile, Michigan

Kevin M. Scholsky, Ph.D.
Senior Polymer Scientist
Polymer Research Department
S.C. Johnson and Son, Inc.
Racine, Wisconsin

Peter J. Tarcha, Ph.D.
Senior Polymer Chemist
Drug Delivery Systems
Abbott Laboratories
North Chicago, Illinois

Curt Thies, Ph.D.
Professor
Biological Transport Laboratory
Department of Chemical Engineering
School of Engineering and Applied
 Sciences
Washington University
St. Louis, Missouri

TABLE OF CONTENTS

Chapter 1

DIFFUSION CONTROLLED SYSTEMS: POLYMERIC MICROCAPSULES

James C. Price

TABLE OF CONTENTS

I. INTRODUCTION

Controlled drug delivery may have originated unknowingly when medicinal su▚ were incorporated into fatty substances for application to the skin. Several thousa▚ elapsed before a concerted effort was made to control drug release in a predictable▚ for topical, oral, or any other dosage route. Now, through microencapsulation with▚ polymers, it is possible to have some control over the site of release, the onset, the i▚ and the duration of action of a drug. Although controlled release is often achieved w▚ devices as coated tablets or matrix tablets, there are incentives for the develop▚ microparticulate systems in spite of greater difficulty and expense for their productio▚ incentives include the need for liquid suspension and injectable dosage forms, as▚ better control of release characteristics, ruggedness, and failure rate.

Control of drug diffusion from the dosage form is a logical approach for dr▚ require frequent administration to maintain therapeutic levels in the body. Howeve▚ limitations are imposed on maintaining controlled drug delivery by the normal physi▚ processes of the body, and by how much drug can be enclosed conveniently in▚ dosage form. For example, retardation of diffusion alone cannot be used to ex▚ duration of release of a drug from an oral dosage form beyond its transit tim▚ gastrointestinal tract. For drugs that require large doses, few patients would be co▚ to swallow a 5- or 10-g tablet or capsule, or even several smaller tablets or capsule▚ time. Drugs that undergo extensive first-pass metabolism are also poor candidates▚ development of a controlled-release dosage form.

Polymers can be used to control the diffusion of drugs by (1) controlling how▚ the drug molecules move through the polymer molecular matrix, or by (2) contro▚ movement of dissolved drug molecules through channels or pores in a matrix perm▚ the dissolution medium. In the first case, the rate of diffusion depends on the solu▚ the drug in the polymer matrix, the size of the drug molecules, and the hindrance of m▚ by the matrix structure. In the second case, the rate of diffusion depends on the avai▚ length, and tortuosity of the pores; the solubility of the drug in the penetrating medi▚ the medium's viscosity. In a given microcapsule, both mechanisms may contribu▚ movement of the drug molecules into the dissolution environment. The extent of cont▚ by each mechanism will depend on the nature of the drug, the polymer, other micr▚ parameters, and the dissolution environment. Control of drug release with a polyr▚ can be accomplished by erosion of the polymer to release the drug, or by a combin▚ drug diffusion and polymer erosion.

II. DIFFUSION

Diffusion of a dissolved substance from a region of higher concentration to a r▚ lower concentration is a spontaneous process that stems from the thermal motion of m▚ and results in a decrease in free energy of the system. The measure of the tender▚ substance to diffuse is usually expressed as the diffusion coefficient, D. The units a▚ cm^2/sec, but may be m^2/sec or others. An expression describing the diffusion coeff▚ two gases can be written as

$$D = 1/3\ y_1 c_1 X_2 + 1/3\ y_2 c_2 X_1$$

where y_1, y_2 are the mean free paths of the molecules, c_1, c_2 are the average spe▚ X_1, X_2 are the mole fractions. The diffusion of a molecule in a liquid is much less ra▚ in gases, and diffusion in solids is usually even slower because of the constraint▚ surrounding molecules. However, flexible polymers such as silicone rubber ma▚ diffusion rates approaching those in mobile liquids.

For a homogeneous polymer, Fick's first law, describing movement of molecules of a substance through a medium, is often stated in the form

$$J = -D \, dC/dx, \tag{2}$$

where J is the permeant flux (g/cm^2/sec), D is the diffusion coefficient, and dC/dx is the concentration gradient in the diffusion medium. The diffusion coefficient, D, is related to the molecular size and the microscopic viscosity of the diffusion environment, as shown by the Einstein equation

$$D = kT/6 \, \pi r \eta, \tag{3}$$

where k is the Boltzman constant, T is the absolute temperature, r is the molecular collision radius, and η is the microscopic viscosity.

For porous membranes in which the diffusing substance diffuses through pores filled with a liquid (usually aqueous), Fick's law is modified[1] to account for the porosity and tortuosity of the pores as follows:

$$J = D' \, K' \, \epsilon \, \Delta C/\tau \, l, \tag{4}$$

where D' is the diffusion coefficient in the liquid phase filling the pores, ϵ is the porosity, τ is the tortuosity, l is the average length of the pores, ΔC is the difference in concentrations of the solutions just inside and outside of the membrane, and K' is the permeant distribution coefficient between the fluid in the pores and the surrounding fluid. K' is one (1) when these liquids are the same.

The permeability P (cm/sec) of a membrane or polymeric shell is defined as

$$P = DK/h, \tag{5}$$

with h being the thickness of the shell, and K the partition coefficient. When the diffusion and the partition coefficients are not independently known, P is sometimes defined as P = DK, and is expressed in the units cm^2/sec, rather than cm/sec.

An alternative way of specifying the characteristics of the shell or membrane is the limiting flux[1],

$$J_{lim} = JhC/C_s, \tag{6}$$

where C is the concentration of the core substance in the solvent behind the membrane, and C_s is the solubility in the solvent. The concept of limiting flux using the fractional solubility, C/C_s, is helpful when comparing diffusion data from different solvents.

Considering Fickian diffusion with sink conditions, the factors affecting the apparent rate of release of core molecules can be reduced to:

1. The diffusion path length
2. The molecular collision radius of the diffusing substance
3. The microscopic viscosity of the diffusion environment
4. The surface area of the dosage form in contact with the sink medium
5. The concentration difference between the start of molecular diffusion and the sink

These factors are expanded upon below.

Diffusion path length — For a polymeric device that shows no change in dimensions for the duration of the diffusion, the diffusion path length is affected by the polyme ratio, the porosity and the tortuosity of the polymer, and, in matrix systems, the p size and positioning of the core substance. These factors offer avenues of explorati modifying the release rate of such devices.

Molecular collision radius of the diffusing substance — Selection of appr derivatives of a drug can offer some degree of modification, but other factors such as sol (and, therefore, concentration difference) will be changed.

Viscosity of the diffusion environment — In porous polymer matrices the pore be small enough to exclude macromolecular drugs from the dissolution environme which case diffusion of molecules from the core will be through an environment of molecules whose momentary structure may be modified by the pore surface. When the are comparatively large, macromolecular substances may modify the immediate e mental viscosity. In any event, it is the microscopic viscosity rather than the bulk vi that determines diffusion rate.

Surface area of the dosage form — A major factor that can be controlled by proc or formulation is the diameter of the microcapsules; however, this will depend on th sizes that are achievable. Other factors, such as surface roughness and imperfection contribute to the total surface area of the dosage form, but are less easily controlled

Concentration difference — Under sink conditions, this factor is controlled solubility of the core in the microcapsule diffusion environment.

III. POLYMERIC MICROCAPSULES

A microcapsule may be defined as any small particle that consists of an activ material whose dissolution and other physical properties are modified by the prese some inert carrier material. Polymeric microcapsules can take many useful form "core" material may be in the form of a distinct single solid mass surrounded by the c it may be dissolved (molecularly dispersed) in the carrier, or the core may be distrib the carrier matrix in the form of solid particles that can be of any size, ranging from a large mass nearly as large as the whole microcapsule, down to colloidal-sized unit "carrier" can take the form of a solid material permeable only to small molecules o or it can be perforated with relatively large pores through which solutions can freely pen

A. RESERVOIR MICROCAPSULES WITH RATE CONTROLLING SHELL

Microcapsules that contain core reservoirs surrounded by shells that limit the diffusion of the drug into the surrounding environment (Figure 1A) are the simp describe. They offer two distinct advantages: the possibility of zero-order release c teristics, and low polymer-to-core ratios (with minimum bulk, lower cost). A disadv is that they are more fragile than matrix microcapsules.

The requirements for zero-order release from the microcapsules are as follows:

1. The shells (membranes) remain intact and unchanged during release.
2. The movement of core molecules through the shell is the rate limiting step dissolution process.
3. The concentration of core molecules inside the limiting shell surface remains co This condition is fulfilled when there is a saturated solution of the core insi shell, and there is an excess of solid core material available to dissolve.
4. All of the microcapsules in a dose should have similar release rates and drug

For microcapsules having shells of practical thickness and finite cores, release core material will likely show three stages:

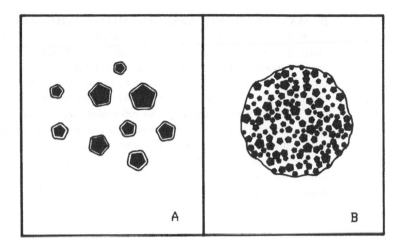

FIGURE 1. Cross-sectional views of microcapsules. Pentagonal shapes represent drug cores. A. Reservoir microcapsules; B. Matrix microcapsule.

1. An initial phase that may exhibit either rapid or delayed release. Rapid release results from diffusion of core molecules out of a saturated shell. A delay or lag time is indicative of equilibration of continuous phase and/or core molecules with the shell or its pores.
2. A zero-order release phase that lasts until almost all the solid or liquid core has been depleted.
3. A final phase where only a solution of the core remains, and whose concentration is constantly decreasing.

Release characteristics in the last phase will be first-order. The duration of the zero-order phase is dependent on the relative amount of the core and the rate of release. It is interesting to note that with this type of system, the microcapsule shells can be solid, granular, porous, rough, or smooth; spheres, cylinders, cubes, or any other shape, and, as long as the above conditions are fulfilled, zero-order release can be achieved from microcapsule populations with uniform characteristics.

The actual rate of release from such microcapsules during the zero-order phase is controlled by the concentration gradient between the inside and outside of the shell, shell thickness, and shell permeability. When microcapsules have shells with near-zero porosity, and movement of the core molecules is by diffusion through the shell matrix, then high solubility of the core material in the shell polymer is favorable for more rapid release, because the concentration difference between the outer wall and the aqueous dissolution environment is higher (assuming that partition coefficients of the high solubility and low solubility cores are similar). When the shell is porous enough to allow movement of environmental solvent to the core, then high solubility of drug in that solvent is favorable for rapid release. Shell thickness can be used to control release rate; however, it has been noted that once the ratio of the outer radius to inner radius reaches about four in a spherical particle, further increases result in little change in release rate.[1] Shell permeability can be influenced by many factors, such as the type of polymer, its molecular weight, the presence of plasticizers (increase), insoluble fillers (decrease), and porosity. The *total* release rate (as opposed to the unit release rate) will depend on the surface area presented by the dose to the environmental solvent, and the combined characteristics of all the microcapsule units in the dose.

B. MATRIX MICROCAPSULES (MONOLITHIC MICROCAPSULES)

Matrix microcapsules can be described as solid polymer systems in which material is distributed more or less uniformly throughout the polymer matrix. The may be molecularly distributed as a solid solution in the polymer, may be large form of micronized particles, or may be in the form of particles whose size is a su fraction of that of the microcapsule. Sometimes the microcapsule can contain a mi core particles from macroscopic to molecular size. An advantage to matrix micro is ruggedness. Dissolution characteristics are less likely to be altered by pressure or al An illustration of this morphology is shown in Figure 1B.

Except for special circumstances, core release from such microcapsules is n order, but a substantial fraction of the release of many such systems is described Higuchi models.[3] For spherical microcapsules a simplified equation is:

$$1 + 2F - 3F^{2/3} = Kt$$

where F describes the fraction of drug remaining, as a function of time, t.

For microspheres having a homogeneous matrix, the equation is

$$K = 6 DC_s/Ar_o^2.$$

Here D is the diffusion coefficient, C_s is the solubility of the drug in the matrix, initial concentration of drug in the matrix, and r_o is the radius of the microsphere.

For microspheres that are not homogeneous (granular),

$$K = 6 DC_s V_{sp}/\tau Ar_o^2,$$

where V_{sp} is the specific volume of the drug and τ is the tortuosity of the porous The specified conditions for these models are that A is substantially greater than C_s a pseudo-steady state results shortly after the extraction begins. Typical dissoluti from matrix microspheres with fairly uniform characteristics[4] are shown in Figure of the same data up to 95% dissolution using the Higuchi relationship for spherica particles are shown in Figure 3. Dissolution rate decreases with increasing particle can be readily shown by substitution into Equation 7 that the 50% dissolution tim 0.5) is proportional to r^2. This is often confirmed by experimental data (Figure 4 release from a matrix system is perhaps more difficult to model than a reservoir-m system because of the greater number of variables to account for. In addition to shell thickness and surface area considerations, drug loading and drug particle size interacting effects on dissolution. At low drug loading, and where drug release is of dissolution into the polymer matrix followed by diffusion through the matri environmental interface, a decrease in particle size of the drug results in an increas of drug release[6] (see Figure 5). At high drug loadings, and where solubility of the the membrane is unimportant, reduction of drug particle size is likely to have the effect,[7] as seen in Figure 6. This is because, at high drug loadings, particles are together, and many are in contact with other particles. As the particles dissolve, th channels in the microcapsule matrix, thus increasing access to the dissolution envir Very small particles dispersed in the polymer are less likely to form continuous cha they dissolve.

IV. PREPARATION OF POLYMERIC MICROCAPSULE

The selection of polymers and method of manufacture of drugs containing micro are limited to avoid exposing patients to toxic substances. These include the bre

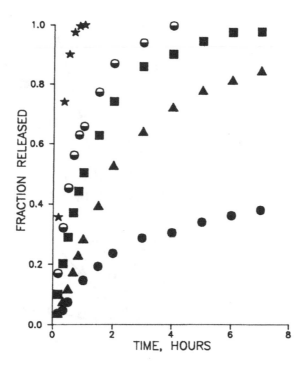

FIGURE 2.   Dissolution profiles of matrix microcapsules showing effect of polycaprolactone:cellulose acetate propionate polymer ratio. Polymer ratio ★ = 3.0:0.0; ◒ = 2.25:0.75; ■ =
1.5:1.5; ▲ = 0.75:2.25; ● = 0.0:3.0. (From Chang, R. K., et
al,[4] Control of drug release rates through the use of mixtures of
polycaprolactone and cellulose propionate polymers, *Pharm.
Technol.*, 10, 29, 1986. With permission.)

products of polymers, or traces of toxic substances such as monomers used for polymerization, or chlorinated solvents used in processing. The polymers most often used for controlled release microcapsules are either natural products or simple derivatives of naturally
occurring polymers; however, the use of polymethacrylates has been investigated.[8,9]

Because of the large surface area presented by microparticulate dosage forms, the permeability of the coating or matrix material of the microcapsules must be lower than that for a
typical coated or matrix tablet. Polymers which swell appreciably in aqueous body fluids
are likely to release the drug core too rapidly to be useful.

Cellulose derivatives with potential to achieve controlled drug release are the esters:
cellulose acetates, cellulose acetate propionates, and cellulose acetate butyrates, all of which
are readily available. At the present time, the most widely used polymer for retarding
dissolution of a drug for oral dosage is ethyl cellulose, a cellulose derivative in which part
of the hydroxyl sites are substituted with ethoxyl groups. It is available in various grades,
whose properties are dependent upon the degree of ethoxyl substitution and the molecular
weight. Commercial grades are available with substitution of 2.25 to 2.60 ethoxyl units per
anhydroglucose unit (44 to 50% ethoxyl content).[10] A cellulose ester derivative that has seen
commercial application is cellulose acetate butyrate, in which hydroxyl sites have been
substituted with acetate and butyryl ester groups. Properties of this polymer vary according
to the relative substitution of acetyl and butyryl groups. The polymers are more hydrophobic
and somewhat less permeable to water with increasing butyryl content. Other cellulose esters
no doubt have potential for controlled release, but are less readily available.

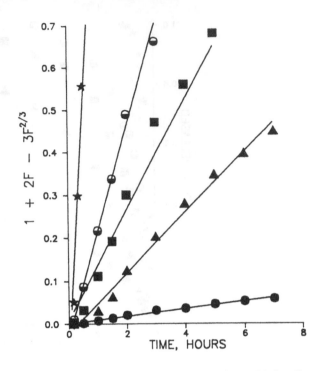

FIGURE 3.   Higuchi spherical matrix dissolution model plots. F = fraction of drug remaining, data and symbols same as in Figure 2. (From Chang, R. K., et al.,[4] Control of drug release rates through the use of mixtures of polycaprolactone and cellulose propionate polymers, *Pharm. Technol.*, 10, 29, 1986. With permission.)

For parenteral use, it is desirable to use a polymer that is biocompatible and bioer⬛ Much work with this type of dosage form has been done using polylactic acid and copo⬛ with polyglycolic acid, which are hydrolytically degraded in the body to hydroxycarb⬛ acids and eventually metabolized to carbon dioxide and water. Bioerodible syste⬛ covered in detail in Chapters 7 and 8.

There are many methods of creating polymer microcapsules. The earliest, most researched, and commercially utilized is coacervation, in which a polymer disperse⬛ suitable solvent is caused to separate out as an insoluble liquid phase that collects ⬛ suspended drug particles or globules. Because of the wide use of this method ⬛ importance historically and commercially, it is discussed in Chapter 4.

Emulsion methods — Several methods of achieving encapsulation rely upon e⬛ fication at some stage of the process, including interfacial polymerization, interfacia⬛ ervation, melt/congeal methods, emulsion polymerization, and emulsion-solvent evapora⬛

Interfacial polymerization, in which polymerization is caused to take place aro⬛ emulsion droplet containing the desired core material, suffers from having to use p⬛ toxic monomers in processing, traces of which may remain with the final product⬛ the microcapsule walls tend to be very thin with high permeability to small drug mo⬛ because of the interfacial nature of the polymerization. Interfacial coacervation ⬛ emulsion droplets can be induced when a polymer solution is brought into interfacial ⬛ with a solvent. This method also tends to produce microcapsules with thin walls⬛ methods were described by T. M. S. Chang and coworkers.[11] Interfacially-produc⬛ crocapsules are usually more suitable for artificial cells or protective coatings than for ⬛ of diffusion of drugs because of the rapidity with which small drug molecules diffuse t⬛ the thin membrane walls.

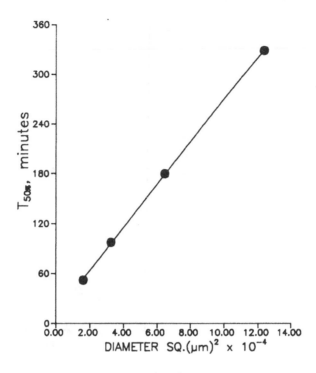

FIGURE 4. Relationship of 50% dissolution time to square of microcapsule diameter. Cellulose acetate butyrate microspheres containing propranolol 0.8:1 drug:polymer ratio. (From Chiao, S. L. C.,[5] Ph.D. Dissertation, University of Georgia, Athens, 1988.)

If a liquid monomer containing core material is emulsified in a nonsolvent medium, the droplets that are formed can be caused to polymerize by means of a catalyst. Thus the core is trapped in the solid or rubbery polymer. Depending on the conditions, the nature of the core and monomer/polymer, the core can be trapped in matrix form as a solid solution, or as single core surrounded by polymer. Many polymers have been used with this method, but most applications have been for nonmedical purposes. However, C. S. Deng reported the preparation of Silastic® silicone rubber microspheres containing phenobarbital in 1972 and dexamethasone in 1976.[12,13] As with interfacial polymerization, the possibility of traces of unreacted monomer or noxious catalysts remaining with the microcapsules is a deterrent to the use of the method for medical purposes.

Methods other than polymerization can be used to harden or solidify a potential encapsulating agent. Thus, sodium alginate and chitosan solutions can be solidified by exposure to calcium chloride or HCl. Chitosan solution can be solidified by exposure to calcium chloride or HCl. Chitosan solution can be solidified by change of pH or by the use of a nonsolvent such as acetone. Likewise, heat can be used to denature some natural polymers such as albumin. A widely used method of preparation of albumin microspheres is simply to emulsify a solution of the albumin in an immiscible oil and then to heat the emulsion until the albumin is denatured. Drugs or other adjuncts that were included in the original albumin solution can be trapped in this manner if they do not partition into the oily phase and are not degraded by the heat in the aqueous environment. Magnetic microspheres are often prepared by this method.[14]

Waxes and low-melting polymers can be used as encapsulating agents with the melt/congeal method. The drug is added to a melted agent, and the mixture is emulsified in a suitable nonsolvent liquid at the same temperature as the melted agent. Then the temperature

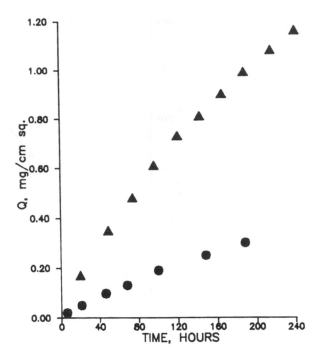

FIGURE 5.   Effect of drug particle size on chlormadinone release from a silicone matrix; low (10%) drug concentration. ● = Macroparticles; ▲ = Micronized particles. (From Haleblian, J. et al.,[6] Steroid release from silicone elastomer containing excess drug in suspension, *J. Pharm. Sci.*, 60, 541, 1971. With permission.)

of the emulsified system is reduced to below the congealing point of the encapsul
solidified particles can then be recovered from the dispersing medium.

The most widely applicable emulsion method for drug encapsulation is emulsion
evaporation. This method has its origins in a process patented in 1939[15] and 1940[16]
gelatin beadlets containing fish oils as a source for vitamins A and D. As originally de
a gelatin solution containing about 20% gelatin was heated to about 65°, and the
was emulsified in the melted gelatin. The resulting emulsion was then emulsified
medium at the same temperature to give a three-phase emulsion in which the gelati
the internal phase in an oily suspending medium. A reduction in temperature conge
gelatin droplets, from which most of the water could then be removed by evapor
alternatively, by the use of some extracting solvent such as alcohol. At the time,
"microcapsule" was not applied to the product and the coating was intended to
the stability and ease of handling, and improve the taste of the oils. Controlled or s
release was not intended or accomplished. As can be seen, the process contains
of both melt/congeal and emulsion-solvent evaporation.

In more recent applications of the method, the encapsulating polymer is diss
acetone, alcohol, or more exotic solvents; the drug is added to form a suspension, e
or solution, and the resulting mix is then emulsified in a medium that is nonsolven
polymer and drug. The solvent for the encapsulating polymer must not be miscible
dispersion medium. After emulsification, the polymer solvent is encouraged to e
with continued stirring, application of heat, reduced pressure, or all three. The s
microcapsules are then recovered from the medium by various means. A patent cov
of the variations of polymer solvent and dispersing media for this method.[17] Micro
that result from the processes are most often matrix microspheres.

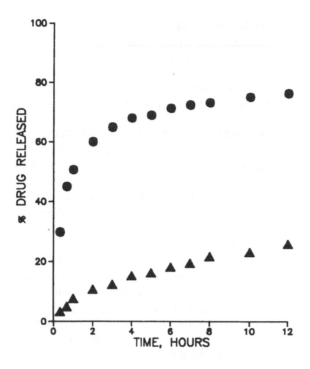

FIGURE 6. Effect of drug particle size on dissolution from cellulose acetate propionate matrix microcapsules containing theophylline; high (50%) drug concentration. ▲ = Micronized drug particles; ● = Macro-particles. (From Shukla, A. J. and Price, J. C., Effect of drug (core) particle size on the dissolution of theophylline from microspheres made from low molecular weight cellulose acetate propionate, *Pharm. Res.*, 6, 418, 1989. With permission.)

V. CHARACTERIZATION OF MICROPARTICULATE DRUG DELIVERY SYSTEMS

Because of the many variables possible during the processing of microcapsules, characterization of the particles is essential both during development of a delivery system and for quality assurance after processing procedures have been established. Physical factors that are important to the delivery characteristics include microcapsule size and size distribution, surface area accessible to the dissolution environment, porosity, density, drug loading, and drug core particle size.

A. MICROCAPSULE SIZE

The rate of drug release of many microcapsule systems is inversely proportional to the square of the particle size. Therefore, any change in mean particle size or size distribution can affect release rate. For microcapsules with diameters above 38 μm, ordinary sieving methods can be used, but it must be remembered that aggregates cannot be detected, and therefore microscopic observation should be carried out on all batches. The distribution of sizes in a batch of microcapsules is likely to be log-normal because of the manner in which the microcapsules are made or the core particles are prepared. In such cases, analysis of the particle counts or separations can be conveniently carried out by standard methods such as Hatch-Choate analysis.[18,19]

B. SURFACE AREA

Surface area per unit weight of smooth, nonporous, spherical microcapsules is in proportional to the statistical diameter, but the presence of pores and irregularities surface of the particles affects surface area presented to the dissolution environme may affect dissolution rate. Nitrogen or krypton gas adsorption can be useful to det surface areas[20] if the microcapsules are relatively free of moisture or volatile substa

C. DENSITY AS A FUNCTION OF POROSITY

Porosity (the fraction or percent of void space in a microcapsule) can greatly af properties. If a substantial portion of the void space is closed off, changes may evident from surface area studies, but would be reflected in the density. Therefo calculating the theoretical density from the proportions of components in the microca and comparing with the actual measured density, porosity can be estimated.

D. DRUG LOADING

Although the theoretical concentration may be close to the actual drug loading ideal conditions, there are several possibilities for nontheoretical encapsulation for a cesses. Loading can vary with microcapsule size (even in the same batch), core size, processing temperature, and processing time, as well as variation in formulatio ponents. In addition to batch analysis, individual particle size fractions should be an separately for drug content. If polymer or other components do not interfere, b microcapsule and drug can be dissolved in an appropriate solvent, and the drug an directly. Sometimes it is more effective to leach out the drug core using a nonsolv the polymer. Alternatively, the polymer can be dissolved off the core with a selective s and the core then dissolved in an appropriate solvent for analysis.

E. DISSOLUTION TESTING

In vitro dissolution testing of microcapsules is a capstone characterization test, the of which are linked to many of the other properties of the microcapsules. Dissolutio should not be regarded as duplicating clinical conditions, but as indicators of how or slowly the microcapsules give up their drug contents, relative to other batches o formulations. When biological absorption is faster than the dissolution process, it n possible to link *in vitro* dissolution to bioavailability. However, it must be remember the presence or absence of food in the gut, or even the type of food present, can alte the dissolution and absorption of a drug from microcapsules or other dosage forms.

With regard to the actual testing procedure, the USP Paddle Method[21] is convenie uses standardized equipment. This and other compendial methods and some noncomp general methods of dissolution testing are covered in Hanson's book on dissolution tes Preparations intended for oral dosage should be tested initially with solutions of at lea pH values, a low pH solution such as Simulated Gastric Fluid, USP; and a slightly a solution such as Simulated Intestinal Fluid, USP. A slightly acid test solution, e.g., p may be appropriate for some drugs. Enzymes are usually omitted from these solutic the tests. Testing at other pH values between pH 2 and 7.5 also may be appropria initial evaluation. Microcapsules intended for environments other than the gastroint (GI) tract should be tested with solutions at a pH appropriate to the dosing environm small quantity of nonionic surfactant, such as polysorbate 80, is often added to the dissc test solution to assure complete wetting of the microcapsules and more closely appro dosing conditions. For most drugs, ultraviolet or visible spectrophotometric absorptio ysis methods are satisfactory. To eliminate uncertainty from light-scattering when susp microcapsules are present, Shively and Simonelli have suggested the use of dual-wave spectrophotometry.[23]

VI. APPLICATION VS. THEORY

If all experiments turned out as planned or predicted, researchers would never have to enter the laboratory, and production of a dosage form would only require the acquisition of appropriate processing equipment, measurement of the formulation ingredients, then processing according to plan. As everyone knows, even the simplest production process can go awry. Microencapsulation processes seldom achieve perfection, and models that describe dissolution from theoretical microcapsules usually do not allow for imperfections. Models do, however, help us to determine the nature of the imperfections, thereby allowing us to attempt to correct them, or perhaps, helping us to decide whether or not we can live with them. Strictly speaking, models describe dissolution from *individual* microcapsules, whereas dissolution tests (or doses) are of *populations* of microcapsules. It is sometimes overlooked that multiparticulate systems are usually made up of a distribution of sizes; the character of the distribution may contribute more to the character of the dissolution curve than the particular type of kinetics exhibited by individual particles. Dappert and Thies gave an excellent discussion of drug release from multiparticulate systems, and pointed out that although individual microcapsules may release at a constant rate, individual release rate constants are often distributed log-normally in the population.[24] In such a population, the release curve will approximate first-order kinetics, frequently observed in multiparticulate systems. It has been well documented by Donbrow and co-workers that dissolution from

populations of microcapsules can follow various types of kinetics, depending on the statistical distributions of parameters such as drug loading or release rate constants of individual particles. Hoffman et al. followed dissolution of individual microcapsules using conductivity and spectrophotometric methods to show constant release rates, which varied from particle to particle, but the overall population gave first-order dissolution profiles.[25,26] Gross et al. developed statistical models for the release kinetics of non-monodisperse multiparticulate microcapsule systems.[27] Donbrow et al. reported experimental and simulated release profiles of individual microcapsules and populations to demonstrate first-order, sigmoid, square root of time, and other kinetics, from particles which individually release at a constant rate.[28]

For some microcapsules, it may be very inconvenient or impossible to follow dissolution of individual particles to confirm the mechanism by which the drug is released. There is also the danger that insufficient numbers of particles are examined so that the results are not representative of the total population. Populations of particles are often polydisperse with respect to size, and may be polydisperse with respect to payload, rate constant, and lag time. If the population sampled is made monodisperse with respect to pertinent parameters, then the population dissolution kinetics will closely approximate the dissolution profile expected from the appropriate model of the microcapsule system. Nearly monodisperse size can be approximated by taking narrow sieve cuts of the population. Analysis of drug content of these cuts can give information about the payload contained in various size fractions and the variation thereof, indicating the uniformity (or monodispersity) of the coating process. Madan et al. reported zero-order release of populations of nearly monodisperse clofibrate microcapsules,[29] and close conformity of matrix microspheres to the Higuchi model for spherical monoliths has been reported for uniform samples.[3]

REFERENCES

1. **Baker, R. W.,** *Controlled Release of Biologically Active Agents,* John Wiley & Sons, New York, 1987.
2. **Sayed, H. A. and Price, J. C.,** Tablet properties and dissolution characteristics of compressed cellulose acetate butyrate microcapsules containing succinyl sulfathiazole, *Drug Dev. Ind. Pharm.,* 12, 577, 1986.

3. **Higuchi, T.,** Mechanism of sustained action medication. Theoretical analysis of rate of releas drugs dispersed in solid matrices, *J. Pharm. Sci.,* 52, 1145, 1963.

4. **Chang, R. K., Price, J. C., and Whitworth, C. W.,** Control of drug release rates through mixtures of polycaprolactone and cellulose propionate polymers, *Pharm. Technol.,* 10, 29, 198

5. **Chiao, S. L. C.,** Formulation and Evaluation of Disintegrating Controlled Release Tablets C Encapsulated Propranolol Hydrochloride, Ph.D. dissertation, University of Georgia, Athens, 19

6. **Haleblian, J., Runkel, R., Mueller, N., Christopherson, J., and Ng, K.,** Steroid release fro elastomer containing excess drug in suspension, *J. Pharm. Sci.,* 60, 541, 1971.

7. **Shukla, A. J. and Price, J. C.,** Effect of drug (core) particle size on the dissolution of theophy microspheres made from low molecular weight cellulose acetate propionate, *Pharm. Res.,* 6, 4

8. **Lehman, K., Boessler, H., and Dreher, D.,** Controlled drug release from small particles en with acrylic resins, *Acta Pharm. Suec.,* 13, suppl., 37, 1976.

9. **Pongpaibul, Y., Price, J., and Whitworth, C.,** Preparation and evaluation of controlled rel methacin microspheres, *Drug Dev. Ind. Pharm.,* 10, 1597, 1984.

10. *Handbook of Pharmaceutical Excipients,* Monograph on Ethylcellulose, American Pharmaceut ciation, Washington, D.C., 1986, 113.

11. **Chang, T. M. S., MacIntosh, F. C., and Mason, S. G.,** Semipermeable aqueous microca Preparation and properties, *Can. J. Physiol. Pharmacol.,* 44, 115, 1965.

12. **Deng, C. S. M.,** Production and Evaluation of Drug Containing Silastic® Microspheres, Maste University of Georgia, Athens, 1972.

13. **Deng, C. S. M.,** Development of Controlled Release Dexamethasone — Containing Silicon Microspheres, Ph.D. dissertation, University of Georgia, Athens, 1976.

14. **Widder, K., Flouret, G., and Senyei, A.,** Magnetic microspheres: synthesis of a novel paren carrier, *J. Pharm. Sci.,* 68, 79, 1979.

15. "Vitamin Preparations," British Patent 490,001, Atlantic Coast Fisheries Company, 1939, thr 33, 814, 1939.

16. **Reynolds, S.,** "Compositions of Gelatin with Vitamin A", U.S. Patent 2,183,084, 1940, throug 2140, 1940.

17. **Kitajima, M., Kondo, A., Morishita, M., and Abe, J.,** "Process for preparing a microcapsu Patent 3,714,065, 1973.

18. **Hatch, T. and Choate, S. P.,** Statistical description of the size properties of non-uniform substances, *J. Franklin Inst.,* 207, 369, 1929.

19. **Hatch, T.,** Determination of "average particle size" from screen-analysis of non-uniform substances, *J. Franklin Inst.,* 215, 27, 1933.

20. **Lowell, S. and Shields, J. E.,** *Powder Surface Area and Porosity,* Chapman and Hall, New Yo

21. *United States Pharmacopeia,* XXII, 1578, The United States Pharmacopeial Convention, Rockv 1989.

22. **Hanson, W. A.,** *Handbook of Dissolution Testing,* Pharmaceutical Technology Publications, S OR, 1982.

23. **Shively, M. L. and Simonelli, A. P.,** The investigation of dual-wavelength spectroscopy for th of dissolved drug in microcapsule suspensions, *Int. J. Pharm.,* 50, 39, 1989.

24. **Dappert, T. and Thies, C.,** Statistical models for controlled release microcapsules: rationale a *J. Membr. Sci.,* 4, 99, 1978.

25. **Hoffman, A., Donbrow, M., and Benita, S.,** Direct measurements on individual microcapsule d as a tool for determination of release mechanism, *J. Pharm. Pharmacol.,* 38, 764, 1986.

26. **Hoffman, A., Donbrow, M., Benita, S., and Bahat, R.,** Fundamentals of release mechanism inte in multiparticulate systems: determination of substrate release from single microcapsules and relatio individual and ensemble release kinetics, *Int. J. Pharm.,* 29, 195, 1986.

27. **Gross, S., Hoffman, A., Donbrow, M., and Benita, S.,** Fundamentals of release mechanism inte in multiparticulate systems: the prediction of the commonly observed release equations from population models for particle ensembles, *Int. J. Pharm.,* 29, 213, 1986.

28. **Donbrow, M., Hoffman, A., and Benita, S.,** Variation of population release kinetics in po multiparticulate systems (microcapsules, microspheres, droplets, cells) with heterogeneity of on three parameters in the population of individuals, *J. Pharm. Pharmacol.,* 40, 93, 1988.

29. **Madan, P. L., Madan, D. K., and Price, J. C.,** Clofibrate microcapsules: preparation and re studies, *J. Pharm. Sci.,* 65, 1476, 1976.

Chapter 2

DIFFUSION CONTROLLED SYSTEMS: HYDROGELS

Richard W. Korsmeyer

TABLE OF CONTENTS

I. INTRODUCTION

A hydrogel is a water-swollen network polymer. Familiar hydrogels include desserts and soft contact lenses. All hydrogels, regardless of their actual origin, ▮ thought of as being composed of hydrophilic monomer units linked to form a water ▮ polymer, and then crosslinked to form an insoluble network. The crosslinks hold▮ network together can be covalent, ionic, or hydrogen bonds; crystals; or simply p▮ entanglements. The physical properties of the hydrogel derive from the nature of the ▮ links, as well as the monomer. In the swollen state, the properties of the hydrogel are s▮ influenced by its water content, which often exceeds its polymer content. The comb▮ of high water content with water insolubility makes these materials well suited to a ▮ of applications such as absorbent materials, membranes for separations, soft tissue r▮ ments, contact lenses, and even to improve moisture retention in soil. The numerc▮ plications of hydrogels in medicine and pharmacy have recently inspired publicatic▮ three-volume set covering many aspects of material properties and applications.▮ specifically, there has been considerable interest in exploiting the unique proper▮ hydrogels in the area of controlled-release technology. The purpose of this chapt▮ review the most important properties of hydrogels as they relate to controlled rele▮ summarize the major techniques of preparation, and to give examples of a few inte▮ applications. In keeping with the theme of this book, the emphasis is more on the m▮ themselves than on the techniques and problems of drug delivery.

II. STRUCTURE AND PHYSICAL PROPERTIES OF HYDROG

The fundamental building block of a hydrogel is the water-soluble monomer. ▮ different monomers can be used, ranging from hydrophilic vinyl-type monomers to ▮ and amino acids. The latter two are obtained from natural sources already in polymeric▮ The monomer is then polymerized, either by nature, as in the polysaccharides and pr▮ or by a synthetic process. The crosslinking of the polymer to form the hydrogel n▮ may be done either during the polymerization, obtaining the hydrogel directly, or af▮ water-soluble polymer has already been formed (see below). In addition to the ▮ chemical characteristics of the parent monomers, the resulting network is characteri▮ the average distance between crosslinks (usually expressed in molecular weight a▮ which has a strong effect on its properties.

A. THERMODYNAMICS AND SWELLING BEHAVIOR

In the dry state, hydrogels (often called xerogels when dry) are generally rathe▮ with properties ranging from "leathery" to "glassy." However, when the material is ▮ in an aqueous medium, water is imbibed, and the gel swells to an equilibrium defi▮ the point at which the swelling pressure is balanced by the retractive force of the ne▮ The swelling pressure is the result of the difference in water activity inside and outsi▮ polymer, and is analogous to an osmotic pressure. Unlike osmotic pressure, the sv▮ pressure is not a colligative property because, owing to the crosslinked structure ▮ polymer, there is really only one molecule in "solution." The final water content d▮ on the hydrophilicity of the polymer and the degree of crosslinking, and can range ▮ well over 90%.

Theoretical treatments of network swelling are based on thermodynamic descripti▮ the two counterbalancing forces. Both polymer solution thermodynamics and netwo▮ chanical properties are areas of active research interest, and all current theories have ▮ shortcomings.[2,3] However, the purposes of this chapter will be served well enough ▮ classical treatment of Flory,[4,5] which is summarized below.

The free energy change due to swelling may be described as the sum of the change due to mixing of the polymer with the solvent, plus the change in elastic free energy due to deformation of the network:

$$\Delta G = \Delta G_M + \Delta G_{el} \tag{1}$$

This is the fundamental assumption (known as the Flory-Rehner[5] additivity assumption) of network swelling theory. Gottlieb[2], and Eichinger and Neuberger[3] have argued that discrepancies between theory and experiment cannot be explained by refinement of solution thermodynamics and elasticity theory (see below) alone, and that this assumption should be reconsidered. The author believes that the additivity assumption is adequate to the purpose of this chapter.

The free energy of mixing is usually described by the Flory-Huggins liquid lattice model which, for a gel, is

$$(\mu_1 - \mu_1^0) = -RT[ln(1 - \upsilon_2) + \upsilon_2 + \chi\upsilon_2^2] \tag{2}$$

where μ_1 is the chemical potential of the solvent υ_2 is the volume fraction of polymer in the gel, and χ is a heat of mixing parameter which gives the polymer-solvent interaction per solvent molecule divided by kT:

$$\Delta H_M = kT\chi n_1\upsilon_2 \tag{3}$$

Note that the mixing of polymer and solvent is thermodynamically favored if $\chi < 0$. Thus, good solvents are associated with low values of χ. Further development of the theory[4] shows that the division between "solvent" and "non-solvent" is at $\chi = \frac{1}{2}$ where the entropy and enthalpy of mixing cancel each other. Many water/polymer systems are close to this borderline value (see below). The theory in its basic form should predict solvent activities for a given polymer solution with a single value of χ. In practice, while solutions of rubber in benzene are well described by a constant χ, the success is not general, particularly for polar polymers and solvents. A practical fix is to allow χ to be a function of concentration for a given polymer-solvent system. Methods of calculating χ for hydrophilic copolymers in water are given by Mikos and Peppas.[6]

The next step is to describe the change in free energy associated with expansion of the network. The classical theory is based on the assumption of the "affine" network, which says simply that microscopic deformations are proportional to macroscopic ones. For an isotropic deformation, this leads to:

$$\Delta G_{el} = (kT\upsilon_e/2)(3\alpha_s^2 - 3 - ln\ \alpha_s^3) \tag{4}$$

where υ_e is the effective number of chains in the network, and α_s is the linear deformation factor of the chains. When a polymer of relaxed volume V_O swells to volume V, α_s is defined by $\alpha_s^3 = V/V_O = 1/\upsilon_2$ (affine assumption).

Equations (2) and (4) form the basis of the classical swelling theory. It is relatively straightforward to combine these two equations into one equation for swelling and then substitute more easily measured quantities for α_s and υ_e. The details are given in the references previously cited and also in Reference 7.

$$\frac{1}{\overline{M}_c} = \frac{2}{\overline{M}_n} - \frac{(\bar{\upsilon}/\bar{V}_1)[ln(1 - \upsilon_{2,s}) + \upsilon_{2,s} + \chi\upsilon_{2,s}^2]}{\left[\upsilon_{2,s}^{1/3} - \frac{1}{2}\upsilon_{2,s}\right]} \tag{5}$$

This is the Flory-Rehner[5] model for a swollen network. An inherent assumptio⬛ derivation is that the relaxed state of the polymer is without solvent. Since hydr⬛ often crosslinked in solution, the dry state is not always the appropriate reference. polymer is crosslinked in solution to a polymer volume fraction, $v_{2,r}$, and then sv⬛ an equilibrium, $v_{2,s}$, the Flory-Rehner equation can be modified accordingly:[8,9]

$$\frac{1}{\overline{M}_c} = \frac{2}{\overline{M}_n} - \frac{\overline{v}/V_1[In(1 - v_{2,s}) + v_{2,s} + \chi v_{2,s}^2]}{v_{2,r}\left[\left(\frac{v_{2,s}}{v_{2,r}}\right)^{1/3} - \frac{1}{2}\left(\frac{v_{2,s}}{v_{2,r}}\right)\right]}$$

The utility of these equations is that they give the interrelationship between t⬛ tities,v_2, χ, and $\overline{M}_c$. This relationship is relevant to drug delivery because diffusion molecules through hydrogels is mostly dependent on v_2 whereas transport of larger m⬛ can also be affected by $\overline{M}_c$.

B. SURFACE PROPERTIES AND BIOCOMPATIBILITY

High interest in the use of hydrogels as biomaterials has led to intense study⬛ surface properties. The importance of surface properties to biocompatibility can b⬛ overstated; it is the interface between the material and the biological environment w⬛ interactions occur. Biocompatibility in its most frequently used sense means the a⬛ the body to tolerate the material without unacceptable histological consequence⬛ extended period of time. For controlled drug delivery applications, the importanc⬛ compatibility depends on the site of administration and varies in proportion to the⬛ of the device. For short-term delivery, e.g., oral dosage forms, biocompatibility ⬛ an issue, and the major concern is overt toxicity. For transdermal devices, irrita⬛ major concern, and may limit useful service life to less than could be achieved by tec⬛ alone. However, toleration of transdermal device may have little to do with the⬛ properties of the polymer, and may, in any given instance, be related to the activ⬛ added penetration enhancers, etc. For a subdermal implant designed to release d⬛ several months, biocompatibility is proportionally more important, although the requ⬛ are still probably less rigorous than for a permanent device in a critical area, such a⬛ valve.

Unlike a crystalline solid, a hydrogel presents a diffuse surface with a more⬛ gradual transition between the bulk gel and the surrounding bulk water.[10] This diffuse⬛ is illustrated schematically in Figure 1. An important feature of the hydrogel surfa⬛ extremely high mobility of the polymer chains. This chain mobility allows the su⬛ adapt to its environment. For example, poly(2-hydroxyethyl methacrylate) has t⬛ chains: one terminated with a methyl group, the other with a hydroxyl. Conta⬛ measurements by Holly and Refojo[11] showed that the polymer surface appears hydr⬛ when measured in air, but hydrophilic when measured in water. The accepted exp⬛ for this is that the side chains can rotate up or down to minimize the interfacial⬛ Thus the methyl group rotates to the surface when the polymer is placed in a hydr⬛ environment, and the hydroxyl group can extend outward when placed in a hyd⬛ medium. The fact that a hydrogel can be either hydrophilic or hydrophobic would⬛ suggest an enhanced potential for interaction with the components of the biologic⬛ ronment. However, in a survey of protein adsorption measurements by Horbett,[12]⬛ served trend was that hydrogels tended to adsorb less protein than the (mostly hydr⬛ controls. Horbett suggests that in the absence of any strong binding sites on the p⬛ the high chain mobility may actually reduce the chance of forming a multipoint atta⬛

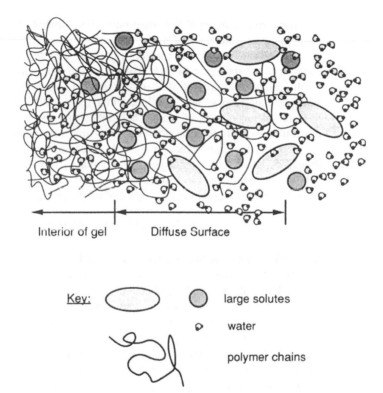

Interior of gel   Diffuse Surface

Key: ⬭   🔘   large solutes

              ◌   water

              polymer chains

FIGURE 1.   Diffuse Surface of a Hydrogel. (Simplified from Ratner.[10])

C. WATER IN HYDROGELS

The condition of water in hydrogels is a subject of some controversy, with somewhat contradictory results reported in the literature. The discussion usually centers on "free" versus "bound" water. Since the distinction is not always clear, the states of water are often described in terms of the observable freezing/melting behavior. Studies on poly(glycerol methacrylate) by Yasuda et al.[13] utilizing DSC, NMR, and permeability measurements showed only two kinds of water based on DSC measurements: a plot of the enthalpy of fusion of water in the gel vs. hydration yielded a straight line with slope equal to the heat of fusion of pure water and an x-intercept corresponding a nonmelting water fraction of 0.36 (g water/g dry polymer). However, their permeability measurements suggested the existence of an intermediate state of water in the gel. While the melting transition of water appeared at a volume fraction of 0.29 (by DSC and NMR), the hydraulic permeability of the gel did not become measurable until the water volume fraction reached 0.43. The authors were cautious in their interpretation of their results, stating: "These observations suggest that water in swollen polymers is different from free water; no distinct state of water can yet be assigned to it. Water seems to change gradually during increasing interaction with polymer molecules."

Haldankar and Spencer[14] studied poly(acrylic acid) by differential scanning calorimetry. They explained their results in terms of a three-state model, where the water in the hydrated polymer was identified as "nonfreezing" (I), "freezing with a constant melting temperature" (II), and "freezing with a melting temperature dependent on water content" (III). In these experiments, the melting point of the type II water was $-17°C$, in close agreement with a result of $-15°C$ by Ohno et al.[15] The melting point of the type III water increased from $-10°C$, gradually approaching $0°C$ at high hydration.

Similarly, Zhang et al.[16] studied poly(vinyl alcohol) by DSC and concluded that three states of water existed in the polymer: "free", "freezing bound water", and freezing". The amount of nonfreezing water and freezing bound water increase addition of substances with high affinity for the polymer.

In contrast, Roorda et al.[17] studied PHEMA gels by differential thermal analy adiabatic calorimetry, and concluded that their results were not consistent with thermodynamic classes of water, but rather that the water molecules were contin distributed over all possible orientations to and interactions with the polymer.

The practical importance to controlled release technology of the state of water drogels is its relation to transport. Water that is tightly bound to the polymer will able to contribute much to solvation of another diffusing species. Conversely, free w the gel provides a good environment for solute transport.

III. METHODS OF PREPARATION

A. FROM WATER-SOLUBLE POLYMERS

One of the easiest ways to make a hydrogel is to take a water-soluble polym crosslink it. Polymers with pendant –OH groups can be crosslinked with a variety of such as glutaraldehyde or adipic acid. For example, a 10 to 20% solution of pol alcohol) reacts smoothly with 0.5 mole% glutaraldehyde at room temperature with of sulfuric acid catalyst to form transparent soft gels. Polymers with pendant anionic can be gelled by addition of cations. A solution of 1.5% sodium alginate can be d into a bath of 1.5% $CaCl_2$ to form hydrogel beads almost instantly. The solution cross method is often advantageous because the starting material can be a well-charact purified polymer, and often the crosslinking conditions can be mild enough to be out in the presence of the active agent. The alginate encapsulation described above h used to encapsulate living cells without damage.

Ionizing radiation, such as ^{60}Co-γ or electron beams[9] can also be used to cr solutions of water-soluble polymers. Radiation crosslinking has the apparent advant introducing fewer chemicals to the system; however, this method often leaves a troubl sol fraction and possibly degradation products.

B. POLYMERIZATION

The polymerization methods for hydrogels are no different from those for or engineering resins. The usual classification of methods applies, namely, addition c densation reactions in any of the standard settings: bulk, solution, dispersion, em latex, interfacial, etc.[18] Some of the more common methods for hydrogels are dis below.

1. Addition Polymerization

Addition polymerization is the familiar mechanism for vinyl and related mon Common hydrophilic monomers which are used to prepare hydrogels by an addition anism include hydroxyethyl methacrylate, hydroxypropyl methacrylate, methacrylic acrylic acid, N-vinyl pyrrolidinone, and vinyl acetate (to be hydrolyzed after polymer to poly(vinyl alcohol)). Properties of the product may be controlled by co-polymerizin hydrophobic monomers such as methylmethacrylate, butyl acrylate, vinyl acetate (w hydrophobic unless hydrolyzed), and others. Copolymers of two or more hydrophilic omers are also useful. Since two different monomers rarely have the same reactivity the composition of the polymer is often different from the monomers in the fee convention and for convenience, most reports describe copolymers in terms of th composition. Addition reactions are usually initiated by free radical initiators such a bisisobutyronitrile (AIBN), acyl- or alkyl peroxides, such as benzoyl peroxide, etc. Redox catalyst pairs can also be used for faster initiation.[18]

2. Condensation Polymerization

Condensation polymerization techniques can also be exploited to form hydrophilic polyurethanes, polyamides, polyesters, etc. Condensation polymers have varying susceptibility to hydrolysis. The hydrolytic stability of the resulting polymers can be controlled by the choice of monomers to obtain products which degrade over a specified time. This controlled degradation can be utilized to control the rate of drug release or merely to eliminate the depleted polymer from the site after use (see Chapter 7).

3. Bulk Polymerization

Bulk or mass polymerization is the reaction of neat monomers. It is the technique of choice to prepare a monolithic block of hard material, which can then be formed by machining techniques. For example, disks can be made by polymerizing in a cylindrical mold and then slicing the resulting rod as desired. When used to form glassy polymers by free radical (addition) reactions, the Trommsdorf effect, an uncontrolled acceleration of the reaction, is sometimes observed. Acrylate monomers are especially susceptible to the Trommsdorf effect. The autoacceleration can usually be tamed by reducing the initiator concentration, lowering the reaction temperature, or improving the heat transfer between the reaction vessel (mold) and the temperature bath.

4. Solution Polymerization

Solution polymerization is especially useful for hydrogels, as the swollen crosslinked gel can be obtained directly. The presence of a large amount of solvent aids control of the reaction. If the amount of solvent exceeds the equilibrium solvent content of the final gel, the gel will exhibit syneresis (the opposite of swelling) as the reaction proceeds. If the solvent is a poor one for the polymer, the gel can precipitate as crosslinked particles instead of a monolithic block.

C. PURIFICATION

For many applications, the hydrogels prepared by any of the above methods must undergo purification before use to remove unreacted monomers, traces of initiator, side products, etc. Solvent extraction is usually the method of choice. For toxicity and safety reasons, water is the best extraction solvent if the gel is highly hydrophilic. Hydrogels which contain hydrophobic co-monomers may be more easily extracted with other solvents. Compressed gases such as carbon dioxide, in the liquid or supercritical state, are useful extraction solvents due to their ease of removal after extraction.[19] They also have the virtue that their solubility parameters depend strongly on density. Thus, the solvent power can be tuned to a specific application. However, they tend to be poor solvents for polar materials, and require the use of expensive high-pressure equipment. Their use may be justified in particular cases if the residual solvent is an important issue.

IV. DRUG LOADING

A. ADDITION OF THE DRUG BEFORE POLYMERIZATION

If the active agent is sufficiently stable and does not interfere with the polymerization, it may then be incorporated into the polymer by mixing it directly with the monomers before polymerization. The product then is obtained in one step in its final form. While this method has the advantage of simplicity, it presents problems for most pharmaceutical applications since it prevents further purification of the material without removing the necessity of proving stability, potency, purity, etc.

B. INCORPORATION OF THE DRUG INTO A PRE-FORMED HYDROGE▌

In most cases, the drug will be incorporated into the hydrogel after polymeriza▌ purification. This is usually done by soaking the gel in a solution of the drug in an ap▌ solvent. Loading kinetics are governed by the same processes that control drug rele▌ below), so it is known in advance that the time necessary to load the polymer w▌ will be in proportion to (not necessarily the same as) the intended release period. ▌ is possible to take advantage of particular properties of the polymer to reduce the▌ time. For example, the effect of pH or solvent type on swelling of the polymer or s▌ of the drug can be used to increase the efficiency of loading. If a loading solven▌ found which swells the polymer more than water alone, then loading will be mo▌ Nonaqueous solvents, such as ethanol or chloroform, will normally have to be ren▌ some specified low level before a device will be approved for human use. It is ▌ very difficult to strip the last bit of solvent from a glassy polymer, therefore to ▌ residual solvent can be an issue. One solvent which exhibits the low toxicity of wate▌ being quite lipophilic and very easy to strip, is compressed CO_2. The use of CO_2 as ▌ solvent to introduce small molecules into a number of polymers has been described b▌ et al.[20,21] and by Sand.[22] The author is not aware of any applications of this tech▌ hydrogels. Owing to the relatively low solubility parameter of even high-density C▌ probably appropriate only for relatively hydrophobic drugs in polymers that have▌ some hydrophobic bulk character.

V. DIFFUSION AND SUSTAINED RELEASE IN HYDROGE▌

Hydrogels can be designed to release drug by various mechanisms, including ▌ of the gel and hydrolysis of the drug from the polymer backbone. However, the most ▌ mechanism is passive diffusion driven by the concentration gradient of the drug. ▌ transport in gels follows the basic laws discussed in Chapter 1. The purpose of the ▌ pages is to give a further development of some aspects of diffusion that are sp▌ controlled release from hydrogels.

A. THE SWOLLEN GEL

1. Diffusion in Swollen Gels

Fick's law (7) governs diffusive transport in swollen gels.

$$j_i = D_{i,eff} \nabla c_i$$

In this and in the following sections we will take this form of Fick's law as a gi▌ put all nonideal effects into the effective diffusion coefficient, $D_{i,eff}$ which will be▌ simply as D. While there are advantages to other mathematical formulations, par▌ for concentrated multicomponent solutions, for the purposes of this chapter the ▌ sophisticated treatments introduce unneeded complications. Therefore, the emphasi▌ on the diffusion coefficient of the drug in hydrogels.

The most important parameter governing the diffusion coefficient in swollen h▌ is the water content. In general, the diffusion coefficient of a solute has a very lo▌ in a dry gel, and increases with increasing water content. Gels which are mostly wa▌ appear little different from water to small diffusing species. Diffusion of small m▌ in polymers and gels is most often treated by the free volume approach. The free ▌ theory was developed by Cohen and Turnbull[23] to describe liquids, and was ad▌ polymers by Fujita.[24] Later developments include application to hydrogels by Yasud▌ aze, and Peterlin,[25,26] and continuing improvements in generality and accuracy by ▌ and Duda.[27-31] In the free-volume model, the volume of the polymer is ▌ssume▌

apportioned between the *occupied volume* of the polymer molecules themselves and the *free volume*, the latter consisting of *interstitial* free volume, inherent in the closest packing arrangement of the molecules, and free *hole* volume. The theories assume that the free hole volume can be redistributed as needed for transport. The free hole volume is often taken to be the difference between the volume of the material at ambient temperature and its volume at absolute zero. For a swollen polymer, the solvent also contributes occupied and free volume to the system.

The general form of free-volume expressions for diffusion coefficients is

$$D = \text{(preexponential term)} \exp\left\{\frac{-\text{ penetrant volume}}{\text{free volume}}\right\} \tag{8}$$

Thus, the diffusion coefficient depends on the size of the penetrant molecule relative to the amount of room it has to move. Most published work concentrates on obtaining correct measures of the penetrant volume and the free volume of the system in terms of measurable quantities.

While the free-volume approach, particularly in its more detailed versions, can have considerable predictive power, full utilization of its predictive ability requires information that is not always available. For applications of hydrogel delivery systems, correlation and extrapolation of data using the simplified form of the theory can often be satisfactory for design and development work. One simple and useful approximation is the one associated with the names of Yasuda, Lamaze, and Peterlin.[25,26] The Yasuda et al. version of the free-volume theory is one of the most useful for most cases of diffusion of small molecules in moderately to highly swollen gels, because it is simple and it incorporates the most important factor (hydration). The form of the Yasuda et al. version of the free volume theory is

$$\frac{D}{D_w} = A \exp\left[-B\left(\frac{1}{H} - 1\right)\right], \tag{9}$$

where D_w is the diffusion coefficient of the solute in pure water, H is the membrane hydration, and A and B are system constants. Thus a plot of log D vs. $1/H$ yields a straight line for a given solute in a given hydrogel.

The proportionality between log D and $1/H$ breaks down for large solutes in highly crosslinked systems,[32] for slightly swollen membranes, and for heterogeneous materials with hydrophobic solutes (where the solute may partition into the polymer itself, rather than the water phase). When approximations are necessary, those based on a sound theory, which balance refinement with simplicity, are preferred. Reference 33 is an excellent guide.

2. Sustained Release from Swollen Gels

Release of a drug from a swollen hydrogel can be described by the solution to the diffusion equation (10) with the appropriate geometry and boundary conditions.

$$\frac{\partial c}{\partial t} = D\nabla^2 c \tag{10}$$

The general approach is as follows: the solution to the diffusion equation gives concentration as a function of position and time. While this solution may be of interest in itself, the controlled-release technologist usually wants to know how fast the active agent will be released from the device. The amount of drug diffused out of the hydrogel at a given time,

M_t can be obtained in either of two ways — by integrating the concentration profile the thickness of the gel to obtain the amount remaining:

$$\frac{M_t}{M_\infty} = 1 - \frac{1}{lc_0}\int_0^l c(x,t)dt$$

or by applying Fick's law at the outer boundary and integrating the flux from the release up to time t:

$$M_t = DA\int_0^t \left(\frac{\partial c}{\partial x}\right)_{x=l} dt$$

A large number of solutions for different cases can be found in the book by Crank completeness, the solutions for the simple cases of slab, cylindrical, and spherical ge are given below.

For a slab of thickness $2l$ initially at a uniform concentration below the solubili of the drug, with the surfaces maintained at a constant concentration, the mass diffused out at time t divided by the mass of drug diffused out at infinite time is

$$\frac{M_t}{M_\infty} = 1 - \sum_{n=1}^\infty \frac{8}{(2n+1)^2\pi^2}\exp\left\{\frac{-D(2n+1)^2\pi^2 t}{4l^2}\right\}$$

The corresponding solution for a long cylinder of radius a is

$$\frac{M_t}{M_\infty} = 1 - \sum_{n=1}^\infty \frac{4}{a^2\alpha_n^2}\exp(-D\alpha_n^2 t),$$

where the α_n are the positive roots of

$$J_0(a\alpha_n) = 0$$

and $J_0(x)$ is the Bessel function of the first kind of order zero. Tabulated values of functions and their roots can be found in mathematical handbooks; some tables are in in Crank.[34] The roots form an infinite series, and the first five values of $a\alpha_n$ are 5.520, 8.654, 11.79, and 14.93.[35,36]

Diffusion from a sphere of radius a under the same conditions follows:

$$\frac{M_t}{M_\infty} = 1 - \frac{6}{\pi^2}\sum_{n=1}^\infty \frac{1}{n^2}\exp(-Dn^2\pi^2 t/a^2)$$

The complete analytical solutions, particularly those involving Bessel functions bit cumbersome for data analysis due to the necessity to sum an infinite series. The approximate solutions are often used. A little-noticed but highly useful approxima given by Etters:[37]

$$\frac{M_t}{M_\infty} = [1 - \exp(-k(Dt/l^2)^a)]^{1/b}$$

where the parameters k, a, b have the following values, according to geometry:

	k	a	b
Sheet	10.5449	1.3390	2.6001
Sphere	9.4380	1.0427	2.1877
Cylinder	5.3454	1.1299	2.30

This equation approximates the analytical solution within 2% over the entire range of the process.

A widely used approximation is the rule that at short time, the amount released is proportional to $\sqrt{t}$. The square-root-of-time law is an exact solution to the diffusion equation in a semi-infinite medium,[36,38] and will apply to a finite medium as long as the initial concentration remains unchanged at the centerline. The short-time rule for a slab is:

$$\frac{M_t}{M_\infty} = 2\sqrt{\frac{Dt}{\pi l^2}} \tag{18}$$

The approximation is good for M_t/M_∞ less than about 0.6. The corresponding short-time solution for spherical geometry is

$$\frac{M_t}{M_\infty} = \frac{6}{\sqrt{\pi}}\left(\frac{Dt}{a^2}\right)^{1/2} \tag{19}$$

and for a cylinder it is

$$\frac{M_t}{M_\infty} = \frac{4}{\sqrt{\pi}}\left(\frac{Dt}{a^2}\right)^{1/2} \tag{20}$$

The $\sqrt{t}$ approximations for cylindrical and spherical geometry are much more approximate and less useful (they apply to shorter times) than for a slab. Some better approximations that are only slightly more complex are given in Crank.[34]

The diffusion coefficient is frequently calculated from a plot of M_t/M_∞ vs. $\sqrt{t}$ at short time. Here the slope is proportional to D and is obtained from Equations (18 to 20) above. Sometimes, if good data are available, calculation of the difusion coefficient using both the short- and long-time (see below) solutions can reveal changes taking place in the hydrogel during the release process.

Less widely used, but often useful, is the approximation that all problems of this type approach first-order kinetics at long times:

$$\frac{M_t}{M_\infty} = 1 - Ae^{-k_1 t} \tag{21}$$

Thus, data from a release experiment will converge to the straight line given by

$$\ln\left(1 - \frac{M_t}{M_\infty}\right) = -k_1 t + \ln A \tag{22}$$

at long times.

This approximation derives from the fact that as t increases, the higher order terms of the summation in Equations (13, 14, and 16) become small enough to discard, leaving only

the first term with its single exponential. Therefore, the diffusion coefficient can be
from the value of the slope, k_1, according to the first term of the exact solutions:

$$k_1$$

slab: $\dfrac{D\pi^2}{4l^2}$

cylinder: $\dfrac{5.784D}{a^2}$

sphere: $\dfrac{\pi^2 D}{a^2}$

The simple solutions to the diffusion equation provide the scaling relationship
time, physical dimensions, and amount released. Thus, they are the basic design e
for controlled release systems. Another major use of this scaling relationship is to
a check on the data: The normalized release curve is defined as a plot of (M_t/M_∞)
dimensionless time (Dt/l^2) or (Dt/a^2). If the normalized release curve changes w
loading or with thickness, then either there is a defect with the devices (perh
uniformity) or else another process in addition to diffusion is occurring.

B. DIFFUSION IN AN INITIALLY DRY GEL

For the case of diffusion in a swollen gel considered above, the system is
equilibrium. The diffusing species has a certain concentration gradient which per
rest of the system slightly, but values of water concentration, density, dimensio
system, etc. remain relatively constant in time and space within the gel. The sit
greatly changed when a xerogel containing drug is placed in water. As noted ab
final polymer volume fraction in the swollen hydrogel may be only 10 or 25%, th
large volume change will take place as the gel imbibes water $(Q = 1/v_2)$. Small
species (i.e., drug) in the gel will diffuse in the presence of an influx of water. T
influx is countercurrent to the direction of transport of drug in a sustained release
As the outer regions of the gel imbibe water, they swell outward, increasing the d
molecule of drug must travel to be released. Most importantly, the diffusivity of
increases dramatically as the polymer chains are separated by the imbibed wa
discussion which follows gives an order-of-magnitude estimate of the effect.

In a fully swollen gel, a small molecule might have a diffusion coefficient of D
cm^2/s, close to its value in pure water. In the corresponding dehydrated material,
molecule might exhibit $D = 10^{-11}$ cm^2/s. If the polymer in its dry state is below
temperature, then the macromolecular chains are essentially immobile (for the pur
this discussion; for a review of molecular motion in glassy hydrophilic acrylic p
see Kolařík[39]). In the glassy state, only very small penetrants, such as gases $(D =$
10^{-9} cm^2/s) and solvent vapors $(D = 10^{-10}$ to 10^{-17} cm^2/s), will have much m
For a drug, D could be vanishingly small.

1. Swelling-Controlled Release Systems

Because the diffusivity of the drug increases over many orders of magnitude as
matrix swells, the release mechanism is controlled primarily by the swelling proce
rather than by drug diffusion in the swollen hydrogel. An additional complicatio
the behavior of glassy polymers placed in a swelling solvent is often not well desc
Fick's law. It was observed[41] that certain polymer-solvent combinations resulted in
curves that were linear with time instead of the decreasing rate predicted by Fic
This phenomenon was dubbed Case-II transport to distinguish it. Case-II transport
be dependent on mechanical relaxation of the polymer chains, rather than on diff

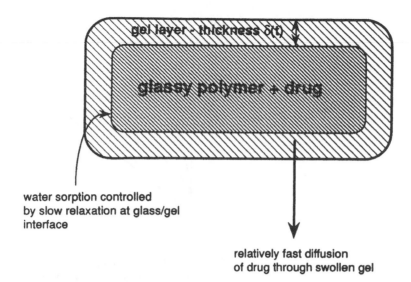

FIGURE 2.   Idealized picture of a swelling-controlled release hydrogel.

solvent. There are tools for prediction of solvent transport mechanisms in terms of dimensionless groups of system parameters.[42,43]

This observation of Case-II transport lead Hopfenberg and Hsu[44] to propose that *swelling-controlled* delivery systems could be designed to release drug at a constant rate. In a swelling-controlled system, the polymer swells relatively slowly, preferably by a Case-II mechanism. The slow swelling process results in the growth of a highly permeable gel layer on the outside of the polymer, while the interior of the polymer remains glassy (see Figure 2). Diffusion of the drug in the gel layer is relatively rapid; thus, the release is controlled by the rate of water sorption. In favorable cases,[44-47] this situation results in a constant rate of release of the drug.

2. Swellable Delivery Systems

The idealized Case-II transport of water in hydrogels seems rare. More often water sorption curves in hydrophilic polymers follow some anomalous behavior, where both diffusion and mechanical relaxation affect the process but neither completely predominates. Some initially glassy hydrogels appear to swell by purely diffusion-controlled kinetics. Initially, glassy hydrogels are still useful for controlled delivery; however, because even though perfect Case-II transport of water leading to perfect zero-order release of the solute may not occur, release from a *swellable* (as opposed to a purely *swelling controlled*) hydrogel can offer improved kinetics relative to an initially swollen hydrogel. The reason is that the reduction in resistance to diffusion of the drug that occurs as the gel swells can partially compensate for the inevitable decrease in driving force for diffusion (∇c) that results from the diffusion process itself.

Empirically, release curves from a variety of swellable dosage forms share some common features. The normalized release curve usually starts with a decreasing rate (concave downward) portion, but then goes through an inflection, and may show a slight upward curvature before returning to decreasing rate as it runs out of drug. In favorable cases, the changes in curvature can average out to give an *overall* rate that is much more constant than diffusion from an initially swollen gel. This effect has also been demonstrated with a simple mathematical model that assumes only that the diffusion coefficients of both water and drug are increasing functions of water concentration.[48,49] The wider range of behavior that can be

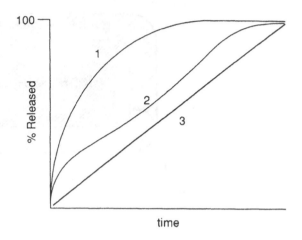

FIGURE 3.   Qualitative drug release behavior of swollen gels
(1); swellable gels (2); and swelling-controlled gels (3).

expected in the presence of significant mechanical relaxations has also been explored
qualitative drug release behavior of swollen hydrogels, swellable hydrogels, and sw
controlled hydrogels is illustrated in Figure 3.

VI. SOME IMPORTANT HYDROGEL POLYMERS

This section outlines the properties of some of the prominent hydrogel homopo
as well as a few selected copolymers. As mentioned above, copolymers of the major hy
monomers, with each other and with many other monomers, can yield a rich spect
materials. It is impossible to cover all the possible copolymers in one chapter. The en
here will be on the major homopolymers. The effect of copolymerization is mainly a bl
of the properties of the two homopolymers, so the reader may (cautiously) infer the pro
of an unknown copolymer by interpolation.

A. PHEMA AND RELATED POLYMERS

Since its development by Wichterle,[51] poly(2-hydroxyethyl methacrylate) or PI
has been one of the best studied of the synthetic hydrogels. It is prepared by radica
merization, usually in the presence of a crosslinking agent. The crosslinking agen
often used is ethylene glycol dimethacrylate or EGDMA. Of course, purification of s
monomers is critical for almost any polymerization. The case of HEMA is addit
complicated because trace amounts of EGDMA are generally present in commercial I
and are difficult to remove completely. Thus, although well-characterized gels can
tained if one purifies the monomer as much as possible and then adds a known amc
crosslinker, preparation of very lightly crosslinked gels may be subject to variability
purity of starting material. Koßmehl et al. give purification procedures for HEMA, m
methacrylate (MMA), butyl methacrylate, and *N*-vinyl pyrrolidinone (NVP).[52]

Gels prepared from pure PHEMA are only moderately water-swellable, attaining
contents of around 40%. However, the interaction parameter χ, increases with inc
swelling, as given by Janáček and Hasa[53]:

$$\chi = 0.320 + 0.904\upsilon_2$$

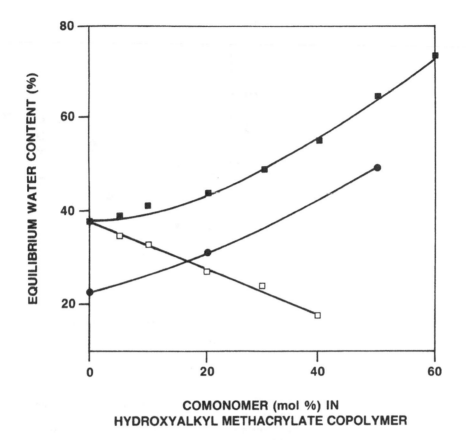

FIGURE 4. Equilibrium water content at 22°C of copolymers of HEMA with MMA and with NVP ■ — HEMA/NVP; □ — HEMA/MMA; ● — Hydroxypropyl methacrylate/NVP. (From Baker et al., Synthetic hydrogels. 2. Copolymers of carboxyl-, lactam- and amide-containing monomers — structure/property relationships, *Polymer*, 29, 691, 1988. By permission of the publishers, Butterworth & Co. Ltd.© 1988.)

Copolymerization of HEMA with methacrylic acid (MAA) can produce materials which swell to a much greater extent.[54,55] Mikos and Peppas[6] found that the χ values for all the P(HEMA-co-MAA) gels, regardless of the copolymer ratio or degree of crosslinking, depended only on the polymer volume fraction, according to

$$\chi = 0.510 + 0.061 v_2 + 0.919 v_2^2 \tag{24}$$

The quadratic expression for χ above was obtained by regression on data obtained from swelling experiments, and covers values of v_2 from 0.15 (PMAA) to ~0.68 (PHEMA). Note that the numerical values of χ given by Equations (23) and (24) differ little in the range of $0.3 < v_2 < 0.7$.

The equilibrium water content of HEMA gels can be extended in both directions without introducing ionizable groups by copolymerizing with either methyl methacrylate (to reduce water content) or *N*-vinyl pyrrolidone (to increase water content), as shown in Figure 4.[56]

B. PNVP

Poly(*N*-vinyl pyrrolidone) or PNVP (sometimes called PVP) was originally developed as a blood plasma extender. Gels of PNVP are more hydrophilic than PHEMA and swell to a correspondingly greater extent. The equilibrium water content of a PNVP gel can easily

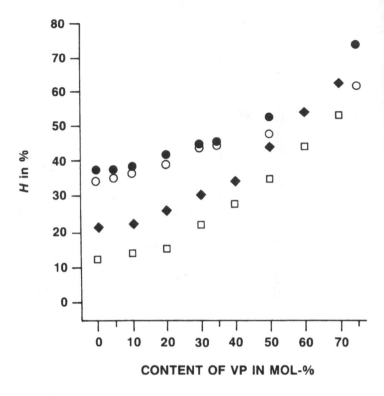

FIGURE 5. Weight percent hydration (*H*) for different copolymers of NVP with HEMA, MMA, and BuMA. All materials crosslinked with 0.2% EGDMA unless otherwise noted. Isotonic sodium chloride at 35°C.[52] ● — NVP/HEMA; ◆ — NVP/HEMA/30 mol%MMA; ☐ — NVP/HEMA/30mol%BuMA; ○NVP/HEMA + 1.0% EGDMA. (From Koßmehl, G., et al., Hydrogels based on *N*-vinyl-2-pyrrolidinone and 2-hydroxyethyl methacrylate, *Makromol. Chem.*, 190, 1253, 1989. With permission of the publisher, Hüthig & Wepf Verlag, Basel.)

be as high as 95%.[57] The interaction parameter, χ, ranges from 0.49 to 0.56 unde conditions.[57,58]

Due to its high hydrophilicity, NVP is often copolymerized with less hydrophi omers. Figure 5 shows the effect on equilibrium water content of copolymerizing N HEMA, MMA, and BuMA. The dynamic swelling of a representative NVP/HEM, ymer is shown in Figure 6.[59] This swelling behavior yields favorable (i.e., partiall release kinetics for swellable controlled release systems, as shown in Figure 7.

C. PVA

Poly(vinyl alcohol) or PVA is obtained from poly(vinyl acetate) by hydrolysi mercial PVA is graded according to the degree of hydrolysis and molecular weigh hydrolyzed PVA has a strong tendency to crystallize. Crystallization inhibits water so and fully hydrolyzed PVA can only be dissolved in hot water. Maximum cold water s occurs around 85 to 90% hydrolysis.[60] The formation of crystallites means that gels can be formed without covalent crosslinks. An extensive discussion of PVA gels, i a good section on crystallinity, can be found in Reference 61. The hydroxyl group polymer also provide excellent sites for crosslinking with such difunctional rea glutaraldehyde or adipic acid. Although the polymer's tendency to self-associate terferes with dissolution, PVA is very compatible with water, as indicated by its which is an increasing function of temperature and v_2, ranging from under 0.45 at and $v_2 = 0.035$ to just over 0.52 at T = 90°C and $v_2 = 0.13$.[61]

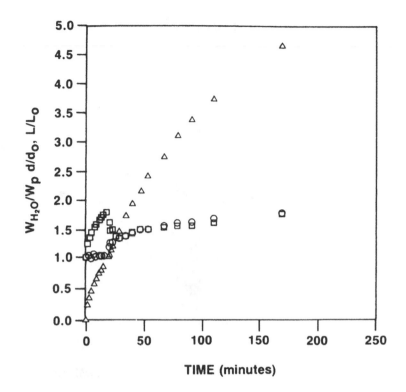

FIGURE 6. Dynamic swelling of a copolymer of NVP with HEMA. △ — weight gain, W_{H2O}/W_p; □ — axial expansion, l/l_O; ○ — radial expansion, d/d_o. (From Korsmeyer, R. W. and Peppas, N. A., Solute and penetrant-diffusion in swellable polymers. III. Drug release from glassy poly (HEMA-co-NVP) copolymers, *J. Controlled Release,* 1, 89, 1984. With permission of Elsevier Science Publishers, Amsterdam.)

An interesting property of PVA is its ability to crystallize at low temperatures in solution. This is in contrast to normal crystallization procedures for most polymers, where the best crystallization is generally obtained at a temperature between T_g and T_m. Watase and Nishinari[62] studied the mechanical properties of PVA gels that had been subjected to repeated freeze-thaw cycles. They found that both the stress at break and the modulus E′, increased with increasing number of freeze-thaw cycles. Elongation at break decreased with the number of cycles. This effect is shown in Figure 8. As would be expected, strength also increased with both molecular weight and degree of hydrolysis.

Crosslinked, semicrystalline PVA has been investigated as a swelling-controlled release system,[63,64] as has the copolymer with ethylene.[47]

D. PEO-BASED MATERIALS

Poly(ethylene oxide) is structurally similar to poly(ethylene glycol), the distinction being that PEG has low molecular weight (100s to 1000s) and PEO has higher molecular weight (10^5 to 10^6). Like PVA, PEO can crystallize; however, the melting point of the crystallites is rather low, and chemical crosslinking is necessary to obtain good hydrogels. Crosslinking can be achieved with a diisocyanate compound.[65] The resulting polymer can be thought of as a polyurethane with a large hydrophilic soft block.

Graham et al. studied release of caffeine[66] and prostaglandin E_2[67] from diisocyanate crosslinked PEO gels. Release from the fully swollen gels followed normal Fickian diffusional kinetics, while release from the initially dry gels was more complex, and showed a period of nearly constant release rate.

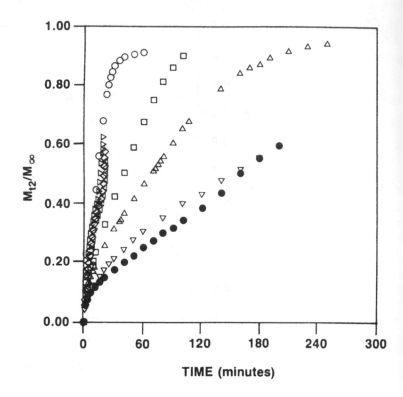

FIGURE 7.   Release of theophylline from an initially dry copolymer of NVP with HEMA. Initial thickness, L_0 and HEMA mole fraction in feed, f_i; ○ — 0.045cm, 0.446; □ — 0.083cm, 0.446; △ — 0.131cm, 0.446; ● — 0.092cm, 0.707; ▽ — 0.131cm, 0.707; ◇ — 0.092cm, 0.211; ◁ — 0.096cm, 0.211;   — 0.088cm, 0.211. (From Korsmeyer, R. W. and Peppas, N. A., Solute and penetrant diffusion in swellable polymers. III. Drug release from glassy poly(HEMA-co-NVP) copolymers, *J. Controlled Release*, 1, 89, 1984. With permission of Elsevier Science Publishers, Amsterdam.)

Small particles composed of PEO and block copolymers with polyproplyene oxi[] been studied by Gander et al.[68] The equilibrium swelling of their materials ranged fr[] to 19, relative to dry polymer. They observed Fickian release of proxyphylline, theop[] and methylcatechin from 400 to 600 μm particles.

A very interesting material was described by Weber and Stadler,[69] who linke[] butadiene (PBD) chains with PEO crosslinks of average length 200 and 600 in a[] ranging from 3.2 to 16.2 wt%. Despite the relatively low amounts of PEO combin[] the hydrophobic PBD, many of these polymers exhibited volume swelling (q =[] greater than 1.25, with some samples approaching 1.5. Transmission electron mic[] showed that the materials contained two phases (as expected), but that the two phas[] both continuous. Materials such as this offer interesting possibilities of loading hydr[] drugs into a water swellable system.

E. POLYSACCHARIDES

In contrast to the synthetic polymers which have been emphasized in this chap[] polysaccharides are natural materials, usually isolated from plants or bacterial fermen[] The polysaccharides are ubiquitous in nature and widely used in industry. A th[] treatment of them is far beyond the scope of this chapter. The interested reader m[] to the recent book by Yalpani.[70] This section will only give a few examples to i[] some of the possibilities of these materials.

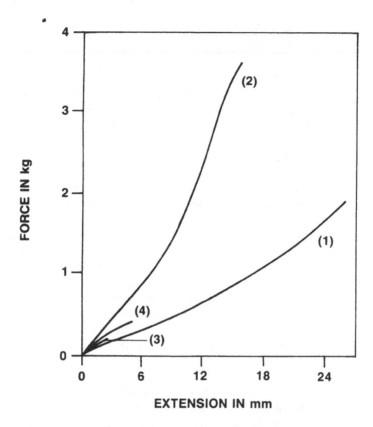

FIGURE 8. Force/Extension plots for cold-crystallized PVA, agarose, and carrageenan gels. (1) — 15wt% PVA gel, degree of polymerization = 1700, degree of hydrolysis = 99.9% freeze/thaw cycles = 0; (2) — 15wt% PVA gel, same as (1), but 3 freeze/thaw cycles; (3) — 2 wt% agarose gel; (4) — 4wt% κ-carrageenan gel. (From Watase, M. and Nishinari, K., Large deformation of hydrogels of poly(vinyl alcohol), agarose and κ-carrageenan, *Makromol. Chem.*, 186, 1081, 1985. With permission of the publisher, Hüthig & Wepf Verlag, Basel.)

Many of the polysaccharides have acid groups: e.g., sulfate groups in the carragenans; and carboxylic acids in gum arabic, xanthan, alginic acid, and zooglan. These charged groups can aid gelation by binding to oppositely-charged molecules (as when alginate is gelled by Ca^{++}) or cause the gel to undergo discontinuous volume transitions.[71] Somewhat unusual among the polysaccharides is the basic polymer, chitosan, which is obtained by deacetylation of chitin, a structural component of crustaceans, arthropods, and fungi.

1. Cellulose

Cellulose, one of the most widely used polysaccharides in pharmacy, can be used to prepare highly swellable gels.[72] These gels are crosslinked by crystallites and/or hydrogen bonds, and thus show irreversible changes on drying.[73] They are highly compatible with water ($\chi = 0.2$), and can be prepared to contain from 0.75 to 6.3 (g water/g dry gel). As with many initially glassy polymers, they exhibit viscoelastic sorption kinetics in water.[74]

2. Agarose and Carrageenan

These linear galactans (some sulfated) are derived from algae and can adopt a helical structure.[70] They can form thermally reversible gels. To put the gels in perspective with the rest of the chapter, they are much weaker mechanically than, for example, PVA gels, as illustrated in Figure 8.[62]

F. POLYPHOSPHAZENES

The polyphosphazenes have seen relatively little application in the hydrogel are
ever, they form a class of interesting materials which may yet see greater expl
Allcock and Kwon[75] have prepared poly[bis(carboxylatophenoxy)phosphazene], a
material ($T_g = -4.7°C$), which can be crosslinked by di- and trivalent cations
sumably cations with higher charges also). They were able to obtain highly swo
including an aluminum-crosslinked sample which contained 9.5 g water/g polyme

G. RESPONSIVE HYDROGELS

A recent application of hydrogels has been the preparation of controlled release
that can respond to changes in their environment to modulate the rate of release of
agent. The area of self-regulated drug delivery systems has recently been revi
Heller.[76] The approach taken for hydrogels is based on exploiting some characteris
swelling phenomenom to make the swelling of the system (and thus the diffusion c
of drug) respond to some particular change in the environment.

For a hydrogel with ionizable groups, the swelling of the gel changes drastica
the state of ionization of the groups changes.

Kou et al.[77] prepared pH-dependent hydrogels from poly(hydroxyethylmethacr
methacrylic acid). The hydration of these hydrogels was a function of pH, yieldi
dependent diffusion coefficient of the model drug (phenyl propanolamine). The de
of the diffusion coefficient on swelling followed the Yasuda free-volume theory.

Siegel et al.[78] prepared copolymers of MMA with N,N-dimethylaminoethyl met
and divinyl benzene to obtain fairly hydrophobic materials which undergo a swell
sition at pH 6.6, absorbing considerable water at lower pH, reaching a water c
88% at pH 3. When these materials were loaded with caffeine, the authors observed
no caffeine release at pH 7, while at pH 3 and 5, the drug was released with near-z
kinetics.

It is impossible to do justice to the subject of hydrogels in the space of one book
The aim has been to provide a summary of the field combined with some choice e
The references given will provide the interested reader with many more theoretic
and more numerous examples, as well as a gateway to a great number of articles of

ACKNOWLEDGMENT

I thank Gary Huvard for calling my attention to Equation 17 and for providing n
values of its parameters in slab and spherical geometry.

REFERENCES

1. **Peppas, N. A.,** *Hydrogels in Medicine and Pharmacy,* CRC Press, Boca Raton, FL, 1986.
2. **Gottlieb, M.,** Swelling of polymer networks, in *Biological and Synthetic Polymer Networks,* K
   Ed., Elsevier, New York, 1988.
3. **Eichinger, B. E. and Neuberger, N. A.,** Differential swelling of elastomers, in *Biological an
   Polymer Networks,* Kramer, O., Ed., Elsevier, New York, 1988.
4. **Flory, P. J.,** *Principles of Polymer Chemistry,* Cornell University Press, 1953.
5. **Flory, P. J. and Rehner, R.,** Statistical mechanics of crosslinked polymer networks. I. Rubberlik
   J. Chem. Phys., 11, 521, 1943.
6. **Mikos, A. G. and Peppas, N. A.,** Flory interaction parameter χ for hydrophilic copolymers
   Biomaterials, 9, 419, 1988.
7. **Peppas, N. A. and Barr-Howell, B. D.,** Characterization of the crosslinked structure of hy
   Hydrogels in Medicine and Pharmacy, Peppas, N. A., Ed., CRC Press, Boca Raton, FL, 198

8. **Flory, P. J.**, Statistical mechanics of swelling of network structures, *J. Chem. Phys.*, 18, 108, 1950.

9. **Bray, J. C. and Merrill, E. W.**, Poly(vinyl alcohol) hydrogels: formation by electron beam irradiation of aqueous solutions and subsequent crystallization, *J. Appl. Polym. Sci.*, 17, 3779, 1973.

10. **Ratner, B. D.**, Hydrogel surfaces, in *Hydrogels in Medicine and Pharmacy*, Peppas, N. A., Ed., CRC Press, Boca Raton, FL, 1986.

11. **Holly, F. J. and Refojo, M. F.**, Water wettability of hydrogels. I. Poly(2-hydroxyethyl methacrylate), *J. Biomed. Mater. Res.*, 9, 315, 1975.

12. **Horbett, T. A.**, Protein adsorption to hydrogels, in *Hydrogels in Medicine and Pharmacy*, Peppas, N. A., Ed., CRC Press, Boca Raton, FL, 1986.

13. **Yasuda, H., Olf, H. G., Crist, B., Lamaze, C. E., and Peterlin, A.**, Movement of water in homogeneous water-swollen polymers, in *Water Structure at the Water-Polymer Interface*, Jellinek, H. H. G., Ed., Plenum Press, New York, 1972.

14. **Haldankar, G. S. and Spencer, H. G.**, Properties of bound water in poly(acrylic acid) and its sodium and potassium salts determined by differential scanning calorimetry, *J. Appl. Polym. Sci.*, 37, 3137, 1989.

15. **Ohno, H., Shibayama, M., and Tsuchida, E.**, DSC analyses of bound water in the microdomains of interpolymer complexes, *Makromol. Chem.*, 184, 1017, 1983.

16. **Zhang, W., Satoh, M., and Komiyama, J.**, A differential scanning calorimetry study of the states of water in swollen poly(vinyl alcohol) membranes containing nonvolatile additives, *J. Membr. Sci.*, 42, 303, 1989.

17. **Roorda, W. E., Bouwstra, J. A., de Vries, M. A., and Junginger, H. E.**, Thermal analysis of water in p(HEMA) hydrogels, *Biomaterials*, 9, 494, 1988.

18. **Odian, G.**, *Principles of Polymerization*, 2nd ed., John Wiley & Sons, New York, 1981.

19. **McHugh, M. A. and Krukonis, V. J.**, *Supercritical Fluid Extraction, Principles and Practice*, Butterworths, Reading, MA, 1986.

20. **Berens, A. R., Huvard, G. S., and Korsmeyer, R. W.**, Application of compressed carbon dioxide in the incorporation of additives into polymers, AIChE Natl. Meet., Supercritical Technology: Applications, Washington, D.C., November 27 to December 5, 1988.

21. **Berens, A. R., Huvard, G. S., and Korsmeyer, R. W.**, Process for incorporating an additive in a polymer and product produced thereby, U.S. Patent 4,820,752, 1989.

22. **Sand, M. L.**, Method for impregnating a thermoplastic polmyer, U.S. Patent 4,598,006, 1986.

23. **Cohen, M. H. and Turnbull, D.**, Molecular transport in liquids and gases, *J. Chem. Phys.*, 31, 1164, 1959.

24. **Fujita, H.**, Diffusion in polymer-diluent systems, *Fortschr. Hochpolym. Forsch.*, 3, 1, 1961.

25. **Yasuda, H., Lamaze, C. E., and Peterlin, A.**, Diffusive and hydraulic permeabilities of water in water-swollen polymer membranes, *J. Polym. Sci.*, *Part A-2*, 9, 1117, 1971.

26. **Yasuda, H. and Lamaze, C. E.**, Permselectivity of solutes in homogeneous water-swollen polymer membranes, *J. Macromol. Sci. Phys.*, B5, 111, 1971.

27. **Vrentas, J. S. and Duda, J. L.**, Diffusion in polymer-solvent systems. I. Reexamination of the free-volume theory, *J. Polym. Sci. Polym. Phys. Ed.*, 15, 403, 1977.

28. **Vrentas, J. S. and Duda, J. L.**, Diffusion in polymer-solvent systems. II. A predictive theory for the dependence of diffusion coefficients on temperature, concentration and molecular weight, *J. Polym. Sci. Polym. Phys. Ed.*, 15, 417, 1977.

29. **Vrentas, J. S. and Duda, J. L.**, Molecular diffusion in polymer solutions, *AIChE J.*, 25, 1, 1979.

30. **Duda, J. I., Vrentas, J. S., Ju, S. T., and Liu, H. T.**, Prediction of diffusion coefficients for polymer-solvent systems, *AIChE J.*, 28, 279, 1982.

31. **Vrentas, J. S. and Chu, C.-H.**, Concentration dependence of solvent selfdiffusion coefficients, *J. Appl. Polym. Sci.*, 34, 587, 1987.

32. **Reinhart, C. T. and Peppas, N. A.**, Solute diffusion in swollen membranes. II. Influence of crosslinking on diffusive properties, *J. Membr. Sci.*, 18, 227, 1984.

33. **Peppas, N. A. and Lustig, S. R.**, Solute diffusion in hydrophilic network structures, in *Hydrogels in Medicine and Pharmacy*, Peppas, N. A., Ed., CRC Press, Boca Raton, FL, 1986.

34. **Crank, J. M.**, *The Mathematics of Diffusion*, Clarendon Press, Oxford, 1975.

35. **Churchill, R. V. and Brown, J. W.**, *Fourier Series and Boundary Value Problems*, 3rd ed., McGraw-Hill, New York, 1978, 193.

36. **Crank, J. M.**, *The Mathematics of Diffusion*, Clarendon Press, Oxford, 1975, 380.

37. **Etters, J. N.**, Diffusion equations made easy, *Text. Chem. Color.*, 12, 140, 1980.

38. **Cussler, E. L.**, *Diffusion, Mass Transfer in Fluid Systems*, Cambridge University Press, New York, 1984.

39. **Kolařík, J.**, Secondary relaxations in glassy polymers: hydrophilic polymethacrylates and polyacrylates, *Adv. Polym. Sci.*, 46, 120, 1982.

40. **Berens, A. R. and Hopfenberg, H. B.**, Diffusion of organic vapors at low concentrations in glassy PVC, polystyrene, and PMMA, *J. Membr. Sci.*, 10, 283, 1982.

41. **Alfrey, T., Gurnee, E. F., and Lloyd, W. G.**, Diffusion in glassy polymers, *J. Polym. Sci.*, C(12), 249, 1966.

42. **Vrentas, J. S., Jarzebski, C. M., and Duda, J. L.,** A Deborah number for diffusion in polyme systems, *AIChE J.,* 21, 894, 1975.
43. **Davidson, G. W. R. and Peppas, N. A.,** Solute and penetrant diffusion in swellable polymers. Deborah and swelling interface numbers as indicators of the order of biomolecular release., *J. C Release,* 3, 259, 1986.
44. **Hopfenberg, H. B. and Hsu, K. C.,** Swelling-controlled constant rate delivery systems, *Poly Sci.,* 18, 1186, 1978.
45. **Korsmeyer, R. W. and Peppas, N. A.,** Macromolecular and modeling aspects of swelling-c systems, in *Controlled Release Delivery Systems,* Roseman, T. J. and Mansdorf, S. Z., Eds. Dekker, New York, 1983.
46. **Korsmeyer, R. W. and Peppas, N. A.,** Dynamically swelling hydrogels in controlled release app in *Hydrogels in Medicine and Pharmacy,* Peppas, N. A., Ed., CRC Press, Boca Raton, FL, 198
47. **Hopfenberg, H. B., Apicella, A., and Saleeby, D. E.,** Factors affecting water sorption in a release from glassy ethylene-vinyl alcohol copolymers, *J. Membr. Sci.,* 8, 273, 1981.
48. **Korsmeyer, R. W., Lustig, S. R., and Peppas, N. A.,** Solute and penetrant diffusion in polymers. I. Mathematical modeling, *J. Polym. Sci. Polym. Phys. Ed.,* 24, 395, 1986.
49. **Korsmeyer, R. W., von Meerwall, E. D., and Peppas, N. A.,** Solute and penetrant diffusion in s polymers. II. Verification of theoretical models, *J. Polym. Sci. Polym. Phys. Ed.,* 24, 409, 198
50. **Lustig, S. R. and Peppas, N. A.,** Solute and penetrant diffusion in swellable polymers. VI volume-based model with mechanical relaxation, *J. Polym. Sci. Polym. Phys. Ed.,* 33, 533, 198
51. **Wichterle, O. and Lim, D.,** Hydrophilic gels for biological use, *Nature,* 185, 117, 1960.
52. **Koßmehl, G., Volkheimer, J., and Schäfer, H.,** Hydrogels based on *N*-vinyl-2-pyrrolidinon hydroxyethyl methacrylate, *Makromol. Chem.,* 190, 1253, 1989.
53. **Janáček, J. and Hasa, J.,** Structure and properties of hydrophilic polymers and their gels. VI. Eq deformation behaviour of polyethyleneglycol methacrylate and polydiethyleneglycol methacrylate prepared in the presence of a diluent and swollen with water, *Coll. Czech. Chem. Commun.,* 3 1966.
54. **Ilavský, M., Dušek, K., Vacík, J., and Kopeček, J.,** Deformational, swelling, and potentiometric of ionized gels of 2-hydroxyethyl methacrylate-methacrylic acid copolymers, *J. Appl. Polym.* 2073, 1979.
55. **Hasa, J. and Ilavský, M.,** Deformational, swelling, and potentiometric behavior of ionized poly(me acid) gels. II. Experimental results. *J. Polym. Sci. Polym. Phys.,* Ed. 13, 263, 1975.
56. **Baker, D. A., Corkhill, P. H., Ng, C. O., Skelly, P. J. and Tighe, B. J.,** Synthetic hydr Copolymers of carboxyl-, lactam- and amide-containing monomers — structure/property relat *Polymer,* 29, 691, 1988.
57. **Davis, T. P., Huglin, M. B., and Yip, D. C.,** Properties of poly (*N*-vinyl-2-pyrrolidinone h crosslinked with ethylene glycol dimethacrylate, *Polymer,* 29, 701, 1988.
58. **Good, W. R. and Cantow, H.-J.,** One and two component hydrogels, 3. Deswelling and con measurements on one component hydrogels, *Makromol. Chem.,* 180, 2605, 1979.
59. **Korsmeyer, R. W. and Peppas, N. A.,** Solute and penetrant diffusion in swellable polymers.] release from glassy poly(HEMA-co-NVP) copolymers, *J. Controlled Release,* 1, 89, 1984.
60. **Toyoshima, K.,** General properties of PVA in relation to its applications, in *PVA — Prope Applications,* Finch, C. A., Ed., John Wiley & Sons, New York, 1973, 555.
61. **Peppas, N. A.,** Hydrogels of poly(vinyl alcohol) and its copolymers, in *Hydrogels in Medi Pharmacy, Volume II: Polymers,* Peppas, N. A., Ed., CRC Press, Boca Raton, FL, 1986.
62. **Watase, M. and Nishinari, K.,** Large deformation of hydrogels of poly(vinyl alcohol), agaros carrageenan, *Makromol. Chem.,* 186, 1081, 1985.
63. **Korsmeyer, R. W. and Peppas, N. A.,** Effect of the morphology of hydrophilic polymeric ma diffusion and release of water soluble drugs., *J. Membr. Sci.,* 9, 211, 1981.
64. **Colombo, P., Caramella, C., Conte, U., Gazzaniga, A., and La Manna, A.,** Surface crossli compressed mini-matrices for drug release control, *Proc. Symp. Controlled Release Bioact. Mat* 11, The Controlled Release Society, New York, 1984, 130.
65. **Graham, N. B., Nwachuku, N. E., and Walsh, D. J.,** Interaction of (polyethylene oxide) with 1. Preparation and swelling of crosslinked poly(ethylene oxide) hydrogel, *Polymer,* 23, 1345, 19
66. **Graham, N. B., Zulfiqar, M., MacDonald, B. B., and McNeill, M. E.,** Caffeine release fr swollen (poly(ethylene oxide) hydrogels, *J. Controlled release,* 5, 243, 1988.
67. **Embrey, M. P., Graham, N. B., McNeill, M. E., and Hillier, K.,** *In vitro* release characteri long term stability of poly(ethylene oxide) hydrogel vaginal pessaries containing prostaglandi *Controlled Release,* 3, 39, 1986.
68. **Gander, B., Gurny, R., Doelker, E., and Peppas, N. A.,** Crosslinked poly(alkylene oxides preparation of controlled release micromatrices, *J. Controlled Release,* 5, 271, 1988.

69. **Weber, M. and Stadler, R.,** Hydrophilic-hydrophobic two-component polymer networks. 2. Synthesis and characterization of poly(ethylene oxide)-linked-polybutadiene, *Polymer,* 29, 1071, 1988.

70. **Yalpani, M.,** *Polysaccharides: Synthesis, modifications and structure/property relations,* Elsevier, Amsterdam, 1988.

71. **Tanaka, T.,** Gels, in *Encyclopedia of Polymer Science,* Vol. 7, 2nd ed., Wiley Interscience, New York, 1987, 515.

72. **Westman, L. and Lindström, T.,** Swelling and mechanical properties of cellulose hydrogels. I. Preparation, characterization, and swelling behavior, *J. Appl. Polym. Sci.,* 26, 2519, 1981.

73. **Westman, L. and Lindström, T.,** Swelling and mechanical properties of cellulose hydrogels. II. The relation between the degree of swelling and the creep compliance, *J. Appl. Polym. Sci.,* 26, 2519, 1981.

74. **Westman, L. and Lindström, T.,** Swelling and mechanical properties of cellulose hydrogels. IV. Kinetics of swelling in liquid water, *J. Appl. Polym. Sci.,* 26, 2519, 1981.

75. **Allcock, H. R. and Kwon, S.,** An ionically cross-linkable polyphophazene: poly bis(carboxylato-phenoxy)phosphazene and its hydrogels and membranes, *Macromolecules,* 22, 75, 1989.

76. **Heller, J.,** Chemically self-regulated drug delivery systems, *J. Controlled Release,* 8, 111, 1988.

77. **Kou, J. H., Amidon, G. L., and Lee, P. I.,** pH-dependent swelling and solute diffusion characteristics of poly(hydroxyethylmethacrylate-co-methacrylic acid) hydrogels, *Pharm. Res.,* 5, 592, 1988.

78. **Siegel, R. A., Falamarzian, M., Firestone, B. A., and Moxley, B. C.,** pH-controlled release from hydrophobic/polyelectrolyte copolymer hydrogels, *J. Controlled Release,* 8, 179, 1988.

Chapter 3

POLYMERS FOR ENTERIC COATING APPLICATIONS

George A. Agyilirah and Gilbert S. Banker

TABLE OF CONTENTS

I. DEFINITION AND HISTORY

An enteric coating is one that resists disintegration or dissolution in gastric med disintegrates or dissolves in intestinal fluids.

The notion that some coatings could delay the release of substances until th emptied from the stomach was first noted in 1867, when it was reported that co protected pills did not dissolve in the stomach.[1] Unna is credited as being the firs gastric insolubility as a basis for medication when he introduced keratin coated 1884.[2-4] Ceppi is reported to have introduced salol as an enteric coating a few years

The realization that certain medicaments needed to be protected against the environment occurred after elucidation of the chemistry and mechanics of the pro digestion by Prout, Beaumont, and Pavlov.[6,7] In 1889 Bourquelot listed four gr medicaments that required gastric protection.[6-8] The groups included drugs attacked by contents, drugs influencing gastric performance, and drugs that irritate the stomach

As soon as it became clear that some types of drugs needed gastric protection, were directed at finding substances that would do the job. Shroeter has listed a nu materials that have been tried or used as enteric coatings together with references investigations.[9] Among the older materials used were formalized gelatin, keratin, salo acid, and sandarac. Most of the earlier materials are no longer used because they perform satisfactorily as enteric coatings, for one reason or another. Keratin, for ex did not withstand gastric digestion.[3] Formalized gelatin proved unreliable becaus merization of the gelatin on storage often resulted in failure of the coatings to rele drug contained in the coated product.[3,7,10] Salol-coated tablets were also found to go the intestine without dissolving.[3] There were also instances when salol-coated tablet in the stomach.[3]

The search for better performing materials has continued through the years. W have a variety of materials, including several new materials, available as enteric and d release coatings, which are discussed in later sections of this chapter. The sear continues for new enteric polymers and polymer forms.

II. PURPOSE OF ENTERIC COATINGS

The function of enteric coatings is primarily protective. This may be either to the stomach from the effect of the drug, or to protect the drug from the effect of the contents. There are a number of drugs which, if directly exposed to gastric mucos result in gastric irritation, and in some cases, actual corrosion of the gastric wall. Suc are enteric coated to protect the individuals taking them from their harmful side Aspirin is an important example of such a drug. Several reports of gastric bleeding fol aspirin medication can be found in the literature.[11-14] Other drugs that fall in this ca are strong electrolytes such as ammonium chloride and potassium chloride.

Enteric coatings also protect drugs from degradation. For example, erythromyc digoxin are unstable in gastric media. Other reasons for enteric coatings are

1.   to better deliver drugs that are absorbed from a region of the intestine, or tha the intestine and require a high concentration of drug to be released there to be ef a (some anthelmintics);
2.   to provide a delayed component for repeat action dosage forms; and
3.   to prevent interaction of certain drugs with pepsin and peptones that would le hindrance of gastric digestion.

III. GASTROINTESTINAL PHYSIOLOGY RELATIVE TO ENTERIC COATING FUNCTIONING AND DESIGN RATIONALE

Enteric coatings rely on the differences in environment between the stomach and intestine for their performance. Understanding the requirements of enteric coatings demands consideration of gastrointestinal (GI) physiology and function.

The most important GI physiological factors affecting the functioning of enteric coatings are

1. The pH of the stomach and intestinal contents
2. Gastric emptying
3. Enzyme activity of the gastrointestinal tract

Based on these regional differences in environment between the stomach and the intestines, there are two mechanisms by which an enteric coating may be made to be resistant to dissolution or hydration in the stomach, yet release rapidly in the upper intestinal tract. These two mechanisms involve the pH change and the enzyme environment change between the stomach and the intestines.

A. pH

The pH of the stomach varies from about 1.0 to 3.5 depending on the presence or absence of food and reflux of intestinal contents into the stomach.[15-19] The pH of the intestine may range from about 3.8—6.6[20] in the small intestine to about 7.5—8.0 in the large intestine.[21] This range results from progressive dilution of acid chyme from the stomach by bicarbonate ions in the pancreatic secretion, which is delivered by the bile duct to the duodenum as well as from intestinal secretions.[16,17]

Based on the pH of the stomach and small intestine, enteric coatings must be designed to resist dissolution at pH values below 4 to avoid disintegration in the stomach, but to begin dissolving at pH 5 and above, and be readily soluble at pH 7. A number of earlier enteric formulations failed to release their contents appropriately because their design was based on the mistaken assumption that the pH of the small intestinal contents was alkaline.

B. GASTRIC EMPTYING

Gastric emptying of coated tablets have been reported to be highly variable, and may take anywhere from 30 min or less to 7 h or more depending on the presence and type of food in the stomach, in addition to other factors.[16,18-20]

Bukey and Brew[18] reported an *average* gastric emptying time of about 6 h. There is general agreement, however, that because of the wide variability in emptying time, an arbitrary gastric emptying time of 1 or 2 h is not a reliable factor on which to base enteric performance. It might be reasonable to assume that any enteric polymer which can resist gastric contents for 6 h is likely to give satisfactory performance in terms of gastric protection in most patients under most circumstances. Although some coatings may be able to resist gastric acid for 1 h, as specified by the compendia, these tablets may not be able to remain intact if held in the stomach for substantially longer periods.

The fact that an enteric tablet has adequate protection against gastric acid does not guarantee that the tablet will be an effective dosage form/drug delivery system, *unless* the enteric coating quickly dissolves/disintegrates on leaving the stomach, when it contacts a new environment.

A general description of gastric motility and activity may be helpful in understanding the manner in which materials are handled by the stomach. The presence of food in the stomach, especially of fatty foods, reduces both the rate of emptying from the stomach and

the level of peristaltic activity. This natural phenomena allows the stomach to und
work of food breakdown, in preparation for gastric emptying and intestinal absor
the stomach nears an empty stage, or operates in an essentially food emptied sta
more vigorous gastric activity occurs, which may be sensed by the individual as
pangs.'' These more vigorous contractions of the stomach are described as "hous
waves. It is for this reason that a solid dosage form which does not disintegra
stomach is much more likely to be expelled in a fasted state promptly than in a
Thus, enteric dosage forms that are administered in the fed state have their greatest
as far as retaining their integrity in the stomach, due to the longer residence tim
more elevated gastric pH that exists in the fed state.

As food is swallowed and enters the stomach, the fundus and body regions of the
relax to accommodate the volume of the meal. As food enters the stomach, it n
layers which are gradually mixed with the gastric secretions in the antrum by the mc
contractions of the stomach. Low-viscosity fluid that is swallowed may move into the
and pass around and surround the more dense solid mass that may be present. The
of the stomach contents will typically begin only after a portion of the gastric cont
become fairly liquid and can readily pass through the pyloris. Peristaltic waves as co
begin in the fundus region, travel down the stomach pre-pyloric area, and then becc
intense as they reach the pyloris. The pyloris is not a valve, as some people may
but is a sphincter. As the antrum leading into the pyloris, and the pyloric sphinc
contracts, the first segment or proximal region of the duodenum relaxes. A mom
the antrum and pyloris relax, and the duodenum regains its tonicity. This type of n
"squeezes" the fluid gastric contents along as the contents move into the duode
the pyloric sphincter recontracts momentarily to prevent regurgitation of intestinal
back into the stomach. This gradual squeezing activity continues to move the conte
and into the further regions of the intestine. The gastric emptying process is influe
by the rate of these antral and pyloric waves as well as by the strength of the con
These peristaltic waves are gentle, and the mixing activity is gentle with a filled
The waves increase in frequency and strength in a more emptied gastric state. It
reported that distention of the stomach is the only natural stimulus known to inc
emptying rate. Fat in any form has the greatest inhibitory effect on gastric empty
inhibitory influence permits more time for the digestion and processing of fat, wh
slowest of all foods to be digested. There may also be a hormonal mechanism w
trigger to reduce gastric motility.

Gastric emptying is generally regarded as occurring by an exponential (first-orde
process. The rate of gastric emptying is probably not strictly linear if plotted fi
especially at the earliest and latest times in the emptying process, but an overall appro
of first-order emptying will usually be fairly accurate.

A few words are appropriate to describe intestinal transit. The rate at which
move along the small intestine is important for both delayed and controlled releas
forms, since drug absorption predominantly occurs in the small intestine. Know
intestinal transit rates and ranges is important to understand the time frame in w
dosage form must operate to release drug and allow drug absorption to produce the
effect. There are two types of intestinal movements — propulsive and mixing mo
The propulsive movements are generally regarded as synonymous with peristalsis
frequency and strength of the intestinal contractions will determine the transit rate
intestine. Intestinal contents move along the intestinal tract at the rate of about 1
sec. At this rate, material will transverse the small intestine in 3 to 10 h.

The small intestine is approximately 7 m in length and is composed of three
first being the duodenum; the second, the jejunum; and the third segment, the ileur
joins the large intestine. The duodenum is the shortest segment, and is only abo

long. The common bile duct and the pancreatic duct enter the duodenum in the first 33 to 40% in organ length (in the first 7 to 10 cm) from the pyloris, where these ducts deliver their contents to substantially neutralize gastric acid that is conveyed with the gastric contents into the upper small intestine. The pH then quickly rises to about 4, even if the contents leaving the stomach were at a pH of about 1. The pH will then gradually increase as the contents move along into the jejunum, which is approximately 3 m long, and then to continue to rise as the material moves through the most lengthy segment of the intestine, the ileum.

The colon or large intestine is about 1.5 m in length, and its principal function is to conduct indigestible materials from the small intestine to the exterior of the body as feces. During the process it removes a large amount of the water content of the materials. The mucosa of the colon is very smooth compared to the small intestine, which is covered with villi and micro-villi. Based on the greatly reduced surface area of the colon, it is not nearly as effective an absorption site as is the small intestine, although the longer residence of some materials in the colon may provide for some absorption of selected ingredients. An enteric dosage form that fails to disintegrate in the small intestine, and is delivered to the colon, will almost certainly deliver no useful quantities of drug, unless the drug is being delivered to the colon for nonsystemic effects.

C. ENZYME ACTIVITY

There are a variety of enzymes in the intestine that help break down various substances. The enzymes which are part of the pancreatic juice are mainly hydrolytic, and include trypsin, chymotripsin, amylase, and lipase. Fats were used in the past as enteric coatings because they are not digested in the stomach due to the absence of lipase, but are digested in the intestine by intestinal lipase. Esterases are also thought to play a role in the disintegration of some of the newer enteric coatings. Pepsin is the only primary enzyme of the stomach.

IV. REQUIREMENTS OF AN IDEAL ENTERIC COATING

Based on the GI physiology outlined above and the purpose of an enteric coating, an ideal enteric coating should possess the following properties:

1. Must resist disintegration or dissolution in the stomach for as long as the dosage form remains there.
2. Must be impermeable to gastric fluids and drug while in the stomach.
3. Must dissolve or disintegrate rapidly in the small intestine.
4. Must be physically and chemically stable during storage.
5. Must be nontoxic.
6. Must be easily applied as a coating.
7. Must be economical, i.e., must not be too expensive.

V. THEORY OF ENTERIC POLYMER PERFORMANCE

A number of materials have been used as enteric coatings. The mode of action can be based on one mechanism or a combination of mechanisms. Some of the earlier coatings contained hydrophilic materials which swelled in the presence of moisture, causing the entire coating to break apart regardless of pH.[20] The idea behind this mechanism was that the coating material would start swelling in the stomach, but break up in the intestine. As Kanig[6] stated, "This type of system could disintegrate too early or too late due to the variability of gastric emptying and would not be reliable."

Other coatings such as Keratin, formalized gelatin, oils, and fats depended on enzymatic breakdown and/or emulsification, aided by bile salts and cholesterol. Coatings based solely

on enzymatic breakdown have not been successful because enzyme breakdown is re
slow.[10,21]

Almost all the currently used enteric materials are synthetic or modified natural p
containing ionizable carboxylic groups. In the low pH environments of the stom;
carboxylic groups remain un-ionized, and the polymer coatings remain insoluble
intestine, the pH increases to 5 and above, allowing the carboxylic groups on the po
coating materials to ionize, and the polymer coatings to disintegrate or dissolve, r
their contents. The main factors influencing the ionization and subsequent disintegr
the coatings are the pKa of the polymeric acids and the pH of the surrounding mediu
relationship between the pH of the medium, the pKa, and extent of ionization of ar
given, in general, by the Henderson-Hasselbach Equation

$$pKa\text{-}pH \;=\; \log \frac{\text{concentration of un-ionized form}}{\text{concentration of ionized form}}$$

It is evident from the above equation that an enteric polymer with a pKa of 4
almost 99.9% un-ionized at pH 1, and 99.0% un-ionized at pH 2 conditions foun
stomach. This same polymer will be almost completely ionized at pH 6. In gene
polymer will be un-ionized and insoluble at pH values 2 units below its pKa, and con
ionized and soluble at pH values 2 units above its pKa. Based on the range of pH
to 3.5[19,21] in the stomach and 3.8 to 6.6[20] in the small intestine, the ideal pKa for
polymers that would prevent their gastric disintegration but help them disintegrat
rapidly in the intestine would be in the range of 3.5 to 5. As noted previously, n
enteric polymer can meet all enteric coating product needs according to the primary ob
for each product, or the needs of the drug(s).

Other factors that influence the disintegration or dissolution of enteric coatings

1. The initial fraction of free carboxylic acid groups on the polymer molecule
    stated that for cellulose acetate phthalate, a free carboxylic group of 9 to 1.
    best for enteric coating.
2. Nature of the core material. Ozturk and others[23] have shown that acidic core m
    may lower the pH of the coating layer relative to that of the bulk, resulting in
    in coating disintegration, whereas basic core materials increased the pH in the
    layer and could lead to premature disintegration in the stomach. These inves
    suggested that the pH-lowering effect of acidic drugs may be offset by cho
    polymer with a lower pKa, whereas for a basic drug, a polymer with a high
    would be desirable to avoid dosage form disintegration during gastric reside
    addition, the water-drawing affinity of the core and its swelling properties on e:
    to water can affect both the performance and reliability of the product. Clea
    nature of the tablet core can greatly affect the performance and reliability of
    coated products.
3. The ionic strength of the dissolution medium also influences coating dissoluti
4. The distance between various carboxyl groups on the polymer backbone also infl
    coating dissolution. Davis and others[25] showed that the pKa of various enteric pc
    increased as the distance between the phthalyl groups decreased, resulting in inc
    disintegration times. Similar results were reported by Delporte using polyvinyl
    phthalate (PVAP) batches of varying combined phthalyl contents as coatings.
5. Coating thickness influences dissolution. The thicker the coating, the longer
    take for the polymer to dissolve.
6. The presence or absence of plasticizers is another important factor that affe
    performance of enteric coatings.[25-27] This factor will be discussed in later sect

VI. ENTERIC COATING MATERIALS

Due to the large number of materials used or proposed for enteric coating, it will not be possible to give an in-depth treatment of all the materials in one chapter. This discussion therefore, is limited to enteric materials that have been widely used, are compendial materials, and have the potential for becoming widely used. The information provided here is largely drawn from technical literature obtained from the manufacturers of the various polymers as well as from the general literature.

A. SHELLAC

Shellac, also called purified lac, is a refined product obtained from the resinous secretion of a tiny insect, *Laccifer lacca* Karr, which lives in the branches of various trees found in India and other countries in that region.[28,29] Shellac is obtained through a series of purification of the secretions. There are two grades of shellac. Orange shellac is produced by a process of filtration in the molten state or by a hot solvent extraction. Bleached or white shellac is prepared by dissolving lac in aqueous sodium carbonate, bleaching the solution with sodium hypochlorite, and precipitating the bleached shellac with 2N sulfuric acid. Refined bleached shellac is shellac with its wax content removed.

On mild hydrolysis, shellac gives a mixture of aliphatic (about 50%) and alicyclic (5 to 10%) hydroxy acids. The major component of the aliphatic acid fraction is aleuritic acid, and that of the alicyclic fraction is shellolic acid (Figure 1). Shellac also contains about 5 to 6% wax and a small amount of lac pigment.[28]

1. Solubility

Shellac is soluble in ethanol, propylene glycol, ammonia solution, and alkaline solutions.

2. Use of Shellac as an Enteric Coating Material

Shellac has been used extensively as an enteric coating alone or in combination with other materials since 1930, when Wruble[30] reported on its use. He found that ammonia solutions of shellac provided the best enteric coatings, among a number of solutions investigated. Goorley and Lee[3] stated that a mixture of shellac and castor oil gave a satisfactory enteric coating. Due to several reported disadvantages, shellac is no longer the material of choice when considering enteric coatings. Gorley and Lee[3] pointed out that tackiness was a disadvantage of applying shellac as a coating. Also being of natural origin, there is the possibility of variation from batch to batch. Luce[31] showed that tablets coated with shellac had substantially increased disintegration times after 6 months of storage, compared to freshly coated tablets. After 12 months storage some tablets failed to disintegrate in simulated intestinal fluid. The delayed disintegration and reduced solubility of shellac on storage is attributed to polymerization resulting from transesterification of the hydroxyl group of one shellolic or aleuritic acid molecule with the carboxyl group of another of the hydroxyl-containing carboxylic acids. This esterification/aging process not only results in polymerization, but also reduces the number of carboxyl groups which provide the enteric solubility properties.

One other disadvantage of shellac as an enteric coating is that it does not dissolve below pH 7.[32] Since the pH in the small intestine, where most drug release is required, is between 3.8 and 6.9, failure of shellac-coated tablets to disintegrate at pH values below 7 is a major disadvantage. The requirement of a high pH for dissolution, coupled with delayed disintegration due to aging, makes it a real possibility that shellac-coated tablets may occasionally go through the gastrointestinal tract without releasing their active ingredients. Even when the active ingredient is released, it is obvious that the onset of action following administration of shellac-coated dosage forms may be greatly delayed. The use of shellac in controlled- or

$$CH_2OH-(CH_2)_5-(CH_2OH)_2-(CH_2)_7-COOH$$

Alleuritic Acid

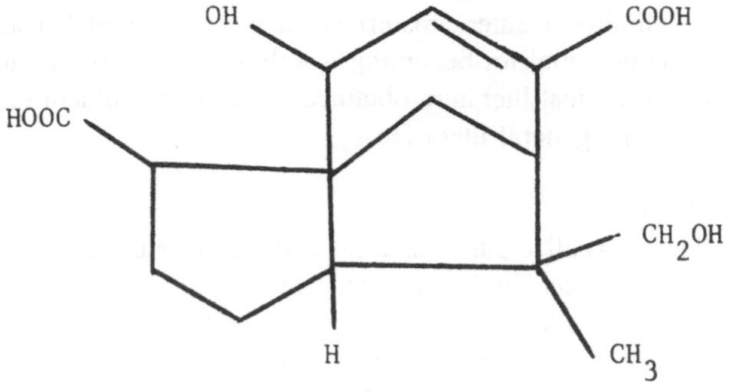

Shellolic Ac

FIGURE 1.   Chemical structures of shellolic and alleuritic acids.

sustained-release products is also risky due to reduced solubility resulting in altere
profiles that are likely to occur on aging.

On the positive side, shellac offers good protection against moisture perme:
and has been widely used as a seal coat for various tablets, especially vitamin tab
to coating with aqueous based compositions. It has also been recommended for inco
in HPMCP coatings to reduce gastric fluid permeation.[33] Making reference to t
shellac in wood finishing operations, Hicks[29] stated that "shellac in liquid form
the task of a sealer, undercoat and finish as no other substance will." In Worl
shellac was used in India for gasproofing clothing and waterproofing ammunition

India and Thailand produce most of the commercial shellac of the world.

B. CELLULOSE ACETATE PHTHALATE (CAP)

Cellulose acetate phthalate was first described as an enteric coating by Hiatt i
The oldest of the phthalate-containing polymers used in enteric coating, it is pre
reacting a partial acetate ester of cellulose with phthalic anhydride. Figure 2 s
chemical structure of CAP.

About half of the hydroxyl groups on the cellulose chain of this polymer are a
and about one fourth is esterified with one of the two acid groups of phthalic ;
other carboxyl group of phthalic acid is free to ionize. The degree of phthalyl su
influences cellulose acetate phthalate solubility in both aqueous and organic solv
therefore its performance as an enteric coating. Aqueous solubility increases with i
phthalyl content.[35] Because the degree of substitution can lead to changes in CAP pi
specifications for CAP composition have been established to ensure more uniform
mance, batch to batch. The NF specifications for CAP are shown below:

Combined phthalyl as $C_8H_5O_3$	30.0—36.(
Combined Acetyl as CH_3CO	19.0—23.!
Free Acid as $C_8H_6O_4$	≤6.0%
Viscosity of a 15% solution in acetone with a moisture content of 0.4%	50—90 cp:

1. Solubility of CAP

Cellulose Acetate Phthalate is insoluble in water, alcohols, hydrocarbons, and ch
hydrocarbons. It is soluble in ketones, ethers, alcohols, esters, and in certain solvent

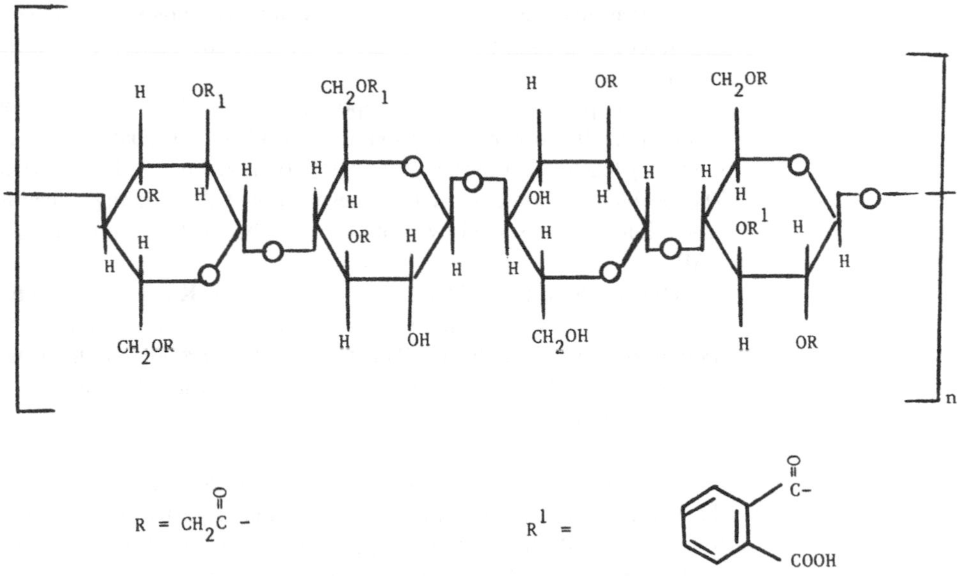

FIGURE 2. Chemical structure of cellulose acetate phthalate.

Its supplier, Eastman Chemical Products, Inc., lists the following as useful solvents and solvent blends:

Acetone
Acetone:ethanol   1:1
Acetone:methanol   1:3
Acetone:Methylene chloride   1:3
Ethyl acetate:Isopropanol   1:1

Other solvents listed in the literature for CAP include methyl ethyl ketone, dioxane, methyl acetate, and ethyl acetate.

2. Properties of CAP as an Enteric Coating Material

There are several reports in the literature about the effectiveness of CAP as an enteric coating material. Hodge and others,[37] after *in vivo* studies on the disintegration of CAP-coated tablets and capsules, concluded that cellulose acetate phthalate-coated tablets and capsules possessed satisfactory enteric characteristics. Ellis and others[38] stated that CAP comes very close to fulfilling the requirements of an ideal enteric coating material. There are also reports to the fact that CAP is a safe, nontoxic material.[36-40]

CAP is a polymeric acid, and behaves like other acidic materials which ionize and dissolve in regions of the gastrointestinal tract depending on the pH of the region and the pKa of the particular polymer samples. There are, however, a number of conflicting reports in the literature as to the mechanism of disintegration of CAP. Bauer and Masucci[41] presented *in vitro* experimental results to show that CAP dissolution in the intestine is due mainly to the hydrolytic action of intestinal esterases, and not due to ionization. Hayashi and others,[24] however, stated that although enzyme action may play a role, it is so slow, and that the main effect on CAP disintegration is ionization. Wilken and others[42] also presented results to show that pancreatin in simulated intestinal fluid had little effect upon the disintegration times of cellulose acetate succinate and cellulose acetate phthalate, and suggested that any effect by pancreatic enzymes was slow and overshadowed by the alkalinity of intestinal solution.

CAP as an enteric coating has significant advantages over shellac and some of the enteric coatings used before it. However, there are certain drawbacks to its use that go unmentioned.

CAP is permeable to water vapor, gastric fluid, and to some ionic substances. reported that in work involving sodium chloride tablets coated with CAP, the sodium c gradually leached out through the intact coating. Luce[43] also reported a similar obser The problem of ionic substances permeating CAP coatings, leading to failure of protection, can be solved by using a seal subcoat that is impermeable, before coatir CAP.

The choice of the right seal coat is important. Kanig[6] reported that when CAP w to coat previously subcoated sodium chloride tablets, a reaction occurred between drogen ion permeating the CAP coating and the carbonate in the subcoating, producir gas, that resulted in rapid rupture of the coating. Luce[43] recommends shellac as a gc coating material.

The permeability of CAP depends on a number of factors, including the presence and amount of plasticizer, and the presence of solid materials. Porter and Ridgway[44] co the permeability to water vapor, and simulated gastric fluid through enteric coatir found that CAP films were more permeable than PVAP films. They showed that inc diethyl phthalate (DEP) plasticizer concentration in CAP films decreased permeabil creasing pigment levels also decreased CAP permeability until pigment levels reache they called the critical pigment volume, beyond which permeability increased agair

Spitael and Kinget[45] showed that the solvent used in making CAP films and the of free film formulation (pouring vs. spraying) influenced the permeability of CAP and caffeine. The films were more permeable when sprayed than when poured. Film from the more volatile acetone were more heterogeneous and porous than those mac a less volatile solvent combination consisting of ethyl acetate and isopropanol.

Cellulose acetate phthalate, like all enteric polymer acid esters, is susceptible to lytic breakdown, during storage, especially under high temperatures and high hi conditions. When this occurs, phthalic and acetic acids are split off, resulting in an i in the free acid content and a decrease in the combined ester content. This is accompanied by an increase in viscosity of the polymer solutions. Such hydrolytic c will bring about changes in CAP enteric coating properties, that usually result in disintegration. The extent of hydrolysis may be obtained by checking the combined p content in combination with the viscosity. A combined phthalyl content of less tha with a sharp increase in viscosity, may mean the polymer will not function properl;

CAP does not dissolve until the pH of the media is more than 6.[36] While thi advantage over shellac, which does not dissolve below pH 7, if a lower pH-releasing is sought, as for example to reduce the onset of action, other enteric polymers r required. Figure 3[46] compares the dissolution rate of CAP as a function of pH, with other enteric polymers.

3. Preparation of CAP Coating Solution

Luce[43] investigated various procedures for making CAP solutions. He reported th; must always be added to the solvent to ensure proper solution preparation. When a solvent is used, CAP should be added slowly with vigorous stirring to about 80% solvent until complete solution occurs. The remaining solvent is then added. In the a mixed solvent, CAP must first be dissolved in the component in which it is most before adding the second solvent. In situations where neither of the mixed solven dissolve CAP, the polymer is dissolved in about 80% of the mixed solvent, and the rem solvent is then added.

Films of CAP are usually brittle and need plasticization. Effective plasticizers fc

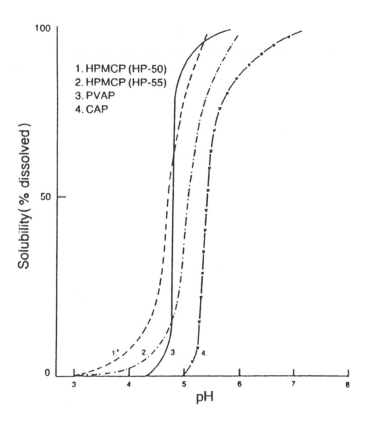

FIGURE 3. Dissolution as a function of pH of various enteric polymers. (From Colorcon Technical Data on Polyvinyl Acetate Phthalate, TD-17, 3M/ 1-81, Colorcon, Inc., West Point, PA. With permission.)

include diethyl phthalate, triacetin, tributyl citrate, and myverol 9—40 (acetylated monoglyceride).[36] The plasticizer is added after the cellulose acetate phthalate is dissolved, usually at a level of 25%, based on the dry weight of CAP. Additives other than plasticizers, such as pigments and detackifiers, may then be added to the coating solutions.

CAP is usually applied in concentrations of 10 to 15% w/v. At least a 5% w/w film level, relative to tablet weight, is required to ensure the integrity of CAP enteric coatings.[43]

Cellulose acetate phthalate has also been used in aqueous systems for enteric coatings. Eastman[47] describes aqueous solutions of CAP and a related polymer, cellulose acetate trimelitate (CAT), prepared by neutralizing the polymers with 30% ammonium hydroxide to form soluble salts of the polymers. In a description of the method, 100 g of the polymer is dispersed in 1 liter of water with stirring, and 18.5 or 27 g of 30% ammonium hydroxide, for CAP and CAT respectively, is stirred into the system until a clear solution results. The solution is then plasticized and is ready for coating. It is recommended that these solutions not be stored for more than 2 d. These solutions contain about 1 M excess of ammonium hydroxide over that required for neutralization but the excess ammonia volatilizes, and the pH drops from an initial value of about 9 to 7.

The other aqueous based system is Aquateric, produced by FMC.[48] It is a spray-dried CAP pseudolatex (see Chapter 9 for a discussion of pseudolatexes) with a particle size under 1 μm. Other components are Pluronic F68, Myvacet 9-40 and Polysorbate 80. In use the powder is redispersed in water with the aid of Tween 80. A plasticizer is usually added to the Tween 80 solution prior to the addition of the Aquateric.

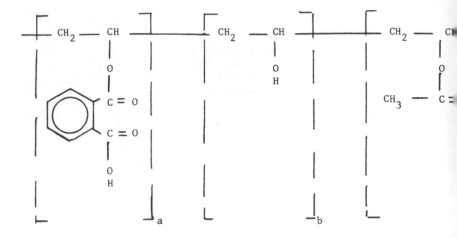

FIGURE 4.   Chemical structure of polyvinyl acetate phthalate (PVAP).

C. POLYVINYL ACETATE PHTHALATE (PVAP)

The structure of PVAP is as shown in Figure 4. It is produced by the esterifi
a partially hydrolysed polyvinyl acetate with phthalic anhydride. In Figure 4, (a)
with (b) depending on the phthalyl content. The acetyl fraction (c) will remain
and depends on the starting raw material.

NF Specifications

Combined phthalyl (as $C_8H_5O_3$)
Free phthalic acid (as $C_8H_6O_4$)
Free acid other than phthalic
Apparent viscosity of a 15% w/w viscosity in methanol at 25 ± 0.2%, using a capillary tube
viscometer

1. Solubility

The following have been identified as good solvents for PVAP.[46]

> Methanol, or Ethanol   95%
> Acetone-Methanol   1:1; Acetone-Ethanol   1:1
> Methanol-Methylene chloride   1:1

PVAP is less than 1% soluble in both acetone and isopropanol.

2. Properties of PVAP as an Enteric Coating Material

The aqueous solubility of PVAP, like the other phthalate-containing polymer
dependent. It is not soluble in low pH media but dissolves quickly at pH 5.[46] Th
PVAP a good enteric polymer. Table 1, which is taken from a paper by Delporte
the relationship between phthalyl content and the disintegration times of PVAP-coate
Since the polymer backbone, polyvinyl alcohol, is water soluble, Delporte attri
observed effect of phthalyl content to the reduction in the ease of solubilizatic
polymer by increasing phthalyl content.

A property of PVAP that makes it a superior enteric polymer in some situatio
it is much less permeable to water vapor and simulated gastric fluid, compared v
and other polymers typically used.[44]

As a phthalate-containing polymer, PVAP is also labile to hydrolysis. Howeve

TABLE 1
The Effect of Phthalyl Content of PVAP on the Disintegration Time of PVAP-Coated Tablets

Phthalyl content %	Disintegration time (min)					
	pH 1.2	pH 3.5	pH 4.5	pH 5.5	pH 6.5	pH7.5
38			22.5	13.5	12.5	10
44.7			55	19.2	23.2	17.5
49.5				22.5	23.2	23.5
53		More than 120 min		25	27.5	24.5
57.3				26.5	30.2	26.5
58.3				30.7	27	18
62.6				60	52	36
65.8				67	56	35

is more resistant to hydrolysis than CAP and HPMCP. Porter[49] compared the hydrolytic stability of CAP, HPMCP, and PVAP when subjected to 60°C and 75% relative humdity for 10 d, and found the amount of phthalyl lost in each case to be 22.0%, 8.0% and 0.3% for CAP, HPMCP, and PVAP, respectively.

Figure 5 compares the viscosities of various enteric polymer solutions. It is clear from the figure that PVAP has the lowest viscosity among the polymers studied, at the same concentration.

PVAP has been approved by the FDA as safe for coating use, following toxicity studies in various animal species and supporting clinical work. Toxicological data obtained from Colorcon[50] shows that the LD_{50} in rats and mice is >8 g/kg of body weight. Values greater than 5 g/kg are usually indicative that a material is practically nontoxic. There is indication that PVAP is not totally devoid of toxicity, however, if consumed over extended periods of time in amounts >1000 mg/kg body weight. Rats fed with 1000 and 3000 mg/kg body weight for 2 years had gastrointestinal irritation. When larger doses were fed to pregnant rats and rabbits, offspring had low body weight. There was also a higher incidence of malformations and greater resorptions. The amount of coating put on an enteric dosage form is typically less than 50 mg per tablet, which poses little or no safety hazards.

3. Coating Preparation

PVAP coating solutions ranging from 10 to 30% can be easily made in any of the recommended solvents or solvent combinations, depending on the coating method to be used. Opaseal, which is a 30% alcoholic solution of PVAP, is typically applied by the ladle procedure, diluted or undiluted.

In spray coating methods, a coating solution of 10% PVAP is used. Colorcon[46] recommends methanol as the most effective solvent for PVAP for spray applications. Jackson[51] reported that unplasticized PVAP films showed varying degrees of cracking, and listed the following plasticizers as effective for PVAP:

- Citroflex 2 (Triethyl citrate)
- Triacetin (Glyceryl Triacetate)
- Citroflex A_2 (Acetyltriethyl citrate)
- Carbowax 400

The above list is in the order of preference based on compatibility and performance tests. The recommendation is to use them at a level of 10% of the PVAP amount. Jackson[51] and Colorcon[46] stated that no advantage was seen when higher concentrations were used, and

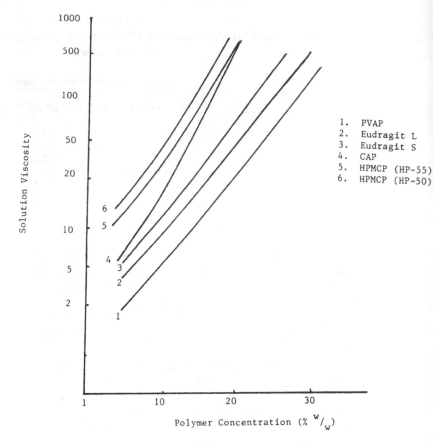

FIGURE 5.   Concentration vs. viscosities of solutions of various enteric polymers in a 1:1 mixture of methanol and methylene chloride. (From Colorcon Technical Data on Polyvinyl Acetate Phthalate, TD-17, 3M/1-81, Colorcon, Inc., West Point, PA. With permission.)

that at 20% plasticizer level, tablets became tacky when stored at 50°. The followir example of a typical coating solution for spray application:

PVAP	10%
Citroflex 2	1%
Stearic acid	2%
Methanol	87%

Stearic acid is included to act as a detackifier. In addition to the recommended deta a pigment may also be added at 10% of the PVAP amount. An 8% coat weight for mented, and 6% for pigmented coating, usually enables coated tablets to meet USP fications.

PVAP can also be applied in aqueous systems. Coateric is a solid coating conc manufactured by Colorcon which is dispersed in water just prior to coating.[49,52] Tl centrate contains PVAP, plasticizer, and pigment.

To make the suspension the solid concentrate is first dispersed by stirring in Ammonium hydroxide is added next in the amount of 4 ml of 30% solution for eve g of Coateric, to stabilize the system from agglomeration. The ammonia combines w of the polymer to form a soluble salt, which stabilizes the system. Much of the an from the salt is lost by vaporization during coating, returning the polymer to its acidi

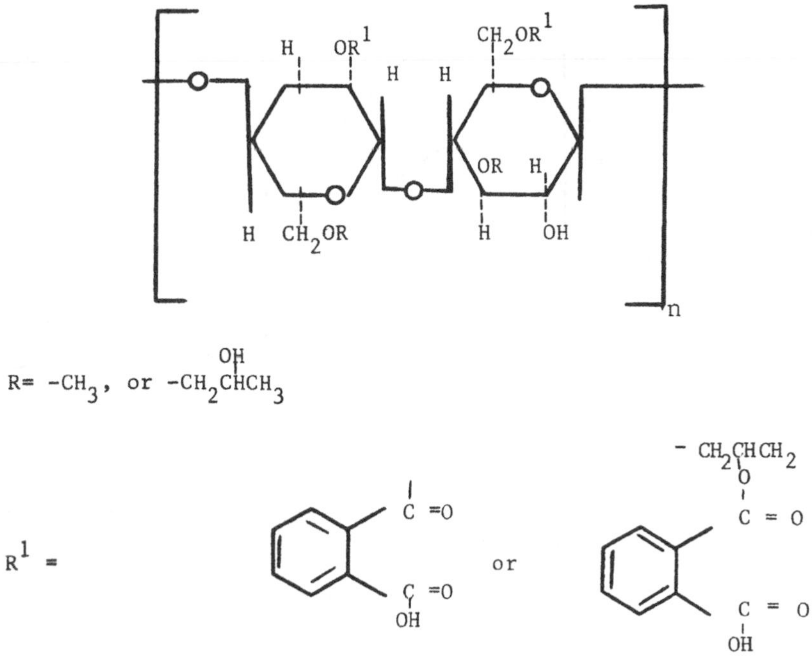

FIGURE 6. Chemical structure of hydroxypropyl methylcellulose phthalate (HPMCP).

D. HYDROXYPROPYL METHYLCELLULOSE PHTHALATE (HPMCP)

Hydroxypropyl methylcellulose phthalate is the newest of the phthalate-containing materials used as enteric coatings. It is prepared by reacting hydroxypropyl methylcellulose with phthalic anhydride.[33] Figure 6 shows the chemical structure of HPMCP.

Two grades of HPMCP are described in the 16th edition of the National Formulary (NF XVI); HP-50 which corresponds to NF 220824, and HP-55 which corresponds to NF 200731.[53] The various grades vary in their degree of substitution. Also available, but not currently described in the NF XVI, is HP-45. A variant of HP-55 is HP-55S, which has a higher average molecular weight of 33,000, as opposed to HP-55 with an average molecular weight of 20,000.[54] HP-55F differs from HP-55 only in the sense that particle size is much smaller.

NF Specifications

	HP-50	HP-55
Free phthalic	$\leq 1\%$	$\leq 1\%$
Phthalyl content	21—27%	27—35%
Methoxy content	20—24%	18—22%
Hydroxypropoxy content	6—10%	5—9%

The viscosity of a 2% aqueous solution of HP-50 is 192 to 288 cps. That of a 15% methylene chloride/methanol 1:1 of HP-55 is 155 to 228 cps.

1. Solubility

All grades of HPMCP are soluble in the following solvent combinations:[33]

Acetone/water (95:5)
Acetone:methanol (1:1)
Methylene chloride/methanol (1:1)

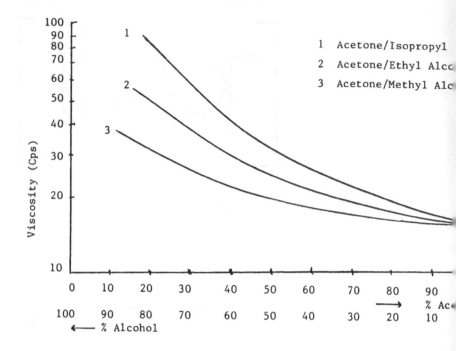

FIGURE 7.   Effect of mixed solvent composition on the viscosity of 10% HP-55 solutions. (From propylmethylcellulose phthalate, Tech. Bull., Appendix 2, Shin-Etsu Chemical Co., Tokyo, 1984. mission.)

Methylene chloride/ethanol   (1:1)
Ethylacetate/methanol   (1:1)
Dioxane

HP-55 is also soluble in acetone, acetone/ethanol (1:1), acetone isopropanol, methylene chloride, and ethyl acetate.

The viscosity of solutions of HPMCP in mixed solvents depends on the solv and their ratio as shown in Figure 7.[34]

2. Properties of HPMCP as an Enteric Coating Material

The mechanism of action of HPMCP is the same as for the other phthalate-c enteric polymers. It is insoluble in water and gastric media, but dissolves by ioni the pH is increased to the levels found in the upper small intestine. The numerical des that follow the HP letters in each product name indicates the pH of dissolution. 1 50 dissolves approximately at pH 5, while HP-55 hydrates and undergoes disso about pH 5.5. These polymers, therefore, dissolve at a lower pH compared to most of the other enteric polymers. Dosage forms coated with HPMCP may, the expected to disintegrate and release more rapidly in the intestine than those co other polymers (all other factors being equal), resulting in a more rapid onset However, a polymer that releases at a pH of 5 could release in the stomach of some in in the fed state. Again, it should be noted that no single enteric polymer known at is ideal for every drug and every coating objective or purpose.

Toxicity studies in rats by Kitagawa and others[55,56] showed that the administ up to 4 to 5 g/kg of body weight of HPMCP showed no evidence of toxicity. Da up to 5 g/kg body weight for 6 months did not elicit any toxic symptoms. Woodwa daily doses of up to 3 g/kg body weight to beagle dogs for 53 weeks. After comp test dogs with the control, he concluded that there was no toxic symptoms due to

Ito[58] also showed that HPMCP has no teratogenic effects. All the above studies show that HPMCP is very safe.

HPMCP is also quite stable. It is not as stable as PVAP, but is more stable than CAP. Pancreatin tablets coated with HPMCP were found to be chemically and physically stable during 4 years of storage in closed containers.[54]

A disadvantage of HPMCP as an enteric coating is that like CAP, it is permeable to moisture and gastric fluids. A manufacturer's comparison of the moisture permeability of two HPMCP grades with CAP found that the amount of water permeating in 24 h through free films was 246, 168, and 213 g/m^2 for HP-50, HP-55, and CAP, respectively.[34]

One method that has been suggested to overcome gastric fluid permeability through HPMCP coatings is to combine HPMCP with shellac in the coating. A 0.1mm thick coating composed of 80:20 HP-55/shellac, reduced the penetration of gastric fluid to below 2%. Double this coating thickness was required to accomplish the same effect when HP-55 was used alone. While shellac does provide a good barrier to water and gastric fluid, and may be useful in HPMCP and other systems, its chemical instability should be remembered and considered in such formulation approaches.

Another problem that has been encountered with HPMCP coating is cracking.[33] Shin-Etsu has investigated this problem and found certain factors that contributed to cracking. The type of tablet being coated was one factor. Cracking usually occurred when the tablets contained microcrystalline cellulose or carboxymethyl cellulose. Also, tablets that were damaged during coating tended to crack. The solvent composition also influenced cracking. Tablets coated with solvent combinations that contained 50% isopropanol cracked, whereas the same kind of tablets coated using other solvent combinations did not crack if the amount of isopropanol was held at 30% or less. The other factor identified was temperature and humidity. Tablets cracked when coated under low humidity conditions, but did not crack when coated under higher humidity conditions.

The right choice of solvent and the inclusion of plasticizers decreased the incidence of cracking. The use of HP-55S could also reduce cracking, since being a higher molecular weight material, it should produce films with a higher resistance to cracking.

3. Coating Preparation

Although a number of solvent mixtures have been listed for HPMCP, the best solvents for HP-50, HP-55 and HP-55S, according to Shin-Etsu and other workers, are methylene chloride/ethanol and ethanol/water combinations. Coatings applied from these solvents are reported to give excellent enteric properties with a glossy finish.[34]

Acetone, acetone/isopropanol, and acetone/ethanol can also be used. Combinations with isopropanol are not good solvents for HP-50 since they produce higher viscosity solutions. Such combinations containing isopropanol sometimes result in cracking, as has been noted. In making HPMCP solutions containing alcohol, the polymer must first be dispersed in the alcohol with stirring. The other solvent is then added slowly with continued stirring.

The concentration of HPMCP used in coatings depends on the kind of solvent used, quantity of coating desired, and whether tablets or granules are to be coated. The concentrations usually range from 5 to 10% for tablet coating, and 4 to 7% for granule coating.

HPMCP coatings can be made without a plasticizer; however, plasticizers may be used to produce more flexible films and to reduce cracking. Suitable plasticizers include glycerin fatty acid esters, monoglycerides, and triethyl citrate.

If another film former is to be added, the material should first be dissolved in a portion of solvent system being used and then added to the HPMCP solution.

Coating levels of 5 to 10% HPMCP relative to dosage-form weight afford good enteric coatings.[33]

Aqueous dispersion of HPMCP can be made with the aid of a wetting agent and plasticized with triacetin for use in enteric coatings.[54]

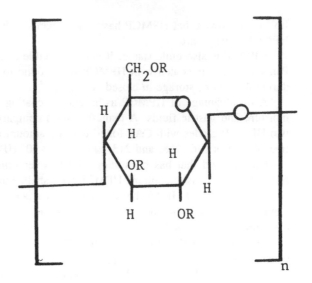

R = H, $-$ CH$_3$, $-$ CH$_2$CH(OH)CH$_3$, $-$ COCH$_3$, $-$ COCH$_2$CH$_2$CO

$-$ CH$_2$CHCH$_3$
$\quad\quad$ |
$\quad\quad$ O$-$COCH$_3$ $\quad\quad\quad\quad$ or $\quad\quad\quad\quad$ $-$ CH$_2$CHCH$_3$
$\quad\quad\quad\quad\quad\quad\quad\quad\quad\quad\quad\quad\quad\quad\quad\quad\quad\quad\quad\quad$ |
$\quad\quad\quad\quad\quad\quad\quad\quad\quad\quad\quad\quad\quad\quad\quad\quad\quad\quad\quad$ O$-$COCH$_2$CH$_2$

FIGURE 8.   Chemical structure of hydroxypropyl methylcellulose acetate succinate (HPMCAS

Stafford[59] also described the use of an aqueous solution of HPMCP in enteric c
In this method, HPMCP is first dispersed in water and then neutralized with a base t
the solution. He reported that for 100 g HPMCP, 11.8 g of 25% aqueous ammoni
g of sodium hydroxide, or 25.3 g triethanolamine is required to fully dissolve HPM

A related substance which has also been described as an enteric coating is Hydroxy
Methylcellulose acetate succinate (HPMCAS).[60]

E. HYDROXYPROPYL METHYLCELLULOSE ACETATE SUCCINATE [(HPMCAS) AQOAT®]

Hydroxypropyl methylcellulose acetate succinate is also manufactured by Shin-
Its chemical structure is as shown in Figure 8.

There are three types of HPMCAS that vary in their degree and type of substituti
solubility at varying pH ranges from 5 to 7. The three types are

- AS-LG (LF), which dissolves at pH 5.0.
- AS-MG (MF), which dissolves at pH 5.5.
- AS-HG (HF), which dissolves at higher pHs and is usually employed in su
release formulations. The G types are granules, and are organic solvent solub
F types are fine powders for making aqueous dispersions.

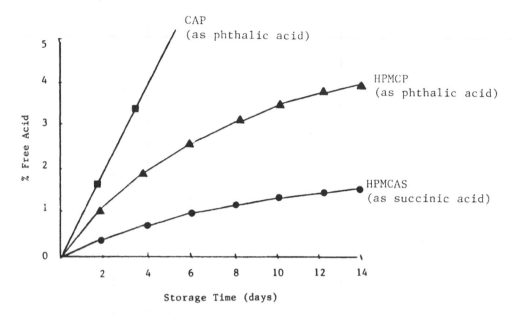

FIGURE 9. Comparison of hydrolytic breakdown rate of CAP, HPMCP, and HPMCAS (Each polymer was stored at 60°C and 100% relative humidity). ■ CAP (as phthalic acid); ▲ HPMCP (as phthalic acid); ● HPMCAS (as succinic acid). (From Nagai, T., Sekigawa, T., and Hoshi, N., in *Aqueous Polymeric Coatings for Pharmaceutical Dosage Forms*, McGinity, J. W., Ed., Marcel Dekker, New York, 1989, 81. With permission.)

Chemical Specifications

	AS-LG AS-LF	AS-MG AS-MF	AS-HG AS-HF
Succinic Acid	Not more than 1%		
Methoxyl content	20—24	21—25	22—26
Hydroxypropoxy content	5—9	5—9	6—10
Acetyl content	5—9	7—11	10—14
Succinoyl content	14—18	10—14	4—8

1. Solubility

HPMCAS is soluble in acetone, methanol, methylene chloride/ethanol 1:1, and ethanol:water 8:2. The recommended plasticizer to be used with HPMCAS materials is triethyl citrate, at a level of 15 to 20% for AS-LF, and 30% for AS-MF and AS-HF.

An aqueous coating dispersion is made by first dissolving the plasticizer in water, followed by dissolution of some hydroxypropyl cellulose (HPC) in the system. The HPMCAS is then added with stirring, followed by a silicone antiforming agent. HPC stabilizes the dispersion.

A comparison of HPMCAS coatings applied from an organic solvent, and from aqueous dispersion, showed that both had similar properties.[53]

Figure 9 shows that HPMCAS films are more stable than CAP and HPMCP films.

Typical coating formulations based on the HPMCAS polymers are as follows:

For granules		**For tablets**	
HPMCAS AS-LF	10%	HPMCAS SM-LF	10%
Triethyl citrate	2%	Triethyl citrate	3%
Talc	5%	Titanium dioxide	2%
HPC-MF	0.05%	HPC-MF	0.05%
Water	82.95%	Water up to	100%

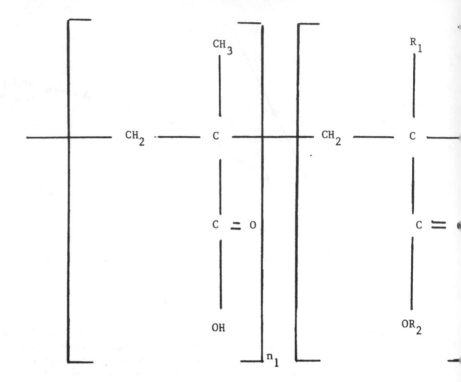

FIGURE 10.   Chemical structure of methacrylic acid copolymers (Eudragits).

F. METHACRYLIC ACID COPOLYMERS (EUDRAGIT)

A variety of acrylic acid copolymers have been described by Rohn Pharma
use in various forms of coatings, including sustained release coatings which are
but permeable throughout the gastrointestinal tract (Eudragit RL and RS), and coat
dissolve in the stomach (Eudragit E).

The types of methacrylic acid polymers used in enteric coatings are methac
methylmethacrylate copolymers (Eudragit L and S), and methacrylic acid eth
copolymer (Eudragit L 30D).[62]

Figure 10 shows the chemical structure of the methacrylic acid copolymer.

R_1 and R_2 are both methyl groups ($-CH_3$) in Eudragit L and S. R_1 is hydroge
R_2 is an ethyl group ($-C_2H_5$) in L 30D.

Eudragit L and L 30D have a methacrylic acid content of 46 to 50.6%, and
n_1/n_2 is about 1:1, whereas Eudragit S has a methacrylic acid content of 27.6
producing an acid to ester ratio n_1/n_2 of approximately 1:2.

Free methacrylic acid and ester monomers in the Eudragit polymers is $\leqslant 0.3$

1. Solubility

Eudragit S and L are soluble in polar organic solvents such as alcohols, aceton
of alcohol or acetone with esters, and chloroform.

Eudragit S, L and L 30D are insoluble in gastric fluids but dissolve in the i
the formation of polymeric salts. They have very low water and gastric fluid pe
Lehman and Dreher[65] studied the release of acetylsalicylic acid from tablets c
Eudragit L, and showed a drug release of only 0.5% to 5.5% after 2 h of exposur
fluid, depending on the amount of coating applied and the batch size of tablets
a 10% coating level, 0.6% acetylsalicylic acid was released after 2 h in gastric
1 kg batch of tablets were coated. This amount increased to 4.1% when a 50 k

tablets was coated at the same coating level. In both cases more than 80% of the drug was released 1 h after the tablets were transferred to USP-simulated intestinal fluid.

Eudragit L 30D dissolves at pH slightly above 5.5. Eudragit L dissolves at pH above about 6, and Eudragit S at a pH above 7.[65,66] The delayed disintegration of Eudragit S could result in incomplete drug release for some drugs; however, advantage could be taken of this delayed release in the formulation of drugs that are targeted to be released in the colon. A mixture of Eudragit L and S could be used to effect dissolution between pH 6 and 7.

The Eudragits have good storage stability against hydrolysis. Eshra[67] found no change in carboxylic acid content after storage at room temperature at 100% relative humidity for 3 months. Lehman[66] also showed that there was very little change in the release of aspirin particles coated with Eudragit L 30D after storage periods ranging from 26 months to 41 months.

One concern over the use of Eudragit coatings has been the possible presence of residual monomers used in their manufacture. Klaus and Lehman,[66] however, have stated that the monomers used in their manufacture have very low toxicity. The LD_{50} values were listed as 7.9 g, 2.2 g, and 1.02 g/kg body weight for methyl methacrylate, methacrylic acid, and ethylmethacrylate, respectively. The amount of total monomers in the Eudragit products for pharmaceutical purposes is usually less than 0.1%.[66] These polymeric substances are not absorbed and not degraded, and are excreted unchanged. No toxicity effects were observed after 2 weeks when rabbits and dogs were fed from 6 to 28 g/kg body weight of dry Eudragit copolymers. Also, no significant changes were observed in rats after chronic toxicity studies over a 3-month period. Thus the Eudragit copolymers appear to be safer than was first thought. They are listed in NF XVI and have been recognized as safe by the Federal Drug Administration (FDA).

2. Application

Eudragit L and S are supplied either as 12.5% solutions in isopropanol (Eudragit L 12.5 and Eudragit S 12.5) or as solid powders (Eudragit L100 and Eudragit S100) that can be dissolved in organic solvents. Also available is Eudragit L 12.5 P. This plasticized material contains 1.25% dibutylphthalate as a plasticizer, in addition to the 12.5% copolymer in isopropanol.[68]

Eudragit L 30D is a 30% aqueous dispersion (latex). When spray dried, the resulting dry powder is designated Eudragit L100-55. Eudragit L100-55 can be dissolved in organic solvent or dispersed in water for coating applications.

The recommended use concentration of Eudragit solutions in organic solvents is from 4 to 7%. Eudragit solutions tend to be sticky. Substances such as talc and magnesium stearate are usually added to reduce tackiness and stickiness. Eudragit films are brittle and need to be plasticized. Suitable plasticizers include polyethylene glycol, propylene glycol, diethylphthalate, dibutylphthalate, and Triacetin. The plasticizers are used at a level of 10% of the dry weight of the copolymers; however, up to 20% could be added without affecting film properties.

The dry Eudragit powders (L100, S100, and L100-55) are dissolved in organic solvents by stirring into an appropriate solvent in which a plasticizer has been added. The resulting solution is clear to opaque. Undissolved residue may be removed by filtration or decantation. Rohm Pharma recommends that if a higher concentration of around 20% is required for any reason, a 4:6 solvent mixture of acetone/isopropanol be used for L100, and a 1:1 solvent mixture of the same solvents be used for L100-55.[69]

Talc or magnesium stearate are usually added to reduce stickiness or tack, as noted, as well as to produce smoother films. Pigments are added for colored coatings. Such additives are dissolved or dispersed in a portion of the solvent and added to the Eudragit solution, after which the whole system is homogenized or milled.

Rohm Pharma gives the following examples of colorless and colored enteric coatings:[64]

Colorless coating	Parts by weight
Eudragit L/S 12.5 solution	489
Talc/mag stearate	12
Isopropyl alcohol	502
Plasticizers	6

Colored coating	Parts by weight
1. Pigment suspension 30% solids	
Isopropyl alcohol	330
Talc/mag stearate	80
Titanium dioxide/color pigment	60
Polyethylene glycol 6000	10
Water	20
2. Eudragit L/S 12.5 solution	400
Diluent	1100
Total	2000

To achieve good enteric properties it is recommended that a coating of 3 to 5 of dry Eudragit L/S film former be applied. This corresponds to a 3 to 5% weight i with 8 mm diameter tablets, with a thickness of 4 mm, and weighing 200 mg.

Rohm Pharma gives the following as average requirements for production of coating:

1.   For 1 kg tablets, 350 g of Eudragit L12.5 is required, while for 1 kg of gr pellets or powders, 800 g of Eudragit L12.5 is required.
2.   50 g Eudragit L100-55/kg of tablets and 150 g/kg of granules.
3.   An average coating level of 4 to 6 mg/cm^2 is required for L30D and L100-55

Eudragit L30D can be used as supplied (30% dispersion), or diluted with water use. The same plasticizers mentioned earlier are suitable. Magnesium stearate is incom with Eudragit L30D and should not be added. Some pigments, depending on their charge, will also be incompatible, and produce latex coagulation.

The following is an example of coating formulation using L30D:[70]

Pigment suspension (30% solid)	Parts by weight
Water	7,000
Talc	2,040
Titanium dioxide	400
Polyvinyl pyrollidone	150
Antifoam agent	10
Eudragit L30D	16,667
Plasticizer	500
Water	15,333
Total	42,500

Eudragit L100-55 is dispersed in water with the aid of a small amount of al dispersion formulation sufficient for coating 10 kg of medium size tablets is descri Rohm Pharma as follows:

300 g of L100-55 is slowly added to 610 g of water with stirring. This is followed by the slow addition of 1 *N* sodium hydroxide solution (4.04 g NaOH) and stirring is continued until a low viscosity milky liqui

A few drops of silicone antifoam is then added to prevent extensive foaming. The resulting dispersion can then be treated as previously described for Eudragit L30D.

VII. EVALUATION OF ENTERIC COATINGS

A. *IN VITRO* METHODS

There are a number of reports in the literature relating to enteric coated products that met *in vitro* compendial requirements, but failed to perform as required *in vivo* because they either disintegrated in the stomach, excessively released their drug content in the stomach, or failed to release adequate amounts of drug in the intestines.[71-76] Madan and Minisci,[72] for instance, noted that 11 out of 17 enteric coated products which met USP gastric resistance requirements released drug in the stomach. Wagner[75] evaluated a commercial enteric coated tablet administered to human volunteers, which was recovered in the feces and found to contain 98% of the administered sodium aminosalicylate still in unreleased tablet form. The coating used in this case was of the "fat/wax" type, which has since been replaced by a carboxylic acid/ester polymer. These reports in the literature all seem to agree that the reason for such a lack of acceptable *in vivo* performance for coated products, which have met *in vitro* requirements, is that current *in vitro* tests do not adequately predict *in vivo* performances.

The British Pharmacopea (BP) test for enteric coated tablets[77] involves performing a disintegration test in 0.1 M HCL for two hours, and then examining the tablets for any evidence of disintegration and cracks. If there are no cracks or disintegration, the tablets have passed the acid resistance test. They are then transferred to a phosphate buffer (pH 6.8), and the test continued for another 1 h. The USP test[78] performs a disintegration test on the tablets in simulated gastric fluid USP for only 1 h, and then examines the tablets for the presence of disintegration, cracking, or softening. Tablets that pass the acid resistance test are then transferred to simulated intestinal fluid for an additional 2 h. The tablets are required to disintegrate in simulated intestinal fluid or phosphate buffer and release the drug to meet the compendial specifications.

The USP also has a dissolution test in which the coated tablets are tested in 0.1 N HCL for 2 h and then transferred to a pH 6.8 buffer for an additional 45 min. Tablets releasing less than 10% drug after 2 h in 0.1 N HCl have met the USP requirements for gastric protection. To meet the requirements at pH 6.8, 80% of the drug must be released to solution within the time specification.

Based on our current knowledge of human gastrointestinal physiology, one can easily see why the above compendial methods have not been able to adequately predict performance *in vivo*. One of the drawbacks of the current methods is that they do not take into account the realities of gastric emptying. As mentioned earlier, gastric emptying may take anywhere from less than 1 h to over 7 h. A coating that resists gastric disintegration for 1 or 2 h as used in the BP and USP tests may not necessarily remain intact, if it is held in the stomach for 6 h or longer, due to delayed gastric emptying. Furthermore, the gastric pH is not as low as 1.2 to 1.5 (or below), as produced by a gastric test media of 0.1 N HCL.

Madan[73] showed that the rate of drug release for some enteric coated products in gastric fluid increased with time. One of the products he studied released less than 1% sodium salicylate in 15 min, but by the end of 1 h the amount released was about 19%, and by the end of 2 h, about 60% of the drug was released. With another product, the amounts released increased from less than 1% in 15 min to about 10% in 1 h to 80% in 2 h.

The above results will tend to suggest that even when an enteric coated product has released less than 10% drug in 2 h, there is the possibility of releasing more if it stays in gastric media for more than 2 h. Since enteric coatings may be permeable to gastric fluid and to dissolved drug, it is important in designing and evaluating enteric products to actually measure the drug that is released to solution in gastric media.

Based on gastric emptying alone, it is suggested that acid resistance tests [be] extended to about 6 h. While *in vitro* tests may not be able to duplicate the variab[le] gastric emptying rates even within a single individual, a product that resists simulat[ed] fluid for 6 h *in vitro* is more likely to have better resistance and more reliability in per[formance] in a population of subjects than one that has proved acid resistant for only 2 h o[r]

The other major factor to be considered when designing *in vitro* tests for enteri[c] is gastrointestinal pH. One of the main reasons why enteric products failed in t[he past] their performance was the mistaken idea that the gastric pH was about 1, an[d the] intestinal environment was alkaline. Compendial tests have recognized that mistak[e] and are now using pH 6.8 instead of 7.5 as the pH for simulated intestinal media[. This is] a step forward. However, based on the current knowledge of gastrointestinal pH o[f 1 to 3.5] in the stomach, and 3.8 to 7 in the small intestine, it is not enough to choose pH 6.8 as test media conditions, especially when designing enteric products.

A coating which performs well at pH 1.2 may not behave in the same way if it e[ncounters] a stomach pH of 3 or higher. Also a coating that allows 80% of drug to be relea[sed at pH] 6.8 in 45 min to 1 h is not necessarily going to release the same amount of the [drug at pH] below 6. It is the opinion of the authors that in order to reduce the possibility of [premature] disintegration and/or drug release, or the occurrence of incomplete drug dissol[ution and] reduced bioavailability, disintegration and dissolution studies should be performe[d at inter-] mediate pHs such as pH 3, 4, 5, and 6, in addition to pH 1.2 and 6.8. This is [especially] important in the design of new products, which will allow a more objective fo[rmulation] approach based on specific product goals. It is also suggested that manufacturers [of enteric] products develop meaningful *in vitro* tests for each such product they produce[, tests that are] relevant to expected performance in human subjects and the therapeutic goals of tha[t product.]

The most reliable evaluations for enteric coated products are *in vivo* evaluatio[ns. As] noted by Kanig,[6] it is not possible to repeatedly use human subjects for routine e[valuation] of each manufactured lot. It is important to design *in vitro* tests to closely resemb[le in vivo] conditions, if results obtained *in vitro* are to be good predictions of *in vivo* perfor[mance. A] good *in vitro* test could at least serve to screen good products from bad ones.

B. *IN VIVO* METHODS

As discussed above, current *in vitro* methods of evaluating enteric coatings [do not] accurately predict *in vivo* performance. It is, therefore, important that enteric coate[d dosage] forms be subjected to *in vivo* evaluations. The *in vivo* methods that have been use[d include] x-ray techniques,[3,20,37] gamma camera scintigraphy,[79] pharmacokinetic techniqu[es, and] radio telemetric methods.[81]

With the X-ray method, the coating material is applied to tablets containin[g barium] sulfate. The tablet is then administered to human volunteers or dogs, and its progr[ess in the] gastrointestinal tract followed by periodic X-rays. Serious disadvantages exist for [this] technique. It is not a continuous monitoring method. Gastric emptying and table[t disinte-] gration will nearly always occur between exposures, making it difficult to obt[ain exact] emptying and disintegration times. Radiation exposure limits which are acceptable [prevent] using frequent X-ray examination. The radiation hazard from this approach may b[e viewed] as unacceptable by human subject review committees under any circumstances. In [addition,] incorporating a sufficient amount of barium sulfate or other radio-opaque material t[o produce] the necessary effect alters the tablet substrate from the desired commercial or test [product.]

In gamma camera scintigraphy, the coated dosage form contains a gamma[-emitting] radioisotope which enables its progress to be followed along the gastrointestinal tr[act with] a gamma camera. This procedure has revolutionized our ability to monitor the per[formance] of all types of delayed and sustained release dosage forms. The level of radiation [exposure] to the subject is low. In some of our studies, even when subjects are used in si[x] repeated tests with different products, the *total* radiation exposure they receive is *less* than the difference in natural radiation a person receives who lives in Denver, compared to a person who lives closer to sea level in the Midwest or on the East Coast. A second advantage of the gamma scintigraphy procedure is that it can be monitored *continuously*. In addition, procedures exist that allow outlining the gastric region with good resolution. The amount of nuclear material added to the tablet is very low, permitting use of a test core tablet that is little changed (or unchanged) in properties and performance, compared to the commercial or development product. Using double label and other techniques, it is possible to monitor both the integrity and permeability of the coating in the stomach, and rate and location of release following gastric emptying. Exact time to emptying, and time to disintegration and release in a population of subjects can be determined. This nuclear method also makes it possible, for the first time, to develop *in vitro* methods which correlate to *in vivo* performance, since it is possible to accurately *measure in vivo* performance. It is confidently predicted that gamma camera scintigraphy will be a basic methodology in the design of many future dosage forms, including site-specific controlled-release products such as enteric forms, as well as bioadhesive and other controlled release systems.

The pharmacokinetic procedure involves withdrawing and assaying blood samples for the presence of drug initially contained in the coated dosage form, at various time intervals after administration. Dressman and Amidon[81] cite the inability of this method to distinguish long gastric emptying times from slow or delayed enteric coat dissolution release as a major disadvantage.

An example of the radiotelemetric method was described by Dressman and Amidon,[81] who enteric coated tablets containing citrate buffer powder components ranging from pH 3 to 5. The coated tablet was tied to a Heidelberg capsule which is capable of transmitting gastrointestinal pH. The capsule and coated tablet were administered to dogs. If the coating remained intact in the stomach, the pH transmitted from the stomach will be similar to that transmitted in a control study without the tablet. If the coating disintegrated in the stomach, a higher gastric pH than the control would be transmitted as the buffer dissolves. Disintegration of the coating in the intestine will result in a decrease of intestinal pH. If the tablet did not disintegrate in the intestinal region, the pH transmitted would be similar to control values.

VIII. RECENT ADVANCES AND FUTURE OF ENTERIC COATINGS

Over the past several decades, major advances have occurred in the enteric/delayed release dosage form arena. The first is the availability of a greatly expanded range of polymers/copolymers having improved chemical stability and offering a range of dissolution pH characteristics. The second is that we have a much better understanding of gastrointestinal human physiology, including ranges in normal gastric and intestinal pH, ranges in gastric emptying times and emptying characteristics, and ranges in intestinal transit times. This new information has been made possible by radiotelemetric pH monitoring and gamma camera scintigraphy for emptying, transit, and other information. The latter technique has revolutionized our ability to accurately measure and monitor the actual *performance* of enteric and other delayed release products. Development of aqueous-based enteric coating formulations and systems is proceeding at a rapid rate. In the future we should be able to develop *in vitro* to *in vivo* performance correlations that will allow us to validate enteric product performance from *in vitro* test data.

REFERENCES

1. Coating of pills, *Am J. Pharm.*, 39, 467, 1867.
2. Unna, Keratinirte Pillen, *Pharm. Zentrahlle*, 25, 577, 1884.
3. **Goorley, J. T. and Lee, C. O.**, A study of enteric coating, *J. Am. Pharm. Assoc.*, 27, 379, 1
4. **Thompson, H. O. and Lee, C. O.**, History, literature and theory of enteric coatings, *J. Am Assoc., Sci. ed.*, 34, 135, 1945.
5. **Yvon, M.**, *Union Pharm.*, 436, 1891, through *Yearb. Pharm.*, 236, 1982.
6. **Kanig, Joseph L.**, Production and testing of enteric coatings, *Drug Stand.*, 22, 113, 1954.
7. **Lesser, M. A.**, Enteric coatings, *Drug Cosmetic Ind.*, 49, 151, 1941.
8. **Bourquelot, E.**, *Pharm. J.*, 48, 1035, 1889.
9. **Shroeter, Louis, C.**, Coating of tablets, capsules and pills, in *Remingtons Pharmaceutical Science* E. W., Ed., Mark Press, Easton, 1965, 595.
10. **Porter, Stuart, C.**, Tablet coating, *Drug Cosmetic Ind.*, 44, 1981.
11. **Vickers, F. N. and Malcolm, S. M.**, Aspirin gastritis: gastro duodescopic observations, *Gastroer* 44, 419, 1963.
12. **Madan, P. L.**, Minimizing the incidence of ASA induced occult gastrointestinal bleeding, *C Assoc.*, 114, 496, 1976.
13. **Weiss, A., Pitman, E. R., and Graham, E. C.**, Aspirin and gastric bleeding: gastroscopic obse *Am. J. Med.*, 31, 266, 1961.
14. **Scott, J. T., Porter, I. H., Lewis, S. M., and Dixon, A. S.**, Studies of gastrointestinal bleedi by corticosteroids, salicylates and other analgesics, *Q. J. Med.*, 30, 167, 1961.
15. **Sjogren J. and Bogentoft, C.**, How useful is enteric coating to improve drug delivery?, in *Opt* of Drug Delivery, Proceedings of Alfred Benzoin Symposium, 17, Bundgaard, Hansen, H., Ba and Helmer, K., Eds., Munksgaard, Copenhagen, 1981, 53.
16. **Delporte, J. P.**, Les Enrobages Enterique, *Pharm. Acta Helv.*, 45, 525, 1970.
17. **Wruble, M.**, A laboratory method for the study and control of enteric coatings, *J. Am. Pharm* 27, 21, 1938.
18. **Bukey, F. S. and Brew, M.**, A study of the emptying time of the stomach with reference to tablets, *J. Am. Pharm. Assoc.*, 23, 1217, 1934.
19. **Chambliss, W. G.**, The forgotten dosage form: enteric coated tablets, *Pharm. Tech.*, 7, 124, 1
20. **Warton, A. G., Kempf, G. F., Burrin, P. L., and Bibbins, F. E.**, A new enteric coating and a method for its control, *J. Am. Pharm. Assoc.*, 27, 21, 1938.
21. **Wagner, J. G.**, Enteric coatings, in *Biopharmaceutics and Relevant Pharmacokinetics*, Drug In Pub., Hamilton, 1971, Chap. 23.
22. **Hiatt, G. D.**, Enteric coating for medicaments, U.S. Patent 2,196,768, April 9, 1940.
23. **Ozturk, S. S., Palsson, B. O., Donohoe, B., and Dressman, J. B.**, Kinetics of release fro coated tablets, *Pharm. Res.*, 5, 550, 1988.
24. **Hayashi, M., Nagal, T., and Jogami, H.**, Factors affecting dissolution rate of cellulose acetate in aqueous solution, *Chem. Pharm. Bull.*, 18, 2350, 1970.
25. **Davis, M., Ichikawa, I., Williams, E. J., and Banker, G. S.**, Comparison and evaluation polymer properties in aqueous solutions, *Int. J. Pharm.*, 28, 157, 1986.
26. **Spitael, J. and Kinget, R.**, Preparation and evaluation of free films: influence of plasticizers upon the permeability, *Pharm. Acta Helv.*, 52, 106, 1977.
27. **Lachman, L. and Drubulis, A.**, Factors influencing the properties of films used for tablet coating of plasticizers on the water vapor transmission of cellulose acetate phthalate films, *J. Phram.* 639, 1964.
28. **Shellac**, in *Handbook of Pharmaceutical Excipients*, American Pharmaceutical Association, Wa D.C., 1986, 251.
29. **Hicks, E.**, *Shellac, Its origin and Applications*, Chemical Publishing Co., New York, 1961.
30. **Wruble, J. S.**, Enteric coatings, *Am. J. Pharm.*, 102, 318, 1930.
31. **Luce, G. T.**, Disintegration of tablets enteric coated with CAP, *Manu. Chem. Aerosol News*, 49, 5
32. **Payne, Michael,** Enteric coating, *Pharm. J.*, 25, 657, 1966.
33. **Kuriyama, I., Nobutok, M., and Nakanishi, M.**, Permeability of double-layer films 1., *J. Pha* 59, 1341, 1970.
34. Hydroxypropylmethylcellulose phthalate, Tech. Bull., Appendix 2, Scin-Etsu Chemical Company 1984.
35. **Malm, C. J. and Fordyce, C. R.**, Cellulose esters of dibasic organic acids, *Ind. Eng. Chem.*, 1940.
36. **Eastman Chemical Products, Inc.**, Eastman CAP Enteric Coating Material, Eastman Publicat 100E, 1988.

37. **Hodge, H. C., Forsyth, H. H., Jr., and Ramsey, G. H.,** Clinical tests of cellulose acetate phthalate as an enteric coating, *J. Pharmacol. Exp. Ther.,* 80, 241, 1944.

38. **Ellis, J. R., Prillig, E. B., and Endicott, C. J.,** Tablet coating, in *The Theory and Practice of Industrial Pharmacy,* 2nd ed., Lachman, L. L., Herbert, A., and Kanig, Joseph, L., Eds., Lea and Febiger, Philadelphia, 1970, chap. 12.

39. **Hodge, H. C.,** The Chronic toxicity of cellulose acetate phthalate in rats and dogs, *J. Pharmacol. Exp. Ther.,* 80, 259, 1944.

40. **Watanabe, N. and Fujii, T.,** Teratolgical study of cellulose acetate phthalate in mice, *Lyakuhin Kenkyu,* 6, 49, 1975 through *C.A.,* 88:99222a, 1978.

41. **Bauer, C. W. and Masucci, Peter E.,** The action of intestinal enzymes upon cellulose acetate phthalate and butyl stearate enteric coated tablets, *J. Am. Pharm. Assoc. Sci. Ed.,* 37, 124, 1948.

42. **Wilken, L. O., Jr., Kochhar, M. M., Bennett, D. P., and Cosgrove, F. P.,** Cellulose acetate succinate as an enteric coating for some compressed tablets, *J. Pharm. Sci.,* 51, 484, 1962.

43. **Luce, G. T.,** Cellulose acetate phthalate: a versatile enteric coating, *Pharm. Tech.,* 1, 27, 1977.

44. **Porter, S. C. and Ridgway, K.,** The permeability of enteric coatings and the dissolution rates of coated tablets, *J. Pharm. Pharmacol.,* 34, 5, 1982.

45. **Spitael, J. and Kinget, R.,** Preparation and evaluation of free films: influence of method of preparation and solvent composition upon the permeability, *Pharm. Acta Helv.,* 52, 47, 1977.

46. Colorcon Technical Data on polyvinyl Acetate Phthalate, TD-17, 3M/1-81, Colorcon, West Point, PA.

47. Aqueous Film Coating of Various Drugs in Tablet Form with Eastman CAP and CAT Enteric Coating Materials, Eastman Tech. Publ. 11, ZFD-121, Eastman Chemical Products, Kingsport, 1988.

48. **Joachim, J., Benhalima, N., Delarbre, J. L., Joachim, G., and Delonica, H.,** Galenic and spectroscopic study of sodium sulfathiozole coated with aquateric, in Aquateric aqueous enteric coating, *Appl. Bull.,* Research Update 4, 1.

49. **Porter, Stuart C.,** The Use of opadry, coateric and surelease in the aqueous film coating of pharmaceutical oral dosage forms, in *Aqueous Polymeric Coatings for Pharmaceutical Dosage Forms,* McGinty, J. W., Ed., Marcel Dekker, New York, 1989, 317.

50. Polyvinyl Acetate Phthalate (PVAP) — A toxicological summary — Obtained from Colorcon, West Point. PA

51. **Jackson, Gerald J.,** Properties and applications of polyvinyl acetate phthalate in tablet coating, presented at the Acad. Pharm. Sci. 19th Natl. Meet., Atlanta, November 16 to 20, 1975.

52. Coateric 0804-06, Complete Colored Aqueous Enteric Coating for Aspirin Tablets, Colorcon Technical Data, PTB-06, July 1988, Colorcon, West Point, PA.

53. Analytical methods and Specifications of HPMCP, Appendix 1, Shin-Etsu Chemical Co., Tokyo.

54. Hydroxypropylmethyl cellulose phthalate, in *Handbook of Pharmaceutical Excipients,* American Pharmaceutical Association, Washington, D.C., 1986, 141.

55. **Kitagawa, H., Satoh, T., Yokoshima, T., and Nanbo, T.,** *Pharmacometrics,* 5, 1, 1971.

56. **Kitagawa, H., Yokoshima, T., Nanbo, T., and Hasegawa, M.,** *Pharmacometrics,* 8, 1123, 1974.

57. **Woodward, G.,** HP50 and HP55, Repeated Oral Administration of Each Test Material to Dogs for 53 Weeks, Final Report by Woodward Research Corporation.

58. **Ito, R. and Toida, S.,** *J. Med. Soc.,* Toho Univ., 19, 453, 1972.

59. **Stafford, J. W.,** Enteric film coating using completely aqueous dissolved hydroxypropyl methylcellulose phthalate spray solutions, *Drug Dev. Ind. Pharm.,* 8, 513, 1982.

60. Hydroxypropyl Methylcellulose Acetate Succinate, Shin-Etsu Technical Bulletin, Shin-Etsu Chemical Co., Tokyo.

61. **Nagai, T., Sekigawa, T., and Hoshi, N.,** Applications of HPMC and HPMCAS aqueous film coatings of pharmaceutical dosage forms, in *Aqueous Polymeric Coatings for Pharmaceutical Dosage Forms,* McGinity, J. W., Ed., Marcel Dekker, New York, 1989, 81.

62. Eudragit Acrylic Resins at One Glance, Rohm Pharma Technical Information (Info o/e), Rohm Pharma, Darmstadt, West Germany.

63. Polymethacrylates, in *Handbook of Pharmaceutical Excipients,* American Pharmaceutical Association, Washington, D.C., 1986, 214.

64. Eudragit L and S, Rohm Pharma Technical Publication, Prospectus (Info L/S — 1/e), Rohm Pharma, Darmstadt, West Germany.

65. **Lehman, K. and Dreher, D.,** Coating of tablets and small particles with acrylic resins by fluid bed technology, Prod. Manuf. Inf., *Int. J. Pharm. Tech.,* 2, 31, 1981.

66. **Lehman and Klaus, O. R.,** Chemistry and application properties of polymethacrylate coating systems, in *Aqueous Polymeric Coatings for Pharmaceutical Dosage Forms,* McGinity, J. W., Ed., Marcel Dekker, New York, 1989, 153.

67. **Eshra, A. G.,** Einfluss von sauer oder basisch reagierenden modellsubstanzen auf die stabilitat von filmumhullungen beim wechsel von organischen auf wassrige herstellungs methoden, dissertation, Frieburg, 1982.

68. Standards Sheet (Info L/S — 7/d), Rohm Pharma, Postfach Darmstadt, West Germany.
69. Eudragit Data Sheets on L100 (Info L — 4/e) and L100-55 (Info — L-5/3), Rohm Pharma, West Germany.
70. Processing of Eudragit Acrylic Resins in the Hi-Coater, Eudragit Technical Procedure Pamphl 1/e), Rohm Pharma, Darmstadt, West Germany.
71. **Morrison, A. B. and Campbell, J. A.,** The relationship between physiological availability o and riboflavin and *in vitro* disintegration time of enteric coated tablets, *J. Am. Pharm. Asso* 49, 473, 1960.
72. **Madan, P. L. and Minisci, Marie,** *In vitro* determination of the resistance of commercial ent to acidic conditions, *Drug Intell. Clin. Pharm.,* 10, 588, 1976.
73. **Madan, P. L.,** *In vitro* evaluation of drug release from commercial enteric coated tablets in acid II. Quantitative evaluation of selected products, *Indian J. Pharm. Sci.,* 41, 99, 1979.
74. **Levy, G.,** Failure of USP disintegration test to assess physiologic availability of enteric coa *N.Y. State J. Med.,* 3002, December 15, 1964.
75. **Wagner, J. G., Wilkinson, P. K., Sedman, A. J., and Stol R. G.,** Failure of USP tablet di test to predict performance in man, *J. Pharm. Sci.,* 62, 859, 1973.
76. **Clark, R. L. and Lasagna, L.,** How reliable are enteric coated asprin preparation?, *Clin. Ther.,* 6, 568, 1965.
77. *British Pharmacopeia,* Vol. II, Her Majesty's Stationary Office, London, 1980, A114.
78. *U.S. Pharmacopeia 21/National Formulary 16,* 16th ed., U.S. Pharmacopeial Convention, Inc. MD, 1985, 1243.
79. **Davis, S. S.,** The use of scintigraphic methods for the evaluation of novel drug delivery systems, *Drug Delivery,* Borchardt, R. T., Repta, A. J., and Stella, V. J., Eds., Humana Press, Clifton, 319.
80. **Lappas, L. C. and McKeeham, W.,** Polymeric pharmaceutical coating materials. II. *In vivo* of enteric coatings, *J. Pharm. Sci.,* 56, 1257, 1967.
81. **Dressman, J. B. and Amidon, G. L.,** Radiotelemetric method for evaluating enteric coatings. *Pharm. Sci.,* 73, 935, 1984.

Chapter 4

COACERVATION: PRINCIPLES AND APPLICATIONS

David W. Newton

TABLE OF CONTENTS

I. TERMINOLOGY AND PUBLICATION HISTORY

Coacervation was coined in 1929 by H. G. Bungenberg de Jong and H. R. [describe separation of aqueous colloid solutions into two immiscible liquid layers.[1] 1930s and 1940s, de Jong authored many reports on coacervation studies of prote vegetable gums, which were published in European journals. This work is summa pages 232 to 482 of Reference 1.

According to the research record of de Jong, *aqueous phase separation* is [synonym of *coacervation; liquid crystals* and *metaphases* are descriptive alternative papers refer to film-depositing nonaqueous phase separation as coacervation in son maceutical sources.[2-4] The earliest commercial application of coacervation was to velopment of "carbonless" carbon copy paper by the National Cash Register Co which resulted from patents by B. K. Green and L. Schleicher in the late 1950s.[2] that was a microencapsulated product, some pharmaceutical reports have referred [ervation and microencapsulation interchangeably.

The first reference to coa(z)cervation in *Chemical Abstracts* was 24: 4061,[9] 1[word was introduced as a general subject with volume 28, page 8174, 1934. Sinc *Chemical Abstracts* has indexed 595 citations under the prefix of *coacervat*. Of the stem has appeared in the titles of 206 enteries. Finally, observation of the phenom coacervation anteceded introduction of the term in 1929. The separation of protein s[into two liquid layers, the lower containing microscopic droplets, was apparently o during, or before, the early 1900s.[1,6,**]

II. PHYSICOCHEMICAL CHARACTERISTICS OF AQUEO SYSTEMS

De Jong classified coacervates as *simple* or *complex*, according to the content o protein or vegetable gum) or two (protein and gum or protein) hydrocolloids. Form simple coacervates was concluded to result from molecular dehydration or "water [in the system, whereas complex coacervates depended on electrostatic attraction cromolecular cations and anions. Some comparative features of the two types are [Table 1.[1,5,7]

Reflecting over 25 years of rigorous plasma protein research, Cohn understa["Natural products rarely exist in a state of maximum purity or concentration."[8] The considering that gelatin is a protein derived from crudely extracting hides and bon acacia is the gum exudate of a tree, the quantity and quality of data reported for coa studies thereof is remarkable.

Coacervates are equilibrium systems composed of both a relatively concentrate dilute solution, which impart opacity on mixing. Microscopic observation (100 ×] settled or centrifuged coacervate layer features primarily either the absence, a spa persion, or a dense sediment of microspheres. Creaming of emulsions physically res the latter case. With either a simple or complex coacervate, the largest particulate the largest molecule, so coacervate layers or drops, unlike aqueous micelles, may flow through porosites barely large enough to permit transport of their constituen cule(s).

---

* Reference to coacervates separating as immiscible *liquids* or *layers*, not *phases*, recognizes that the f[of the same state and constituency, albeit in unequal proportions.
** According to page 338 of Reference 1, immiscible droplets were observed in mixed protein solutions

TABLE 1

Comparative Characteristics of Complex and Simple Coacervates of Type A Gelatin*

	Characteristics of coacervates	
Factor	**Complex**	**Simple**
Gelatin, weight %[a]	<3[b]	>2
Optimum pH	3—4.5 (<IEP)[c]	1—10 (Na_2SO_4)
		7—10 (ethanol)
Inducing agent	Stoichiometric proportions of po- lyanionic macromolecule	Water-miscible solvent (40—60% ethanol); inorganic salt[d] (7—10% Na_2SO_4)
Inorganic salts	Suppressant	Inducing
Direct current	Disappearance	No change

[a] Total percentage in mixture of coacervate and supernatant liquids at 40—50°C.
[b] Coacervation may occur imperceptibly at concentrations less than 0.1%.
[c] Acid-extracted or Type A gelatin has an isoelectric pH range of 7—9; it is a net polycation at lower pH values.
[d] Percentage compositions in mixtures of coacervate and supernatant liquids.

* Adapted from De Jong, H. G. B., in *Colloid Science*, Vol. 2, Kruyt, H. R., Ed., 1949, 257. With permission of the publisher, Elsevier, New York.

The physicochemical variables affecting the occurrence and nature of coacervates include:

1. Concentration and intrinsic properties of macroions and microions
2. pH
3. Temperature
4. Dielectric constant
5. Mixing proportions or intermolecular stoichiometry of components

The specific water-solute and solute-solute relations in coacervates remain unproven, but reduced hydration of the macromolecules, thereby concentrating them in the dense, viscous coacervate, is the empirical hallmark.

A. SIMPLE COACERVATES

While there are references to other colloids, gelatin has been the most common subject of patents and papers on simple coacervation.[1,2,5-7,9] Usually, gelatin coacervation is induced by the addition of sodium sulfate (Na_2SO_4) or ethanol, after the earlier reports by de Jong. The supernate will contain more water and ethanol or salt than the coacervate, but the coacervate will contain 3 to 60 times as much gelatin. Coacervation ceases upon adequate dilution of such systems with water, and its pH-dependency with ethanol compared to Na_2SO_4 (Table 1)[7] suggests slight differences between mechanisms of action.

Simple coacervation may be effected with macromolecular nonelectrolytes (methylcellulose, polyvinyl alcohol), polyanions (acacia, pectin), polycations (gelatin), or polydipolar ions (isoelectric gelatin).[1,5,7] Judging from these electrochemically dissimilar solutes, *simple* appears to belie the physicochemical situation.

It is possible that the liquid phase separation of solvent-salt solution mixtures[10] and mixtures of lithium citrate and neuroleptic amine salt solutions[11] are thermodynamically similar to coacervates. The lower amine-rich, water-insoluble, and ethanol-soluble layer of the latter systems contain microdroplets,* but the largest constituent ion has a formula weight of only 407.

* The microscopic observation of droplets in the viscid lower phase was made belatedly in 1989 by the author.

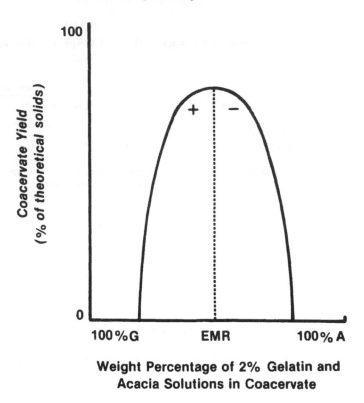

FIGURE 1.   Theoretical coacervate yield measured as the percentage of solids vs. the wt% of 2% isohydric acacia and gelatin solutions. The equivalent mixing ratio, EMR, produces the neutrally charged coacervate, with net positive and negative coacervates to the left and right, respectively (Adapted from De Jong, H. G. B., in *Colloid Science,* Vol. 2, Kruyt, H. R., Ed., 1949, 358. With permission of the publisher, Elsevier, New York.)

B. COMPLEX COACERVATES

Complex describes more phenomenologically than constituitively these much gated, lesser elucidated, liquid systems. De Jong concluded that complex coacer concentrated solutions of undissociated ion pairs, for which a maximum yield occ the ions are present in an electrically neutral equivalent mass or mixing ratio.

At this mixing proportion the positive gelation ions . . . unite with the negative arabinate ions in their equivalent weights corresponding to the given pH; here neither an excess of the one nor of the o component is present. For this equivalent mixing proportion [ratio, EMR] it is appropriate to speak of sal a salt (gelatin-arabinate), however, which separates out with a fairly large amount of water not as a phase but as a typical liquid. The equilibrium [supernatant] liquid — in which the colloid ratio is the the coacervate — then takes on the significance of the saturated solution of this colloid-colloid salt.[1]

This explanation is theoretically depicted in Figure 1, where the EMR de electrically neutral coacervate, not a 1:1 weight mixture of gelatin and acacia.[1,1] parative graph based on duplicate samples of 14 weight ratios from 0.02 to 50:1 of ge sulfate:heparin sodium is shown in Figure 2.[13] The occurrence of maximum coace a gentamicin:heparin weight ratio of approximately 0.8:1 corresponds to a respec lecular ratio of approximately 1:0.015 to 0.2.[14,15,**]

** Analysis of heparin sodium, USP resulted in molecular fractions ranging from 3,000 to 37,500 D

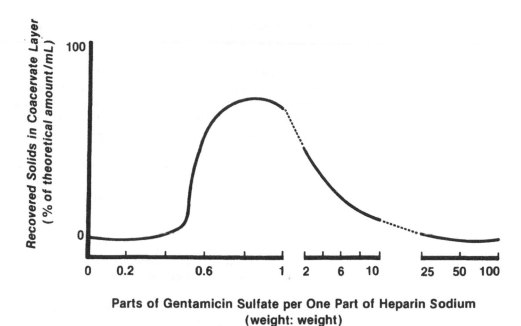

FIGURE 2. Effect of the weight ratio of gentamicin sulfate to heparin sodium on the yield of solids from the coacervate layer of 100 mg/ml solutions. (Unpublished data from the author.)

Gelatin-acacia coacervates were first reported by de Jong,[1] and numerous subsequent studies are cited in Reference 5. The systems gelatin-pectin,[16] gelatin-carbomer,[17] and gelatin-carboxymethylcellulose[18,19] have also been investigated. As with the more important case of aqueous solubility in general, research on complex coacervation since that of de Jong has not yielded a uniformly predictive quantitive theory.[12]

The intermolecular forces that maintain coacervates, the effect of inorganic salts on them, and their spherical occurrence as concentrated solutions continue to stimulate interest. Though de Jong regarded complex coacervates to form by electrostatic or salt bonds, subsequent research evidence suggests a more complicated situation. For example, a nonrepulsive electrosteric interaction between unlike ions could promote reinforcement by van der Waals intermolecular forces in the complex.[20] Such hydrophobic interactions are vital to maintaining the tertiary structure of dipolar proteins.[21,22] Similarly, nucleic acid conformation results from intermolecular hydrogen bonding. Yet, dilute salt solutions perturb neither of these, but dissolve coacervates.

Alternatively, complex coacervates may be stabilized by statistically favored ion-induced dipole forces: "... polarization of dissociable protons — gives rise to intermolecular forces .... The fluctuating [resonating] charge force will be present only when groups are partially dissociated ... in limited ranges of pH."[21]

Accordingly, the pH-dependent minimum equivalent weight (EW) of the polycation coincides with maximum coacervation when combined with the polyanion in ratios that are conducive to both maximum intermolecular nonrepulsion and ion-induced dipole attraction. The plausibility of ion-induced dipoles and the requirement of low EW of the polycation in complex coacervates is suggested by the following observations:

1. Coacervates are stable on dilution with deionized water, which should effec
    ciation of solely electrostatic complexes.*
2. Coacervation of the oppositely charged polyion solutions results in no apparent
    expansion,[1,13] which is otherwise expected from interionic association;[21]
3. Decreasing [permanent] charge on gelatin and acacia with increasing sodium
    concentration does not fully account for the suppression of coacervation;[12]
4. Higher inorganic salt concentration is required to dissolve complex coacer
    clupeine, a lower EW polycation, than those of gelatin; thus, a greater ionic
    is necessary to suppress interpolyionic forces;
5. Stable microdroplets occur with low EW polycations, e.g., gentamicin-hepa
    clupeine-phosphatide,[1] compared with readily coalescing droplets in gelatin-a
6. After some 50 pages, de Jong profoundly challenged his apparent, but electi
    ically incongruous,** direct ionic bonding hypothesis in this sole passage
    413: " . . . [that] gelatin-gum arabic coacervate is a Newtonian liquid . . . d
    a fuller explanation. The direct contacts postulated [up to here] . . . can ha
    static . . . [or] permanent. We must conceive these contacts as dynamic . .
    now and again let go to make afresh other contacts."[1]

The monoexponential increase of solute in the supernates of gelatin-acacia co
systems with increasing potassium chloride concentration shown in Figure 3[23] appe
itatively identical with decreasing electrophoretic mobility of gelatin and acacia ca
added sodium chloride.[12] The Debye-Hückel suppression of interionic association wi
ionic strength, (I), applies also to dipolar ions. But the logarithm of the activity co
is proportional to I, not $I^{0.5}$, in the latter case.[10]

De Jong proposed that salts suppress coacervation by direct ion shielding, cl
charge, not referring to the antedating Debye-Hückel effect.[1] Recent quantitative
have not elucidated the specific mechanism.[12,24,25]

Precise prediction of coacervation according to both ingredients and conditions
ently not possible; not all polycation-polyanion combinations coacervate. The co
variables of pH, and concentration and mixing ratio of gelatin and acacia, show com
patterns in Figures 4 and 5.[1] The data of de Jong, adapted in Figure 5, likely repres
of tedious protein nitrogen and other assays, dedicated to quantifying the colloid fr
The gelatin and acacia contents in coacervates were 10 to 40 times those of the sup

With type A gelatin and acacia, otherwise favorable pH and mixing ratios fail
coacervation when their concentrations exceed approximately 4%.[1,5,26] It has been su
that this unproven phenomenon results from the same mechanism as inorganic sa
tion.[1,12] Dissociation of complex coacervates may be causally similar to the salti
solubility increase of some proteins by low salt concentrations, which results fr
dipole attractions that increase protein polarity; and thus hydration.[10]

De Jong proposed that most of the water in a coacervate was occluded or ph
immobilized between, e.g., gelatin and acacia molecules.[1] The microscopic observat
densely packed microspheres spontaneously reform when water is overlaid on gent

---

* Gelatin and acacia, like other hydrophiles that form complex coacervates, are efficient hydrogen bon
  and acceptors as well as polyions. These two electrochemical properties favor intramolecular and interm
  mesomers and tautomers, resulting in aqueous "melts" instead of saturated solutions in equilibrium
  excess solid phase. A statistical result of intermolecular resonance would be the observed decrease of
  water molecules of hydration, an entropy effect that similarly accounts for a tenfold water-solubility of
  over cyclohexane.

** The author is unaware of essentially ionic, undissociated compounds of formula weights as large a
  and acacia that exhibit such high aqueous concentrations as those in complex coacervates (5-15%
  Jong probably suspected likewise, but lacked research evidence to impugn ionic bonding in complex coa

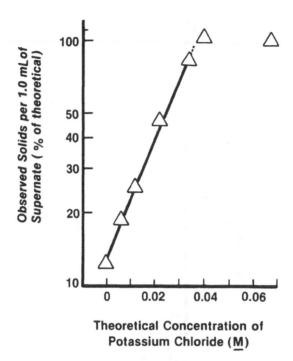

FIGURE 3. Effect of added potassium chloride concentration on the yield of solids from the supernatant layer of coacervates containing equal volumes of 3% type A gelatin and acacia at pH 4.0 and 40°C. (Unpublished data from the author.)

heparin coacervate, which was previously dried to an amorphous, glassy film, suggests the ordered hydration of a complex to effect solution.[13].*

C. MICROSPHERES

The diffuse or dense occurrence of droplets in coacervates is fascinating, yet has received little explanation. The opacity appearing with coacervation is attributed to the formation of microspheres. Because the components of the supernate are not intermolecularly associated as in the coacervate, different refractive indexes result in turbidity of the mechanically agitated system.[1.5] While essentially pure aliquots of the supernate or intercoacervate liquid may be obtained following centrifugation, the coacervate cannot be completely separated from it in its native state.

The gelatin-acacia coacervate requires controlled rate stirring at 40 to 50°C to obtain microspheres.[5,26] In contrast, discrete droplets less than 25 μm in diameter occur in static gentamicin-heparin complex coacervates.[13]

Spontaneous, stable liquid microspheres likely derive from the strongly attracted, minimally hydrated, three-dimensional intermolecular complexes. High surface tension is favored thermodynamically by the minimum surface area to volume ratio of the sphere, and there is high interfacial tension between the coacervate and the coexisting supernate. The apparent exact volume additivity of the polyion solutions in producing the microspherical coacervate, like other gross features, is analogous to that of oil-in-water emulsions.

---

* The apparent nominal droplet size of gentamicin-heparin coacervate remains unchanged after prolonged centrifuging, which further argues against the water content being not electrochemically attracted.

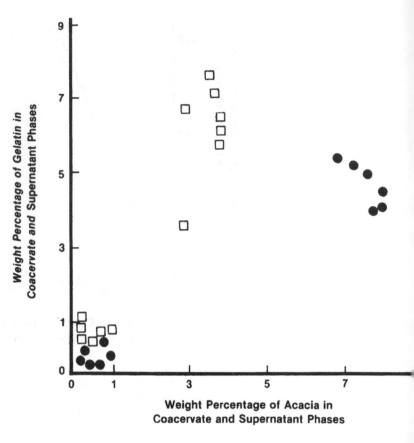

FIGURE 4.   Wt% of acacia and gelatin in the coacervates (values >3%) and supernates (val
<2%) of systems plotted against gravimetric mixing ratios of gelatin:acacia ranging from 0.5:1—
in 2% solutions. □, pH 4.0; ●, pH 3.0. (Adapted from De Jong, H. G. B., in *Colloid Scien*
Vol. 2, Kruyt, H. R., Ed., 1949, 359. With permission of the publisher, Elsevier, New York

III. PHARMACEUTICAL APPLICATIONS AND POSSIBILI

To date, the singular public pharmaceutical objective of coacervation has been to
microcapsules. Unlike traditional hard and soft gelatin capsules, which are filled
powders or fluids for oral ingestion, microcapsules resulting from aqueous and non
phase separation are not uniform hollow chambers. They are matrices of polymer
initially deposited *in situ* as concentrated liquid microglobules or flexible films, resp

A. NONAQUEOUS MICROENCAPSULATION
Nonaqueous phase separation casts polymer films about suspended solid or li
ticles. It is based on differential polymer solubility. The separated phase is not of
ingredients and state as the equilibrium solution from which it deposits, unlike
coacervates.

Pharmaceutical microencapsulation is used to control the stability and *in vivo*
site of release of drugs. The film formation is achieved by[2-5] (1) adding a poor s
incompatible polymer to the first solution, the latter obeying Flory-Huggins the
controlled solvent evaporation; and (3) temperature adjustment. The morphology
range of recovered microcapsules or nanoparticles is predominantly controlled by
and degree of aggregation of the surrounded drug particles, in concert with agita
related physical variables.

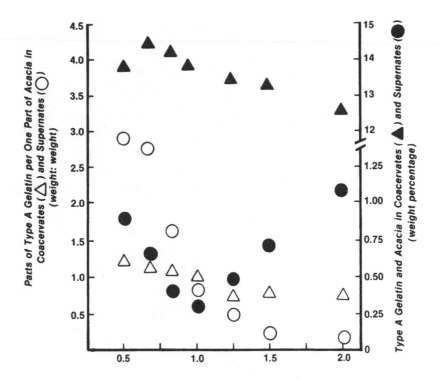

FIGURE 5.   Weight ratio of gelatin/acacia [left ordinate] and total weight percentage of gelatin + acacia [right ordinate] in coacervates and supernates plotted against gravimetric mixing ratios of gelatin: acacia in pH 3.5, 2% solutions (Adapted from De Jong, H. G. B., in *Colloid Science*, Vol. 2, Kruyt, H. R., Ed., 1949, 360. With permission of the publisher, Elsevier, New York.)

B. AQUEOUS MICROENCAPSULATION

As the title of this book includes polymers, the relationship of coacervates to polymers is briefly revisited here. Coacervates are polymeric in that they usually contain one or more macromolecules comprised of small (FW<300) monomers. Complex coacervates may also be considered association colloids, but not like aqueous surfactant micelles.

Simple and complex coacervates are effective wetting agents, readily spreading over most suspended solids and emulsified oils.[1,5,26,28,29] References 28 and 29, the first reports on drug coating via coacervation, appeared coincidentally in 1964 with *International Pharmaceutical Abstracts* by the American Society of Hospital Pharmacists. By June, 1988, *International Pharmaceutical Abstracts* had cited 58 titles under *coacervat(es/ion);* most of them are summarized in Reference 5.

The recovery of free-flowing powders from gelatin coacervates that disperse as discrete microspheres on suspension in aqueous solutions requires controlled stirring and temperature reduction, aldehyde denaturation of the gelatin, and dehydration with 1- or 2-propanol.[5,26,30] Some reports by L. A. Luzzi et al., and R. E. Phares et al., during the late 1960s in the *Journal of Pharmaceutical Sciences* noted the problem of fused masses instead of discrete microcapsules.[5] Distinct microspheres of approximately 30 μm diameter, containing 15% w/w sulfamerazine are pictured in Figure 6.[26] Takenaka et al. retrieved 20 μm microspheres from gelatin-acacia coacervates, which contained 60% w/w of sulfamethoxazole.[31]

Particle size control has been a principle objective of coacervation to obtain medicated

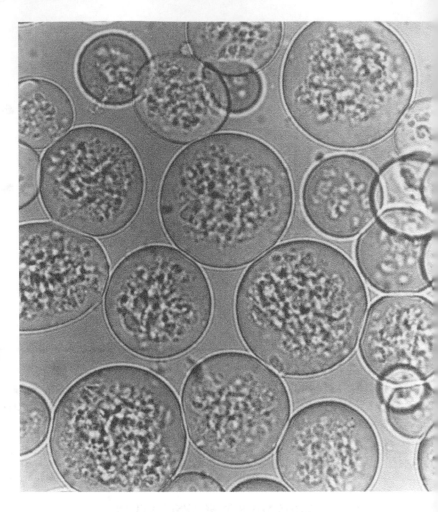

FIGURE 6.   Discrete microspheres from formaldehyde-treated gelatin-acacia coacervate micro[ ] lobules. The mean diameter and sulfamerazine content were 30 μm and 15% w/w, respective[ ] (From Newton, D. W., et al., Characteristics of medicated and unmedicated microglobules recover[ ] from complex coacervates of gelatin-acacia, *J. Pharm. Sci.,* 66, 1327, 1977. With permission [ ] the publisher, American Pharmaceutical Association, Washington, D.C.)

microcapsules.[5,32] Routine recovery of discrete spheres of a particular mean diame[ ] which the standard deviation is less than 10% of that mean, would avail (1) precise [ ] uniformity and dissolution performance, and (2) potential product applications to [ ] enteral and other nonoral routes.

Targeted drug delivery was an early objective of simple coacervation applied to [ ] controlled particle size in an injectable dosage form. Whitmore photographed gel[ ] crocapsules containing streptomycin within phagocytic white blood cells of a m[ ] However, the too-rapid clearance of micrometer- and nanometer-sized particles f[ ] bloodstream by macrophages in the lungs, liver, and spleen[34] continues to thwart [ ] potential of this technology.

The particle size of coacervate microcapsules is dependent on (1) the thermod[ ] limits of the coacervate system, (2) the agitation rate and formulation variables [ ] systems, e.g., gelatin-acacia, and (3) the size of the dispersed solid or liquid partic[ ] coated. Though not by coacervation, albumin microspheres smaller than erythrocyt[ ] been produced.[35]

The few studies to date of denatured gelatin microcapsules produced by coacervation show no prolonged dissolution *in vitro* or *in vivo* in intestinal fluid.[5,26] The condensation reaction of amino groups with aldehydes, the historic tanning and embalming effect, which renders gelatin insoluble, also remains a product liability.[5,31,36] Furthermore, gelatin, albumin, and other practical coacervate coating proteins are potentially allergenic and nephrotoxic.

Complex coacervates of type A gelatin (IEP = 8.2) and acacia at pH 7.5 to 9.5, containing hemoglobin, have been claimed as a safe, functional substitute for erythrocytes.[37] However, such coacervation in this pH range has not been previously achieved,[1,12,26] and there has been no commercial success of a desirable synthetic blood substitute.[38,39]

In summary, aqueous coacervation has proven inferior to nonaqueous phase separation as a drug microencapsulation technique. Microencapsulation has been applied commercially to orally administered pharmaceuticals and, investigationally, to magnetic microspheres. Future applications of aqueous coacervation may involve the original liquid coacervates.

C. AQUEOUS NON-MICROENCAPSULATION

Two early reports for the use of undenatured or fresh coacervates featured their possible simulation of *in vivo* drug distribution equilibria.[40,41] Otherwise, the suggestion that complex coacervates might be used directly as the drug, not as a pharmaceutical formulation aid, has received no or little attention.

Dissolution of the gelatin-acacia coacervate by subphysiologic concentrations of added potassium chloride (Figure 3) suggests that coacervates of certain drugs might be developed for clinical applications. The relatively high concentration of drug(s) in a complex coacervate could be released at a rate or location controlled by the permeability, selectivity, or capacity of a delivery system for physiologic electrolytes. Likewise, modified drug absorption via neutrally charged complex coacervates that are selectively stable in tissue fluids is a little-studied potential application. It is tempting to suspect that the latter is a natural mechanism of transmembrane diffusion.

While not per se identified as coacervation, reports of heparin incompatibility with gentamicin and morphine in solutions for intravenous infusion suggested it.[42,43] These led to the recent observation of microspheres in duplicated admixtures.* The heparin-morphine coacervate incompatibility is interesting. Morphine is a monoamino compound, and the interaction occurred in water, but not in 0.9% sodium chloride injection[43] (0.15 M, the ionic strength of plasma).

IV. BIOLOGICAL IMPLICATIONS

The past 25 years have witnessed little success and practically no innovation in pharmaceutical possibilities for aqueous coacervates. Perhaps microencapsulation via coacervation has not been adequately investigated, or it merely represents a novel scientific achievement that has no commercial pharmaceutical merit. Given this record, future research may focus on elucidating the biological existence and functions of coacervates as unique solutions.

A. LIFE DEVELOPMENT

Acknowledging the 1924 to 1971 works of A.I. Oparin, Fox reviewed complex coacervates with the following perspective: "These microsystems are . . . presumable models of the origin of the protocell . . . Ease of formation suggests such units would have arisen early in primordial organic evolution."[44] This theory, thus, depicts life statistically emerging

---

* The microscopic observation of droplets in the viscid lower phase was made belatedly in 1989 by the author.

from the increasingly ordered formation of low molecular weight monomers, and heteropolymers — primordial cells from primordial soup. The concentration molecules by the microglobules comprises a critical life-determining event.

B. MASS TRANSPORT AND PHARMACOLOGIC MECHANISMS

The routine *in vivo* complex coacervation of drugs and endogenous hormones phenomenon based on the pertinent observations of de Jong,[1] and Fox and Opa neutrally charged optimum coacervate could either flow through pores or diffus the membranes and cytoplasm of cells, possibly dissociating and then reformin coacervates there. The extraction of undissociated ion pairs from aqueous phases roform may model possible *in vivo* complex coacervate function. For exampl facilitated transport could represent the diffusion of variable nonpolar complex c of the same protonated chemical through membranes and cytoplasm.[45] Interesti tonated amines are also superior substrates for ion-pair extractions.

Prominent natural intracellular complex coacervates include heparin-protein[46] to that formed in blood when protamine is given clinically to antidote hepari polynucleotide-protein.[1,44] The stability of both of these coacervates is dependent chloride and pH.

Oparin has shown the following reactions to proceed more efficiently in coac as in living cells — than in their less concentrated and structured aqueous soluti

1.   Starch synthesis from glucose-1-phosphate and its subsequent hydrolys tose,'' . . . which then diffused out of the droplet into the medium.''
2.   The synthesis of polyribonucleotides;
3.   Photosynthesis.

In each of these reactions, the low molecular weight monomers were diffusabl the coacervate and supernate.

Speculating beyond the research of Oparin, Ecanow attributed a variety of co normal and pathological biological phenomena to unobserved complex coacerva submitted that complex coacervates facilitate the high velocity and sophistication o for which the classic anatomic "hard-wired computer model" brain is inadequat

The release, conservation, and pharmacologic alterability of physiologic events by hormones or neurotransmitters also seem too concurrently diverse, frequent, to be the sole result of nascent biosynthesis and passive diffusion described by F An opinion on the biogenic amine theory of mental function, popularized in t seems appropriate at this juncture:

> . . . We have been told that depression, mania, and schizophrenia are merely . . . foul-ups of biog — as if nothing else were happening in our heads but the dull trickling of neurotransmitters . . . the of [mind] . . . lack the convenient dimensions of physical science.[48]

Morphine is chemically similar to endogenous adrenergic agonists,* and it coacervates. Complex coacervates are exquisitely, if variably, sensitive to disso pH, inorganic ions, and direct electric current. Hence, these and related collecti teristics of coacervates suit a plausible, if unelucidated, process by which phar events could be facilitated.

---

* Like morphine, catecholamines and serotonin have protonated amino groups and nondissociate hydroxy groups at physiological pH.[49]

TABLE 2
Idealized Chronologic Complex Coacervate Mechanism of Hormone (Neurochemical) Release and Reuptake

1. Nerve action potential via direct electric current
2. Dissociation of neuronal synapse coacervate zones[a]
3. Flux of extracellular Na^+ into neuron
4. Transient perturbation of intraneuronal electrolytes
5. Dissociation of intraneuronal protein-hormone coacervate
6. Flow of concentrated hormone from neuron
7. Coacervation of hormone with receptor protein during synaptic Na^+ deficit
8. Efficacy or nonefficacy of hormone-receptor coacervate
9. Efflux of Na^+ from neuron during repolarizartion
10. Dissociation of receptor-hormone coacervate by Na^+
11. Re-entry of hormone into neuron and recoacervation therein
12. Recoacervation of neuronal synapse zones

The idealized chronology shown in Table 2 depicts a facile complex coacervation mechanism for the neuronal release and reabsorption of hormones, be they either monomers or polymers. It intends no exclusivity, i.e., it is synchronous and interdependent with both energy-giving phosphorylation reactions and fiber-conducted currents. Furthermore, it implies that homobiotics and foreign chemicals or drugs might elicit, or not elicit, responses based partly on their coacervation effects at various steps.

REFERENCES

1. **De Jong, H. G. B.,** Crystallisation-coacervation-flocculation; Reversal of charge phenomena, equivalent weight and specific properties of the ionised groups; Complex colloid systems; Morphology of coacervates, in *Colloid Science,* Vol. 2, Kruyt, H. R., Ed., Elsevier, Amsterdam, 1949, chap. 8—11.
2. **Bakan, J. A.,** Microencapsulation, in *The Theory and Practice of Industrial Pharmacy,* 3rd ed., Lachman, L., Lieberman, H. A., and Kanig, J. L., Eds., Lea & Febiger, Philadelphia, 1986, 412.
3. **Benita, S. and Donbrow, M.,** Effect of polyisobutylene on ethylcellulose-walled microcapsules: wall structure and thickness of salicylamide and theophylline microcapsules, *J. Pharm. Sci.,* 71, 205, 1982.
4. **Kawashima, Y., Lin, S. Y., Kasai, A., Takenaka, H., Matsunami, K., Nochida, Y., and Hirose, H.,** Drug release properties of the microcapsules of adriamycin hydrochloride with ethylcellulose prepared by a phase separation technique, *Drug Dev. Ind. Pharm.,* 10, 467, 1984.
5. **Deasey, P. B.,** *Microencapsulation and Related Drug Processes,* Marcel Dekker, New York, 1984, 61.
6. **McBain, J. W. and Kellogg, F.,** Salting out of gelatin into two liquid layers with sodium chloride and other salts, *J. Gen. Physiol.,* 12, 1, 1928.
7. **Khalil, S. A. H., Nixon, J. R., and Carless, J. E.,** Role of pH in the coacervation of the systems: gelatin-water-ethanol and gelatin-water-sodium sulfate, *J. Pharm. Pharmacol.,* 20, 215, 1968.
8. **Cohn, E. J., Strong, L. E., Hughes, W. L., Jr., Mulford, D. J., Ashworth, J. N., Melin, M., and Taylor, H. L.,** Preparation and properties of serum and plasma proteins. IV. A system for the separation into fractions of the protein and lipoprotein components of biological tissues and fluids, *J. Am. Chem. Soc.,* 68, 459, 1946.
9. **Phares, R. E. and Sperandio, G. J.,** Preparation of a phase diagram for coacervation, *J. Pharm. Sci.,* 53, 518, 1964.
10. **Edsall, J. T. and Wyman, J.,** *Biophysical Chemistry,* Academic Press, New York, 1958, chap. 5.
11. **Theesen, K. S., Wilson, J. E., Newton, D. W., and Ueda, C. T.,** Compatibility of lithium citrate syrup with 10 neuroleptic solutions, *Am. J. Hosp. Pharm.,* 38, 1750, 1981.
12. **Burgess, D. J. and Carless, J. E.,** Microelectrophoretic studies of gelatin and acacia for the prediction of complex coacervation, *J. Colloid Interface Sci.,* 98, 1, 1984.

* The literature of membrane physiology and pharmacology refers to such zones as gates or channels.

13. **Newton, D. W.,** unpublished data obtained in 1988 and 1989 from research funded by Abbott Lab North Chicago, IL.

14. **Rosenkrantz, B. E., Greco, J. R., Hoogerheide, J. G., and Oden, E. M.,** Gentamicin s *Analytical Profiles of Drug Substances,* Vol. 9, Florey, K., Ed., Academic Press, New York, 1!

15. **Nachtmann, F., Atzl, G., and Roth, W. D.,** Heparin sodium, in *Analytical Profiles of Drug Su* Vol. 12, Florey, K., Ed., Academic Press, New York, 1983, 215.

16. **McMullen, J. N., Newton, D. W., and Becker, C. H.,** Pectin-gelatin complex coacervates. I. Det of microglobule size, morphology, and recovery as water-dispersible powders, *J. Pharm. Sci.,* 1982.

17. **Elgindy, N. A. and Elegakey, M. A.,** Carbopol-gelatin coacervation: influence of some variabk *Dev. Ind. Pharm.,* 7, 587, 1981.

18. **Koh, G.-L. and Tucker, I. G.,** Characterization of sodium carboxymethylcellulose-gelatin comp ervation by viscosity, turbidity and coacervate wet weight and volume measurements, *J. Pharm. Ph* 40, 233, 1988.

19. **Koh, G.-L. and Tucker, I. G.,** Characterization of sodium carboxymethylcellulose-gelatin comp ervation by chemical analysis of the coacervate and equilibrium fluid phases, *J. Pharm. Pharm* 309, 1988.

20. **Tomlinson, E. and Davis, S. S.,** Interactions between large organic ions of opposite and unequa III. Enthalpy-entropy linear compensation and application of solvophobic theory, *J. Colloid Inter* 76, 563, 1980.

21. **Kauzmann, W.,** Some factors in the interpretation of protein denaturation, *Adv. Protein Chem* 1959.

22. **Hughes, M. N.,** *The Inorganic Chemistry of Biological Processes,* John Wiley & Sons, New Yc 6.

23. **Newton, D. W.,** unpublished data, 1989.

24. **Yoshida, N. and Thies, C.,** The effect of neutral salts on gelatin-gum arabic complexes, *J. Colloid Sci.,* 24, 29, 1967.

25. **Tainaka, K.-I.,** Effect of counterions on complex coacervation, *Biopolymers,* 19, 1289, 1980.

26. **Newton, D. W., McMullen, J. N., and Becker, C. H.,** Characteristics of medicated and unm microglobules recovered from complex coacervates of gelatin-acacia, *J. Pharm. Sci.,* 66, 1327,

27. **Schott, H.,** Polymer science, in *Physical Pharmacy,* 3rd ed., Martin, A., Swarbrick, J., and Ca A., Eds., Lea & Febiger, Philadelphia, 1983, chap. 22.

28. **Luzzi, L. A. and Gerraughty, R. J.,** Effects of selected variables on the extractability of coacervate capsules, *J. Pharm. Sci.,* 53, 429, 1964.

29. **Phares, R. E. and Sperandio, G. J.,** Coating pharmaceuticals by coacervation, *J. Pharm. Sci.,* 1964.

30. **Nixon, J. R., Khalil, S. A., and Carless, J. E.,** Gelatin coacervate microcapsules containing sulfa their preparation and the *in vitro* release of the drug, *J. Pharm. Pharmacol.,* 20, 528, 1968.

31. **Takenaka, H., Kawashima, Y., and Lin, S. Y.,** Micromeritic properties of sulfamethoxazole sules prepared by gelatin-acacia coacervation, *J. Pharm. Sci.,* 69, 513, 1980.

32. **McMullen, J. N., Newton, D. W., and Becker, C. H.,** Pectin-gelatin complex coacervates. II. microencapsulated sulfamerazine on size, morphology, recovery, and extraction of water-disper croglobules, *J. Pharm. Sci.,* 73, 1799, 1984.

33. **Whitmore, J.,** A Study of a Pharmaceutical Dosage Form Produced by Coacervation (Micro Ph.D. dissertation, University of Florida, Gainesville, 1966.

34. **Singh, M. and Ravin, L. J.,** Parenteral emulsions as drug carrier systems, *J. Parenter. Sci.* 40, 34, 1986.

35. **Gupta, P. K., Gallo, J. M., Hung, C. T., and Perrier, D. G.,** Influence of stabilization ter on the entrapment of adriamycin in albumin microspheres, *Drug Dev. Ind. Pharm.,* 13, 1471, 1

36. **Fraenkel-Conrat, H., Cooper, M., and Olcott, H. S.,** The reaction of formaldehyde with pr *Am. Chem. Soc.,* 67, 950, 1945.

37. **Ecanow, C. S. and Ecanow, B.,** U.S. Patent 4,439,424, 1984.

38. **James, F. E.,** Researchers step up efforts to develop synthetic blood, *The Wall Street Journal (N* p. 17, September 4, 1987.

39. **Robinson, J. R.,** Biological sciences and the future of pharmaceutics, *Pharm Technol.,* 12, 5° 1988.

40. **Javidan, S., Haque, R.-U., and Mrtek, R. G.,** Microbiologic determination of drug partiti Gelatin-acacia complex coacervate system, *J. Pharm. Sci.,* 60, 1825, 1971.

41. **Takruri, H., Ecanow, B., and Balagot, R.,** Water as a nonpolar partition medium, *J. Pharm.* 283, 1977.

42. **Trissel, L. A.,** *Handbook on Injectable Drugs,* 5th ed., American Society of Hospital Pharmacists, Bethesda, MD, 1988, 329.
43. **Baker, D. E., Yost, G. S., Craig, V. L., and Campbell, R. K.,** Compatibility of heparin sodium and morphine sulfate, *Am. J. Hosp. Pharm.,* 42, 1352, 1985.
44. **Fox, S. W.,** The evolutionary significance of phase-separated microsystems, *Origins Life,* 7, 49, 1976.
45. **Albert, A.,** *Selective Toxicity,* 5th ed., Chapman and Hall, London, 1985, 310.
46. **Uvnas, B.,** The role of the heparin protein complex in the storage of histamine in mast cells, in *Heparin: Structure, Cellular Functions, and Clinical Applications,* McDuffie, N. M., Ed., Academic Press, New York, 1979, 243.
47. **Ecanow, B.,** Interstitial conduction and the emergent mind, *J. Pharm. Sci.,* 71, VIII, 1982.
48. Anonymous, The shell game in neuropharmacology, *Drug Ther.,* 7, 110 (March), 1977.
49. **Newton, D. W. and Kluza, R. B.,** pKa values of drug substances and pH values of tissue fluids, in *Principles of Medicinal Chemistry,* 3rd ed., Foye, W. O., Ed., Lea & Febiger, Philadelphia, 1989, 861.

Chapter 5

POLYMERIZED LIPOSOMES AS DRUG CARRIERS

Steven L. Regen

TABLE OF CONTENTS

I. INTRODUCTION

Naturally occurring and synthetic phospholipids, when dispersed in water, forr like structures called vesicles (or liposomes). These particles are comprised of alte lipid bilayer and aqueous compartments arranged in a concentric fashion. When su to ultrasound, or when repeatedly extruded through porous membranes, such mu partment (or multilamellar) vesicles (MLVs) break up and form unilamellar vesicles a single aqueous phase and a single lipid bilayer. Typically, unilamellar vesicles prepared having diameters ranging between 300 and 1000 Å. The bilayer is typicall range of approximately 50 Å in thickness, and contains between 2,000 to 40,0 molecules per liposome (Figure 1). In contrast to micelles, which are in rapid equi with their monomers, liposomes exist as relatively stable structures which can be isolated, and characterized by electron microscopy.

The encapsulation of a drug within the aqueous compartment or the hydrophobic of a liposome provides a flexible means for significantly altering its pharmacoc behavior and therapeutic efficacy.[1,2] While liposomes have been considered as drug for many years, it is only recently that clinical evaluations of certain liposomal dru been undertaken. Some of the drugs which are now actively being explored as li formulations include: Adriamycin (Doxorubicin), PLAT 23, and Vincristine, inject ticancer drugs; Amphotericin B, an injectable antifungal drug; Albuterol, an inhale chodilator; PLAT 23 and Vincristine, anticancer drugs; Gentamicin, a bactericidal an and Indomethacin, an anti-inflammatory agent.[3]

One of the limitations of conventional liposomes is that they are not very stable and *in vivo*.[4] On standing, liposomes tend to aggregate and fuse with one another, r in the formation of larger structures which eventually precipitate from solution. This instability may, in some instances, pose serious constraints on the commercial man of liposome formulations of interest.[4] From a pharmocological standpoint, the *in v* blility of liposomes has also been of concern. Processes such as lipid-exchange v membranes, and direct removal and net transfer of lipids from liposomes, which are to occur, may influence the therapeutic efficacy of a liposomal drug. If, for exam lipid content of a circulating liposome is modified, it is likely that is release charac will also be altered.

Over the past 10 years, we, and several other groups, have reported the synthe variety of polymerized forms of liposomes (Figure 2). The driving force behind this work has been based on the goal of creating analogous classes of drug carri exhibit (1) improved *in vitro* and *in vivo* stability, and (2) controllable release charact The subject of polymerized liposomes has now been extensively reviewed.[5] In this we do not present yet another general review on this subject, but, instead, focus specific liposomal system whose *in vitro* stability and permeability characteristics ha defined, and whose *in vivo* utility as a drug carrier has been evaluated.

II. POLYMERIZABLE PHOSPHOLIPIDS

While a large number of polymerizable, vesicle-forming surfactants have no synthesized, relatively few phospholipid types have been reported. In the phosphatidy series, those having a conjugated diacetylene moiety within the *sn*-1 and/or *sn*-2 (e.g., **1**) have been the most popular (Figure 3).[6-8] When assembled into an organized these lipids are polymerized by direct exposure to ultraviolet light (254 nm). This photopolymerization proceeds through a topotatic process in which the diacetylene are converted into an intensely colored (blue or red) polymer. Here, a close and alignment of the diacetylene moieties is essential for polymerization to occur. The mo

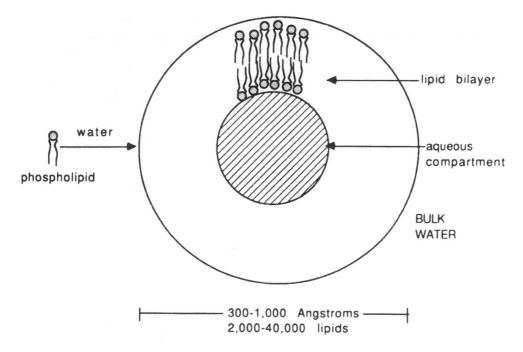

FIGURE 1.   Stylized illustration of a phospholipid bilayer vesicle (liposome).

structure of the resulting polymeric backbone consists of sequential double, single, triple, and single carbon-carbon bonds (Figure 4).

A second class of polymerizable phospholipids that has been used to prepare polymerized liposomes employs a conjugated diene as the polymerizable moiety. Direct exposure to ultraviolet light (254) nm, or thermally-induced free radical polymerization yields a polymer backbone whose structure is believed to consist primarily of a poly-1,4-*trans* backbone.

A third type of phospholipid which can be polymerized by exposure to ultraviolet irradiation contains methacrylate groups positioned at the terminus of each of the *sn*-1 and/or *sn*-2 chains of the molecule. In this case, a poly(methacrylate) backbone is generated.

While detailed biodegradability studies have not yet been carried out for polymerized liposomes derived from any of the above mentioned phospholipids, it appears likely that they will all be non-biodegradable by virtue of their all-carbon backbone. If this is the case, the chronic parenteral use of such drug carriers may result in tissue accumulation and possibly long-term side effects. In an effort to prepare polymerizable lipids that would be biodegradable, phosphatidylcholine molecules **4** and **5** were recently introduced (Figure 5).[9] Here, polymerization is carried out by oxidation of the thiol moieties which affords disulfide linkages. The fact that disulfide bonds are commonly found in biopolymers suggests that polymerized liposomes that bear a disulfide-containing backbone may be biodegradable. No definitive experiments, however, have yet been reported which establish their biodegradability.

In this chapter, attention is focused on one unique class of polymerizable phospholipids that has been specifically designed so that polymerization can be carried out under extremely mild conditions (exposure to ultraviolet light, heat or chemical oxidants is not required), yielding a disulfide-based polymeric backbone. Mild polymerization conditions are of special importance if one wishes to incorporate a thermally-, UV-, or redox-sensitive drug within a liposome. Figures 6 and 7 illustrate the synthetic routes which have been used to prepare lipids **6** and **7**, respectively. These phospholipids, which bear a lipoic acid at the end of one

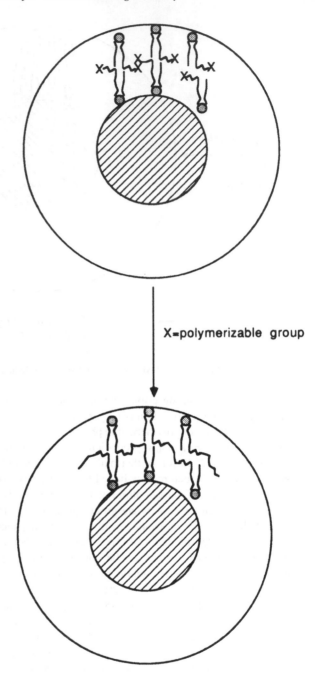

FIGURE 2.   Stylized illustration of a polymerized liposome.

or both aliphatic chains, can be polymerized in liposomal form via a ring-openin
that is initiated by dithiothreitol (Figure 8).[10]

III. SYNTHESIS OF POLYMERIZED LIPOSOMES

A variety of methods have been devised for preparing unilamellar and mul
vesicles. For general reviews on this subject, the reader is referred to a three-volu

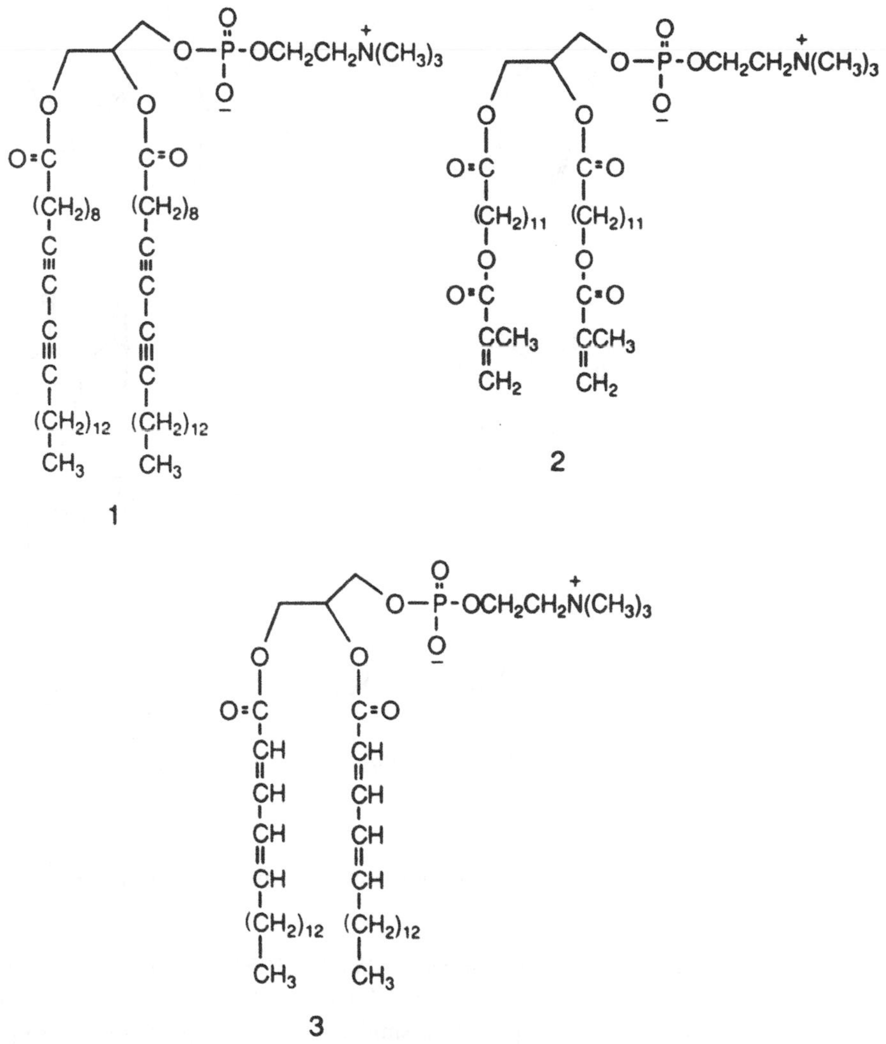

Structure 1:

O=P
O−P−OCH$_2$CH$_2$N$^+$(CH$_3$)$_3$
O$^-$

O=C   C=O
(CH$_2$)$_8$ (CH$_2$)$_8$
C   C
||| |||
C   C
| |
C   C
||| |||
C   C
(CH$_2$)$_{12}$ (CH$_2$)$_{12}$
CH$_3$ CH$_3$

1

Structure 2:

O
||
O−P−OCH$_2$CH$_2$N$^+$(CH$_3$)$_3$
O$^-$

O=C   C=O
(CH$_2$)$_{11}$ (CH$_2$)$_{11}$
O   O
O=C   C=O
CCH$_3$ CCH$_3$
|| ||
CH$_2$ CH$_2$

2

Structure 3:

O
||
O−P−OCH$_2$CH$_2$N$^+$(CH$_3$)$_3$
O$^-$

O=C   C=O
CH   CH
|| ||
CH   CH
CH   CH
|| ||
CH   CH
(CH$_2$)$_{12}$ (CH$_2$)$_{12}$
CH$_3$ CH$_3$

3

FIGURE 3. Unsaturated phosphatidylcholines commonly used in forming polymerized liposomes.

on liposome technology.[11] One of the more popular methods for preparing well-defined large unilamellar vesicles, and which does not require organic solvents or micelle-forming detergents, is based on an extrusion procedure.[12] Experimentally, a thin phospholipid film is coated onto the walls of a glass surface and is hydrated with an appropriate buffer. After the film peels off the glass in the form of multilamellar vesicles, the resulting dispersion is then extruded through Nuclepore polycarbonate membranes (Figure 9). The LUVETs (large unilamellar vesicles by extrusion technique) which are formed show high trapping efficiencies. Figure 10 shows a ^{31}P NMR spectrum of LUVETs produced from **6**, in the presence of a paramagnetic shift reagent. Examination of the integrated spectrum reveals that the number of lipids present in the outer leaflet of the bilayer, appearing at 17 ppm (relative to a triphenylphosphine reference), is similar to the number of lipids located in the inner leaflet (5 ppm).

Captured volumes for liposomes can be calculated by dividing the fraction of a water-soluble "impermeant" solute that has become entrapped within the aqueous compartment, by the lipid concentration that is present in the dispersion (Figure 11). Using [^{14}C] sucrose

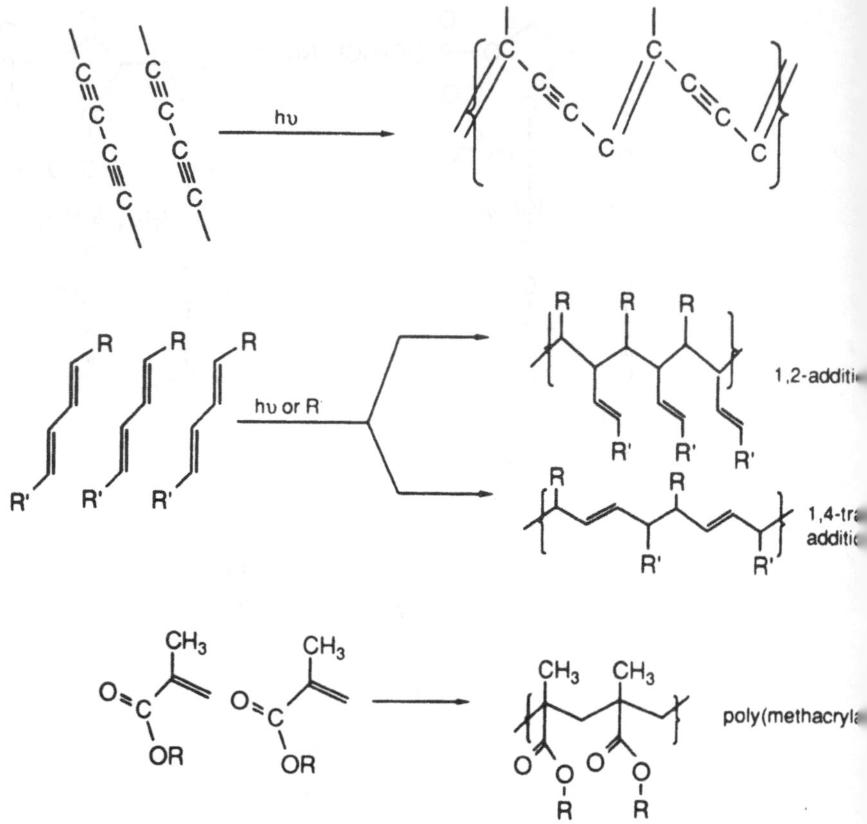

FIGURE 4.   Schematic representation of poly(acetylene) [*top*]; poly(butadiene) [*middle*]; and poly(meth
[*bottom*].

as the solute, for example, LUVETs (1000 Å diameter) of **6** have been shown to
captured volume of 2.1 ± 0.1 L/mol. Such a value compares favorably to captured
that have been reported for similar LUVETs prepared from soya phosphatidylcholin
[^{14}C] inulin as the solute, and a similar Nuclepore membrane.[10]

Polymerization of liposomes derived from **6** and **7** is normally carried out using a
amount of dithiothreitol (DTT) as an initiator, and is monitored by following eit
disappearance of the 1,2-dithiolane moiety (333 nm), or the phospholipid monomer
layer chromatography. Analysis by dynamic light scattering, transmission electron
copy, and gel filtration confirm that polymerization does not lead to a significant ch
the size or size-distribution of these liposomes.

The precise polymeric structure of membranes derived from **6**, and mixtures c
7, remains to be established. In particular, the extent of crosslinking and the extent
and outer monolayer vs. inner-outer bilayer polymerization has not been determined
12 illustrates how **6** is capable of producing linear as well as crosslinked polymeri
branes. Whereas an intermolecular reaction leads to crosslinking, intramolecular c
generates macrocyclic phospholipids that are incorporated into the backbone. Poly
liposomal membranes of **7** are soluble in chloroform. In contrast, those derived fro
completely insoluble. Since **7** can only produce linear polymers, these solubility pr
infer that **6** yields a crosslinked network. Exactly how much crosslinking has oc
however, is not presently clear. Freeze fracture electron microscopy has been us
qualitative evidence for polymerization across phospholipid bilayers produced f

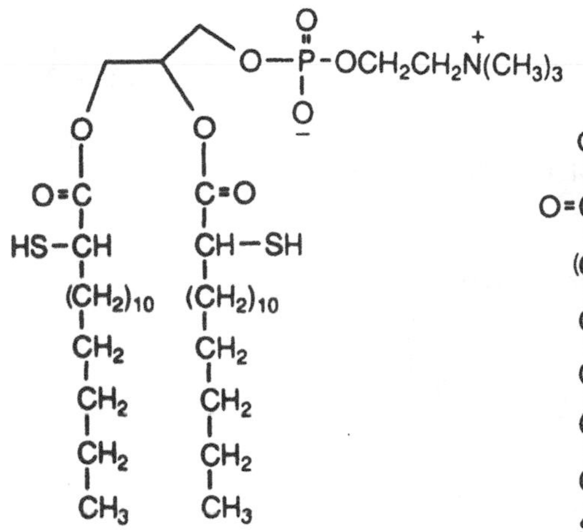

FIGURE 5.   Thiol- and disulfide-bearing polymerizable phosphatidylcholines.

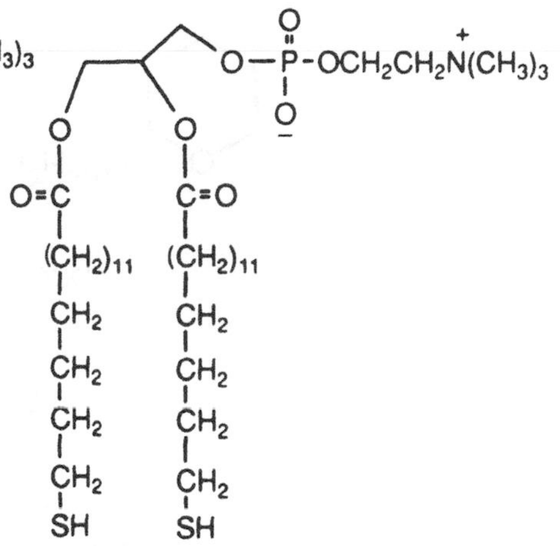

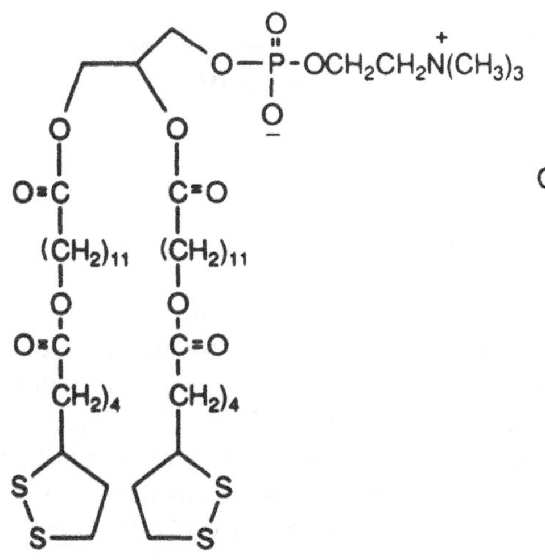

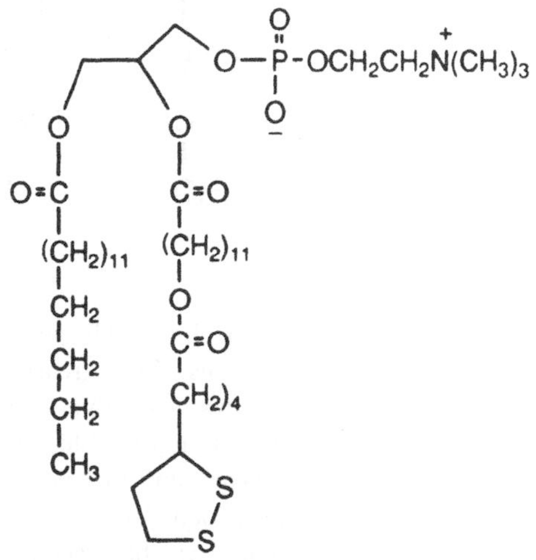

Whether or not polymerized liposomes formed from **6** and **7** yield related structures (Figure 13) remains to be established.

IV. PERMEABILITY CHARACTERISTICS

The permeability characteristics of both polymerized as well as monomeric forms of LUVETs (1000 Å-diameter) of **6** and **7** have recently been defined using [^{14}C] sucrose as the permeant.[10] In brief, it has been shown that membranes derived from **7** are less permeable toward sucrose than those prepared from **6**; increasing the mole percentage of **7** in mixed bilayers results in decreased permeability. Whereas homopolymerization of **7** significantly increases bilayer permeability (by a factor of approximately 9), homopolymerization of **6** significantly *decreases* membrane permeability (by a factor of approximately 50). Moreover, increasing the mole percentage of **6** in mixed polymerized liposomes resulted in reduced

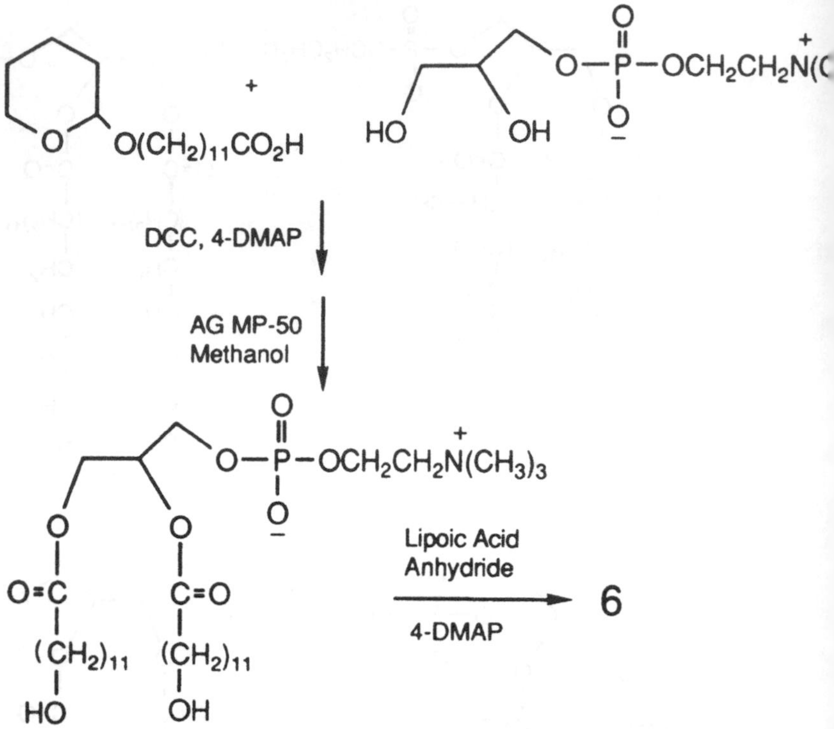

FIGURE 6.   Synthetic route used to prepare **6**.

permeability. The permeability properties of these monomeric bilayers have been ra
in terms of the greater packing efficiency of **7**. Monolayers studies that were carr
the gas-water interface have shown that **7** produces a more tightly packed monol
6. It is reasonable, therefore, to expect that **7** would also produce a more tight
bilayer, and that permeation through such a membrane would be relatively slow
to account for the permeability properties of the polymerized analogs, a "polymer b
hypothesis has been proposed (Figure 14). Specifically, it has been suggested that
or polymer boundaries within the membrane serve as the primary avenue for rele
entrapped sucrose. Because **7** can only produce linear polymers, the resulting
should contain many individual polymer molecules, and thus possess many polym
aries. In contrast, polymerized liposomes derived from **6** should consist of essen
crosslinked polymer molecule and should contain far fewer boundaries. Similarl
crease in permeability that is observed as one increases the molar composition of
polymerized membranes can be accounted for by a decrease in the number of such bc
It is noteworthy that this boundary hypothesis has direct analogy to the lipid r
structure that exists at its gel-to-liquid crystalline phase transition temperature (T
latter case, boundaries ("packing faults") that separate gel and liquid crystalline ¡
believed to contribute significantly to the permeation characteristics of the membra

V. STABILITY CHARACTERISTICS

Polymerized liposomes show, in general, greater stability compared to cor
monomeric liposomes in terms of their shelf life and also their ability to withstar
solvents and detergents.[5] Polymerized liposomes prepared from **6**, that were stored a
dispersions, have been found to have shelf lives in excess of 12 months. These

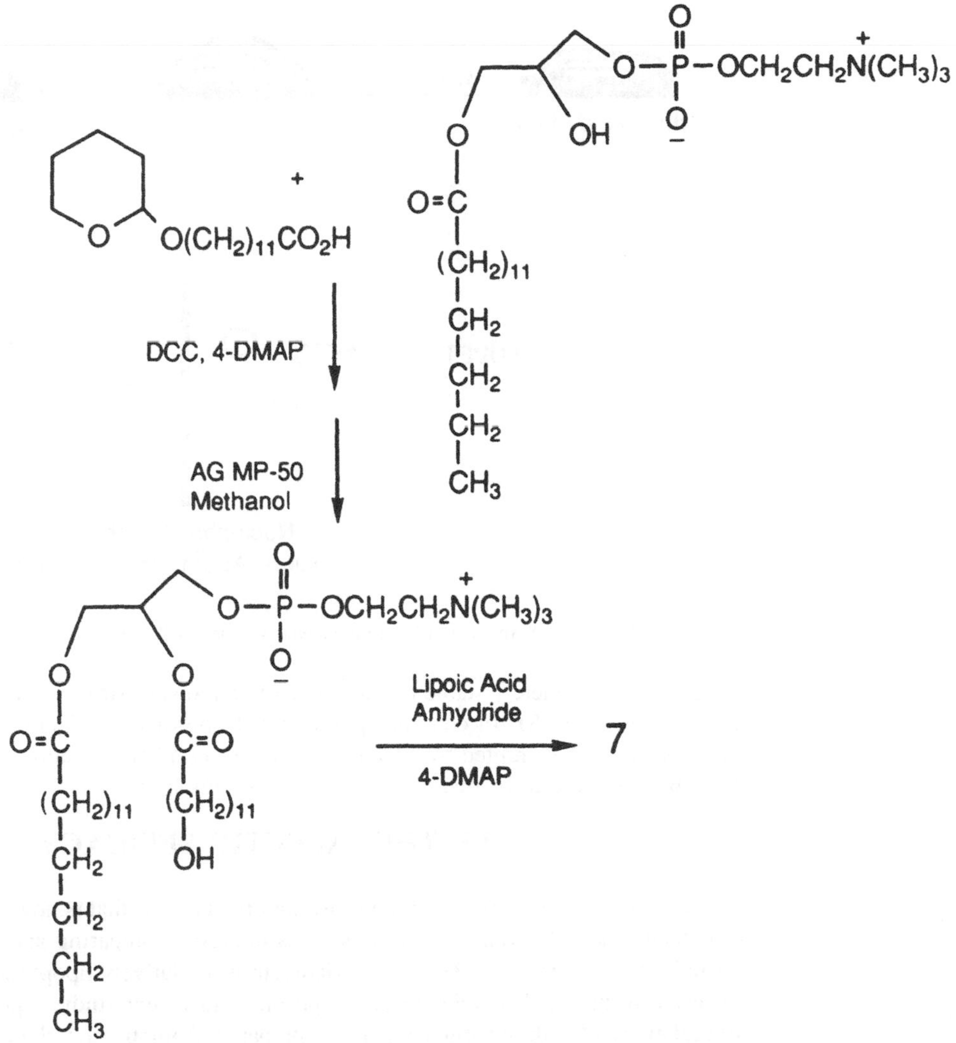

FIGURE 7.   Synthetic route used to prepare 7.

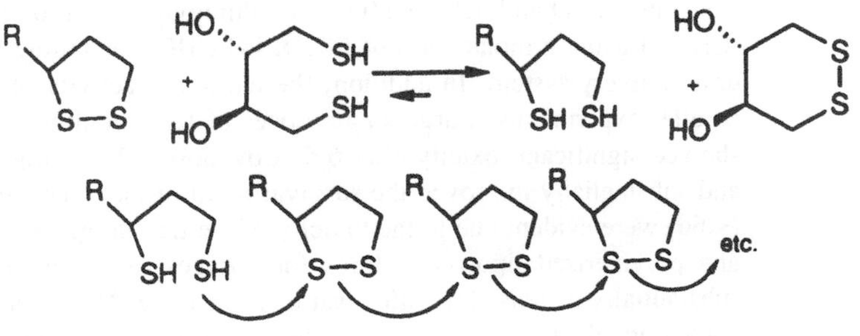

FIGURE 8.   Schematic representation of a dithiothreitol-initiated ring-opening polymerization of lipoic acid.

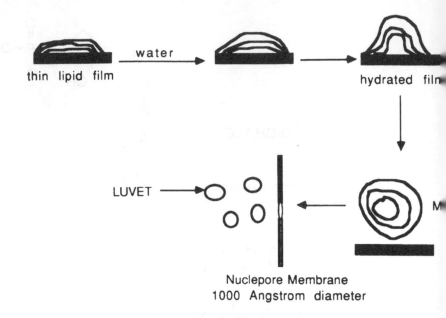

thin lipid film

water

hydrated film

LUVET

Nuclepore Membrane
1000 Angstrom diameter

FIGURE 9.   Formation of large unilamellar vesicles by the extrusion technique (LUVETs).

appear to be completely stable toward ethanol and toward strong detergents such as dodecylsulfate (SDS). In contrast, polymerized liposomes of **7** are disrupted by S also appear to be disrupted by ethanol.[13] The greater inherent stability of liposomes from **6** is believed to be due to the presence of crosslinking.

VI. THERAPEUTIC EFFICACY

Adriamycin (ADR) is one of the most important agents that is now used for the tr of human cancer. Currently, there is serious interest in preparing and evaluating lip formulations of this drug. Because Adriamycin is a relatively lipophilic molecule, i to reside in the lipid membrane of a liposome. In recent studies, polymerized lip formulations of Adriamycin have been prepared from **6**, and their therapeutic evaluated against a leukemia.[14] Specifically, female BDFI mice were injected, intr neally, with P388 murine leukemia cells, and were then treated with polymerized lip ADR. For purposes of comparison, "conventional" monomeric analogs were also p from egg phosphatidylcholine (PC), dipalmitoylphosphatidlglycerol (DPPG), and cho (CHOL) using a molar ratio of PC:DPPG:CHOL equalling 4:1:5, and were evalua drug delivery system. In addition, the antitumor activity of the free drug was exam parallel experiments. Large single doses of free, nonliposomal bound ADR (8–20 showed significant toxicity after 6 d. Low doses (2 to 4 mg/kg) were found to be n and substantially improved the survival of all of the mice studied. At 8 mg/kg, earl (<6d) were evident due to the toxicity of the free drug. In contrast, using both conv and polymerized liposomal drugs (at dosages of 6 mg/kg and 8.5 mg/kg, respe substantially increased the life span of these mice. No difference was observed betw conventional liposomal drug and the free drug in the range of 2 to 4 mg/kg; bo equally effective in tumor growth suppression, resulting in 100% survival of the mic these preliminary studies, it is clear that both polymerized liposomes derived fro well as conventional liposomal formulations, can reduce the toxicity of ADR and an increase in the mean survival time of mice that have been injected intraperitonea P388 murine leukemia cells.

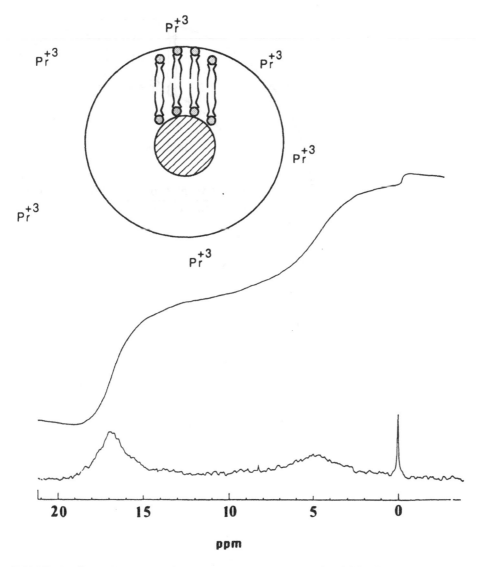

FIGURE 10. ^{31}P NMR spectrum of a 58 mM liposomal dispersion of LUVETs of **6** (monomeric form) containing 2.0 mM Pr^{+3}.

Based on a considerable amount of effort that has been spent over the past 10 years in the design and synthesis of a variety of polymerized liposomes, viable systems for *in vivo* evaluations are now in hand (e.g., liposomes derived from **6**). While it is clear that poly-merized liposomes are more attractive than conventional monomeric liposomes, from a pharmaceutical (i.e., manufacturing) standpoint it remains to be determined whether or not greater therapeutic efficacy can be found for a given application. More *in vivo* studies will be needed to answer this question.

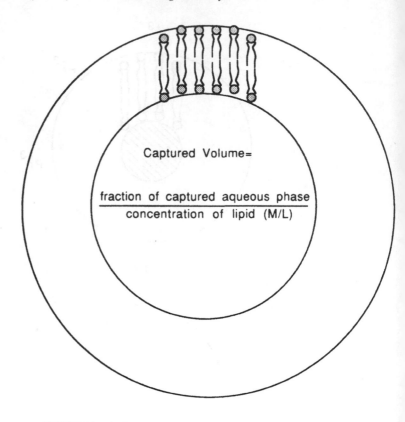

FIGURE 11.   Stylized illustration of a LUVET showing a captured volume.

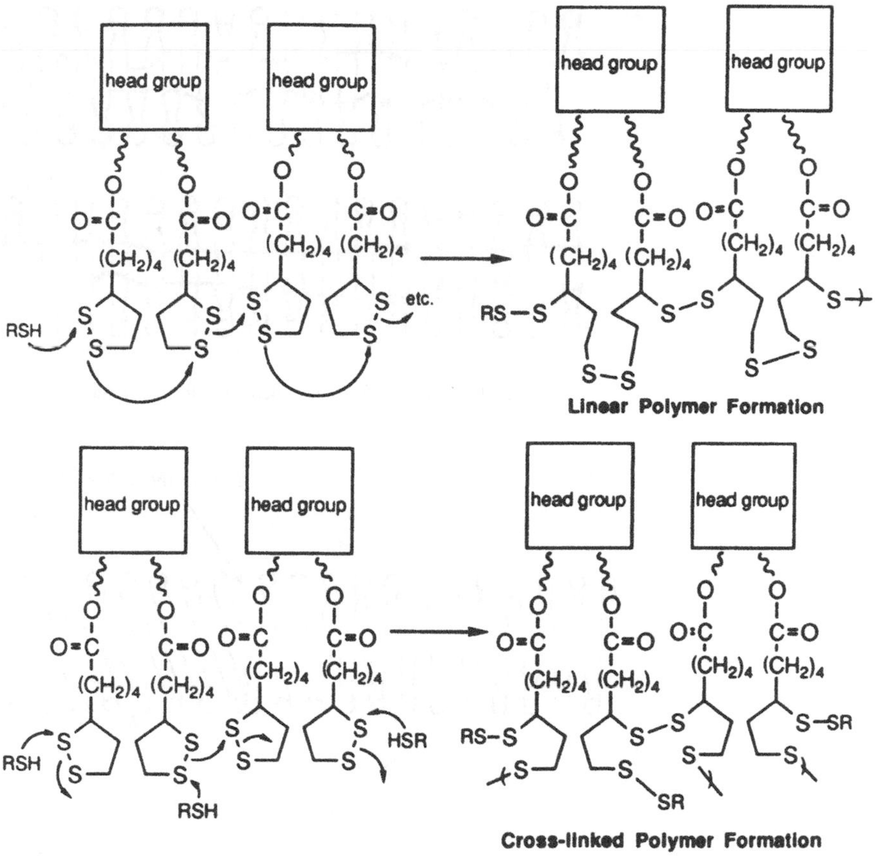

FIGURE 12.   Schematic representation of linear vs. crosslinked polymer formation via **6**.

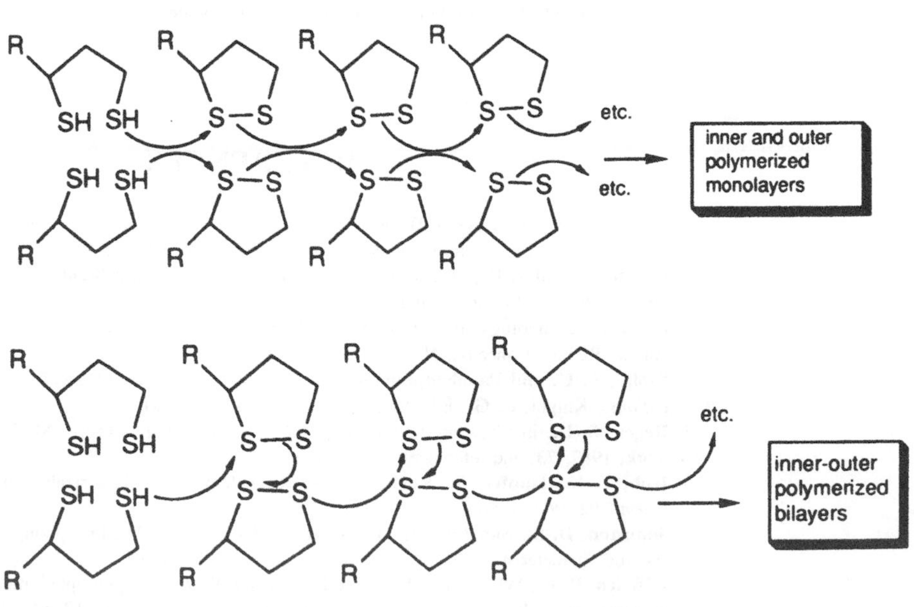

FIGURE 13.   Schematic representation of inner and outer monolayer vs. inner-outer bilayer polymerization.

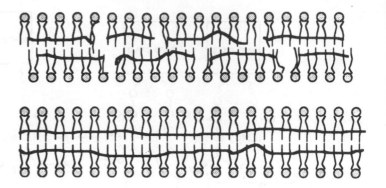

FIGURE 14.   Stylized illustration depicting the "polymer boundary" hypothesis.

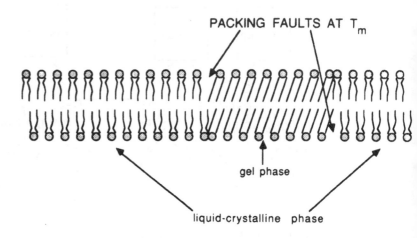

FIGURE 15.   Stylized illustration of a lipid bilayer at the phase-transition temperature, T_m, which shows packing faults within the membrane.

REFERENCES

1. **Juliano, R. L. and Layton, D.,** in *Drug Delivery Systems: Characterization and Biomedical Ap* Juliano, R. L., Ed., Oxford University Press, New York, 1980, 189.
2. **Papahadjopoulos, D., Heath, T., Martin, F., Fraley, R., and Strobinger, R.,** in *Targeting* Gregoriadis, G., Sinior, J., and Trouet, A., Eds., Plenum Press, New York, 1982, 375.
3. Liposome Technology, Inc., 1988 Annual Report, Menlo Park CA.; The Liposome Company, Annual Report, Princeton, NJ.
4. **Szoka, F. C. and Papahadjopoulos, D.,** in *Liposomes: From Physical Structure to Therape* *cations.,* Knight, C. G., Ed., Elsevier, Amsterdam, 1981, 51.
5. **Regen, S. L.,** in *Liposomes: From Biophysics to Therapeutics*, Ostro, M. J., Ed., Marcel De York, 1987, 73, and references cited therein.
6. **Hub, V. H., Hupfer, B., Koch, H., and Ringsdorf, H.,** Polymerizable phospholipid analog *Chem.,* 92, 962, 1980.
7. **Johnston, D. S., Sanghera, S., Pons, M., and Chapman, D.,** Phospholipid polymers — syr spectral characteristics, *Biochim. Biophys. Acta,* 602, 57, 1980.
8. **O'Brien, D. F., Whitesides, T. H., and Klingbiel, R. T.,** The photopolymerization of lipid-d in biomolecular-layer membranes, *J. Polym. Sci. Polym. Lett. Ed.,* 19, 95, 1981.

9. **Samuel, N. K. P., Singh, M., Yamaguchi, K., and Regen, S. L.,** Polymerized-depolymerized vesicles. Reversible thiol-disulfide-based phosphatidylcholine membranes, *J. Am. Chem. Soc.,* 107, 42, 1985.

10. **Stefely, J. S., Markowitz, M. A., and Regen, S. L.,** Permeability characteristics of lipid bilayers from lipoic acid derived phosphatidylcholines: comparison of monomeric, cross-liked and non-cross-linked polymerized membranes, *J. Am. Chem. Soc.,* 110, 7463, 1988.

11. **Gregoriadis, G.,** *Liposome Technology: Preparation of Liposomes,* Vol I, CRC Press, Boca Raton, FL, 1984.

12. **Hope, M. J., Bally, M. B., Webb, G., and Cullis, P. R.,** Production of large unilamellar vesicles by a rapid extrusion procedure. Characterization of size distribution, trapped volume and ability to maintain a membrane potential, *Biochim. Biophys. Acta,* 812, 55, 1985.

13. **Stefely, J. S.,** Lipoic Acid Based Polymerized Liposomes, Ph.D. thesis, Marquette University, 1990.

14. **Hume, L. R., Stefely, J., Regen, S. L., and Juliano, R. L.,** Stability and therapeutic efficacy of antitumor drugs incorporated in disulfide-bridged polymerized liposomes, *J. Pharm. Sci.,* submitted for publication.

Chapter 6

BIOADHESIVE POLYMERS AND DRUG DELIVERY

David A. Pecosky and Joseph R. Robinson

TABLE OF CONTENTS

I. INTRODUCTION

Natural and synthetic bioadhesive polymers that can adhere to hard or soft tissu been used for many years in dentistry, orthopedics, ophthalmology, and in surgica dures.[1-6] Among these "bioadhesive" polymers, monomeric alpha-cyanoacrylate which bind to tissues through covalent bonds, have been the most investigated in the Despite their lack of approval by the FDA, this group of "instant" or "super" glu enjoyed utility in a number of applications, such as in the repair of osteochondial fr for hemostasis, and as soft tissue adhesives.[9,10] In dentistry, alpha cyanoacrylate est been used as adhesives for sealing extraction wounds and as peridontal dressing other synthetic polymers such as polyurethanes, epoxy resins, polystyrene, acryla natural-products,[1] adhesives were also extensively investigated as bone glues.[11,12] Th others have proven to be great technological assets. They may also be a partial or c solution to a number of drug delivery problems, e.g., where existing pharmaceutica forms do not allow sufficient residency time at an absorption site for maximal and absorption of a therapeutic molecule. This improvement in absorption efficiency wc result in a concomitant improvement in the particular therapy or, alternatively, l decrease in extraneous drug load in the body, which may contribute to untoward side

The majority of bioadhesive polymers studied for drug delivery adhere to e tissues and perhaps to the mucus coat present on the surface of these tissues. Th type of bioadhesion is also referred to as "mucoadhesion". Mucus-coated tissue i not surprisingly, in most nonparenteral routes of administration. These targeted epithelial tissues include the eye, mouth, gastrointestinal tract, nasal area, rectum, tract, and vagina.

A brief review of the various structural and physicochemical properties of bio, polymers are presented here along with a discussion of adhesive interactions. Centr overall theme will be the use of bioadhesive polymers with drug delivery as the goal.

II. MECHANISMS OF BIOADHESION

A. GENERAL

Since bioadhesive delivery systems are currently being developed to deliver mucosal epithelial tissue sites, it is clear that adhesion requires interaction of t possibly three, interactive regions: the bioadhesive material, the mucus layer, and e cells.

Mucus is a highly viscous material synthesized and secreted by either goblet specialized exocrine glands in various regions of the body.[13] Characteristically, n composed of a number of components: glycoproteins or mucins, water, electrolytes, ir salts, proteins, lipids, mucopolysaccharides, sloughed epithelial cells, enzymes, and bacterial products, and various other materials depending on the origin of the n

The most important component of mucus is also the basic component of all m the glycoproteins. Glycoproteins consist of a protein core with oligosaccharide sid attached in the glycosylated regions, primarily via the serine and threonine ami along the polypeptide backbone,[14-16] as shown in Figure 1.[17]

The positions and relative amounts of amino acids in the glycoprotein backb important to the matrix structure of the mucus, since they confer the overall tertiary s and folding of the glycoprotein.

The oligosaccharide side chains, which are covalently linked in the glycosylated of the glycoprotein, number from 160 to 200 per protein,[18-20] and can be 50 to 80 mucin weight.[21,22] The oligosaccharides are hydrophilic, and form a protective co

**OLIGOSACCHARIDE SIDE CHAINS WITH
TERMINAL SIALIC ACID (pKa OF 2.6)**

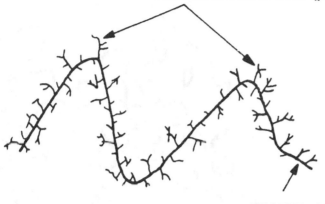

PROTEIN CORE

FIGURE 1. Schematic structure of mucin. (From Pigman, W., *The Glycoconjugates*, Vol. 1, Horowitz, M. I. and Pigmen, W., Eds., Academic Press, New York, 1977. With permission.)

the glycoprotein backbone, which aids in protecting the glycoprotein from the enzymatic action of proteases.[23,24] Mucins, in general, are polydisperse with respect to molecular size, and random with respect to oligosaccharide sequence and chain lengths.[13]

The mucus glycoproteins overlap and interpenetrate each other. Investigators have speculated that this network of glycoproteinacious material is held together by disulfide bonds and secondary forces such as hydrogen bonding and various other molecular associations.[25,26,93,94] Regardless of which form of chain interaction is dominant, the glycoproteins are responsible for the basic network, which is known as mucus. Figure 2 illustrates a schematic representation of the interpenetrated mucus network; the heavily glycosylated regions of the glycoproteins can be seen along with "naked" regions, which consist of highly charged amino acids. It is assumed that crosslinking via disulfide bridges between mucin molecules occurs here.[20,27,28] These and other intermolecular interactions create the extended and random gel network, which imparts to mucus secretions their characteristic viscoelastic properties.

Future investigations into the structure, function, and properties of mucus and the mucosal epithelial cell regions will lead to better understanding of the mechanisms of bioadhesion, and therefore, better design of polymeric bioadhesive delivery systems.

B. CHEMICAL AND PHYSICAL INTERACTION OF ADHESION

Adhesion refers to the state in which two dissimilar bodies are held together by intimate interfacial contact such that mechanical force or work can be transferred across the interface.[29] The interfacial forces holding the two surfaces together may be due to van der Waals' forces, chemical bonding, physical entanglement, or electrostatic attraction. The actual mechanical force of adhesion is determined by the sum of the interfacial forces, and by the mechanical properties of the interfacial zone and the two bodies.

Thermodynamic adhesion addresses the equilibrium of interfacial forces and energies associated with reversible processes. Chemical adhesion refers to adhesion involving chemical bonding at the interface. The term "bioadhesion" is used to describe two materials, at least one of which is biological in nature, held together for an extended period of time, particularly by interfacial and mechanical forces.[30]

Of the interfacial forces mentioned, chemical or covalent bonds are believed to be the

"Naked" Protein Regions

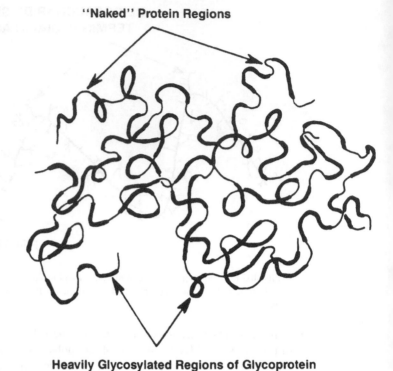

Heavily Glycosylated Regions of Glycoprotein

FIGURE 2.   A schematic representation of a randomly entangled mucus network.

least common in mucoadhesive systems. The five principal interfacial forces in
muco- or bioadhesion are: van der Waals' interactions, hydrogen bonding, ele
interaction, mechanical interlocking of substantial portions of the interface, and hy
interactions.

Van der Waals' forces are short range intermolecular forces between unchar
cules. These forces are comprised of a number of interactions including dispersion
or London) forces, resulting from instantaneous changes in the charge distributi
nonpolar molecules; dipole (dipole-dipole) forces resulting from the orientation of
dipoles in two molecules; induction (dipole-induced dipole) forces arising from a
dipole in another molecule; and hydrogen bonding. Hydrogen bonding seems to pl
role in bioadhesion.

A hydrogen bond is formed between a proton acceptor and a hydrogen atom
to a highly electronegative atom or group. Dipole-dipole attraction accounts for m
properties of a hydrogen bond.[29] Hydrogen bonds will only form when both the
receptor groups are available. Ketones and esters have acceptor atoms but no do
therefore, have few or no hydrogen bonds. However, they will form hydrogen
hydrogen donors can be brought into proximity or to an interface where groups are e

The strength of hydrogen bonds can be estimated as somewhere between van d
forces and primary (covalent) bonds.[31] The importance of hydrogen bonding as ar
mechanism is further evidenced by the phenomenon of autoadhesion of polym
have been subjected to surface oxidation by immersion in acids.[32,33]

The role of hydrogen bonding between adhesive surfaces has been investig
respect to wettability, surface roughness, and adhesive strength.[2,31]

III. PROPOSED THEORIES OF BIOADHESION

To be adhesive, bioadhesive material must first be in an adhesive state. This refers to the condition of the polymer as it is delivered to the desired site of adhesion. The adhesive state depends on which combination of the following adhesive mechanistic theories are germane for the subject bioadhesive delivery system. The bioadhesive may come in many forms, such as a solid or gel, and require some degree of hydration prior to becoming optimally adhesive. It may require a certain pH range to allow ionization of various groups, should electronic or charge density play a predominant role in its bioadhesive abilities. There are physical considerations, too. The bioadhesive system must establish intimate contact with the mucosal tissue, followed by formation of adhesive interactions. There are currently five accepted theories of bioadhesion.

A. ELECTRONIC THEORY

This theory describes adhesion due to electrical interaction of the bioadhesive polymer and the mucosal tissue. The bioadhesive polymer and the mucus glycoproteins are composed of various electronically active groups. There exists the possibility of electron transfer across the interface, which may in turn lead to formation of a double layer of electrical charge at the bioadhesive interface. Thus, the property of bioadhesiveness is presumed to exist due to attractive forces across the electrical double layer.[34,35] This is similar to the capacitance theory, wherein a capacitor is charged when two different surfaces come in contact, and discharged when they are separated.

B. FRACTURE THEORY

This theory attempts to relate the detachment force of separation of two surfaces after adhesion to the adhesive bond strength. Equation 1 allows calculation of the adhesion fracture strength, σ[36]

$$\sigma = (E\epsilon/L)^{1/2} \tag{1}$$

where ϵ is Young's modulus of elasticity, E is the fracture energy, and L is the critical crack length upon separation of the two surfaces. The work of fracture, G_c, of an elastomeric network increases with the molecular weight, M_c, of the network strands.[37-39] This direct relationship is given by:

$$G_c = K (M_c)^{1/2} \tag{2}$$

where K is a constant relating to the density of the polymer, the effective mass, length, and flexibility of a single main-chain bond, and the bond dissociation energy.

As the length of the free macromolecular strands involved in the interaction network increases,[37] or as the degree of crosslinking becomes smaller,[39] thus resulting in longer free strands, the work of fracture increases. This is consistent with the predictions of Lake and Thomas.[37]

Actual mechanical strengths of macromolecular interactive networks have been measured.[40] Here, the interactive network involved entanglement of elastomeric macromolecules. This research concluded that the work of rupture across the plane of entanglement is approximately proportional to the inferred density of entanglement. Moreover, the greater the molecular weight of the free strands of macromolecules comprising the entangled interface, the greater the work of rupture appears to be.[40]

C. ADSORPTION THEORY

The adsorption theory has been investigated and discussed in depth by Kinlo Huntsberger.[42] The primary adhesive or bonding forces involved in adsorption of a hesive polymer to a mucosal tissue are van der Waal's forces and hydrogen bond Norde and Lyklema[45-47] found that adsorption occurs when both protein and poly surfaces are negatively charged, and the maximum adsorption increases with in negative charge density of the polystyrene lattice surface. Upon adsorption, the electr of the protein molecule and the adsorbent surface overlap each other, permitting redist and transfer of charge.

The interfacial bonding force at the contact surface of polystyrene is theorize primarily due to London dispersion forces, e.g., van der Waals' forces.[48] These fo purported to exist between the repeat units of the polymer on the two sides of the inte At solid-liquid interfaces, almost all absorbed macromolecules were found to form layers, with the layer thickness varying with the square root of their molecular we It is clear that formation of adsorptive interfacial bonds depends greatly on the pr of the macromolecule, i.e., molecular weight, chemical structure, flexibility of th segment, and charge density. Charge density was also found to be important in a bioadhesive polymer systems studied by Park and Robinson.[67] The technique used studies involved localization of a lipid-soluble fluorescent probe, pyrene, in the lipi of the cell membrane. Addition of a polymer which binds to the cell membrane con the lipid bilayer, causing a change in fluorescence. The degree of change in fluo is proportional to the degree of binding. It appeared from this work that charge d an important element of bioadhesion, and that polyanions are preferred over pol with respect to toxicity and bioadhesion. Moreover, carboxylated polyanions appear than sulfated polyanions when both bioadhesiveness and toxicity were considered.

D. WETTING THEORY

As with the other theories, this theory draws on the knowledge accumulated for n adhesive systems. The ability of an adhesive to spread over the adhesive surface or case, the biological surface, is important to formation of an adhesive interface. Th equation gives the basic relationship between thermodynamic work of adhesion and in tension.

$$W_{AB} = \gamma_A + \gamma_B - \gamma_{AB}$$

where W_{AB} is the thermodynamic work of adhesion, γ_A and γ_B are surface tensic γ_{AB} is the interfacial tension.[49] These surface energies can be related to an *in vitr* known as the contact angle, θ. The Young equation relates these interfacial tensior contact angle.

$$\cos\theta = (\gamma_{SV} - \gamma_{SL})/\gamma_{LV}$$

Therefore, when $\theta > 0$ the bioadhesion system would not spread readily over tissue, whereas when $\theta = 0$, the system would completely wet the tissue.[49] F wetting conditions with respect to surface tensions can be represented as follows:

$$\gamma_{SV} \geq \gamma_{SL} + \gamma_{LV}$$

A number of researchers have examined the wetting theory of adhesion with re possible contributing variables such as dispersion and polar components in the surf energies of materials.[50]

$$\gamma_i = \gamma_i^d + \gamma_i^p \tag{6}$$

where i can be either the bioadhesive delivery system or the mucosal tissue. The superscripts designate the dispersion and polar components of the overall surface tension, respectively. These components may be examined by combining equation 6 with the previous statements for surface tension.[51,52]

$$\gamma_{SL} = \gamma_S + \gamma_L - 2(\gamma_S^d \gamma_L^d)^{1/2} - 2(\gamma_S^p \gamma_L^p)^{1/2} \tag{7}$$

Others have examined surface and interfacial tension with respect to the spreading coefficient, S, of a liquid adhesive.

$$S_b = \gamma_{SV} - \gamma_{SL} - \gamma_{LV} \tag{8}$$

where S_b is the spreading coefficient of the bioadhesive delivery system in liquid form. The subscripts solid, liquid, and vapor can be adapted to the applicable study system. For example, SV can represent the interfacial surface tension between the mucosal tissue or mucus and the general milieu surrounding the tissue, SL can represent the interfacial surface tension between the mucosal tissue or mucus and the bioadhesive polymer, and LV can represent the interfacial surface tension between the bioadhesive polymer and the surrounding milieu. For favorable bioadhesive conditions the spreading coefficient should be positive.[53,54]

Cultured human endothelial cells have been studied for interactions with polymeric surfaces with respect to wettability.[55] Optimal adhesion of human endothelial cells was generally found with moderately wettable polymers.[55] Cell adhesion was found to increase with increasing contact angle of the polymer surfaces within a series of cellulose polymers. This demonstrated that the surface is important to the ultimate adhesive bond strength.[56] The mean field theory was used in several studies to examine the interfacial properties of immiscible polymers.[57-59] The square root of the polymer-polymer interaction parameter was theorized to be proportional to the polymer interfacial tension.[57-59] High values for the work of adhesion were found to correspond to polymers with structural similarities. These structural similarities yielded low polymer-polymer interaction values, which translate to small interfacial tensions.

E. DIFFUSION OR INTERPENETRATION THEORY

Interpenetration or diffusion is considered to be of primary importance in bioadhesive systems. This theory refers to the interpenetration of the bioadhesive polymer chains into the mucus to a sufficient enough depth to create semi-permanent adhesive bonds. This concept was first introduced as the "diffusion theory" by Voyutskii.[60]

The interpenetration process is illustrated in Figure 3, where the molecules of the bioadhesive polymer and the mucus glycoprotein network diffuse into each other based on their macromolecular diffusion coefficients. The mean diffusional pathways, S, for various macromolecules can be estimated from:

$$S = (2tD)^{1/2} \tag{9}$$

where D is the diffusion coefficient, and t is the contact time or time for bioadhesion.[61]

The range of diffusion coefficients for high molecular weight polymers diffusion through the mucus glycoprotein network has been estimated to be in the range of 10^{-10} to 10^{-16} cm^2/sec.[62-64] The rate of penetration of the macromolecular strands of the bioadhesive polymer and the mucus substrate is directly dependent on the individual diffusion coefficients of the mucosal glycoprotein structure into the polymer matrix, and of the polymer strands into the

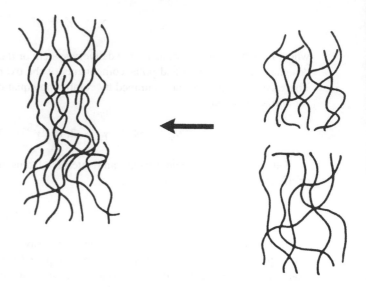

FIGURE 3.   Schematic representation of interdiffusion (interpenetration) of two polymer solutions.

mucosal matrix. Moreover, these individual diffusion coefficients are also functi
flexibility and "openness" or diffuseness of the bioadhesive polymer and the m
coproteins. The diffusion coefficients of various polymer systems have been found t
significantly with increasing degrees of crosslinking.[62]

Leung and Robinson[65] studied the effect of the expanded nature of the mucu
by examining the shear stress of the mucin-mucin interaction. This study found
an increased "openness" of the mucin network, there was a corresponding increas
stress. Furthermore, the polymer-mucin tensile stress was found to increase with
degrees of hydration of the bioadhesive polymer, using copolymers of acrylic
methyl methacrylate as the model system.[65] As the equilibrium degree of hydration
there was a corresponding increase in the expanded nature of the network.[65] Thi
is further supported by comparing the mucus network with crosslinked polyacr
PAA, a bioadhesive polymer that has been shown to be a good adhesive in the pr
mucus.[54] Both mucin and crosslinked PAA consist of a network of macromolecu
are generally negatively charged at physiologic pH. Both readily hydrate in aqueou
and form expanded networks. Both also have a significant number of carboxyl g
each crosslink between two adjacent chains.[54]

A bioadhesive polymer needs to have characteristics other than the structural
just mentioned to allow for good adhesion to biological surfaces. Thus, there
structural similarities between the bioadhesive polymer and the tissue or mucus. T
the difference in solubility parameters of the bioadhesive polymer system and the gly
system, the better the potential adhesive bond between the two.

IV. PHYSICAL STRUCTURE AND PROPERTIES

Early studies by Park and Robinson attempted to classify cationic, anionic, a
polymers by measuring and comparing the adhesiveness of a series of polymers u
culture-fluorescent probe technique.[66,67] This technique examines the change in flu
of probes such as fluorescein isothiocyanate and pyrene, which were incorporated i

TABLE 1
Results of Polymer Binding to Cultured Cell Monolayer

	Polymer	E/M[a]
Cationic polymer	Polylysine	0.08—0.24
	Polyvinyl methyl	0.03—0.13
	Polybrene	0.03—0.18
Anionic polymer	C.M.C.	0.21
	Polyacrylic acid	0.76
	Polyglutamic acid	0.18
	Dextran sulfate	0.01
	Lambda-carrageenan	0.14
Neutral polymer	Dextran	0.08—0.12
	Polyethylene glycols	0
Mixed charge polymer	Gelatin	0.29

[a] The higher (E/M) value implies higher binding affinity to the cell membrane.

conjunctival epithelial cells. These cells were then mixed with solutions of potentially bioadhesive polymers, in the case of pyrene, and the excimer/monomer ratio (E/M) measured as a function of time.[66,67] The "excimer" refers to the complex molecule formed by a photoexcited molecule. The actual parameter used in distinguishing binding potentials was the change in the ratio of excimer to monomer, ΔE/M. Large changes in this ratio correspond to a strong binding potential which would indicate a good bioadhesive candidate.[66,67] Table 1 illustrates some of the results of these studies.[66]

For the polyanionic polymers, the change in fluorescence was found to depend on the number of charged groups. Polymers with carboxyl groups demonstrated a large decrease in fluorescence, whereas polymers with sulfite or sulfonate showed a small change, with the exception of polystyrene sulfonate. Polymer structures that contain both carboxyl and sulfate groups display intermediate changes in fluorescence.[66,67]

Neutral polymers were found to show a relatively large decrease in fluorescence. This would suggest strong interaction of these polymers with the cell surface or probes. It is strongly suspected that neutral polymers disrupt the membrane bilayer to some extent by intercalation and, as a result, the adhesive phenomena may not be entirely due to the polymer binding to the cell surface.[66,67]

In general, polycationic polymers do not appear to be ideal candidates for bioadhesion to cell surfaces because of toxicity. Studies have indicated that polycationic polymers tend to cause openings or holes in the cell membrane.[68,69] Moreover, membranes were frequently found fused, possibly due to neutralization of the negative charge on the cell surface and/or formation of polymeric cation bridges which crosslink opposite membrane surfaces.[69] These effects were related to charge density of the cationic polymer. Polyanionic polymers seem preferable to polycationic or neutral polymers when both bioadhesiveness and toxicity are considered.

Polycarbophil, which is a polyacrylic acid (PAA) lightly crosslinked with divinyl alcohol, is an example of a linear polymer connected via crosslinking to form a water-swellable, insoluble polymer system.

The bioadhesive strengths of a series of crosslinked, water-swellable polymers with differing charge densities have been examined.[70] The general structures studied are illustrated in Figure 4, and the results presented in Table 2.[70] The synthesis of these polycarbophil analogs was accomplished using a free radical polymerization reaction.[70,71] When two different monomers were used, their distribution in the final polymer was dictated by their reactivity ratio.

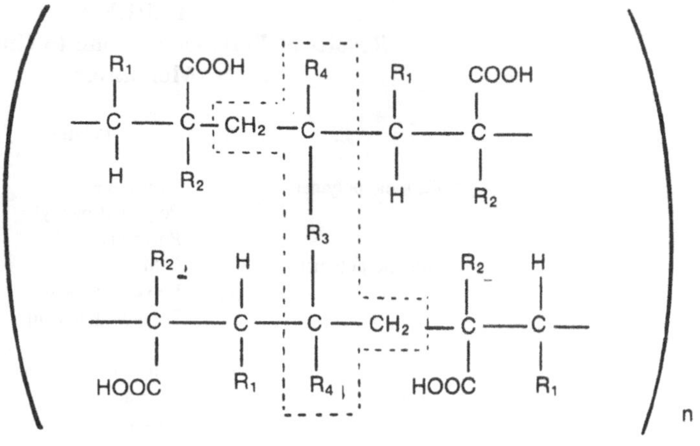

Polymer	R_1	R_2	R_3	R_4
1	H	H	-CHOHCHOH-	H
2	H	H	$(p)-C_5H_4$	H
3	H	CH_3	-CHOHCHOH-	H
4	H	CH_3	$(p)-C_5H_4$	H
5	H	$-CH_2COOH$	-CHOHCHOH-	H
6	COOH	H	-CHOHCHOH-	H
7	H	H	$-CH_2CH_2-$	CH_3
8	H	CH_3	$-CH_2CH_2-$	CH_3

1: Commercially available as polycarbophil (USP XX)

FIGURE 4.   Structures of crosslinked swelling polymers. (From Ch'ng H. et al., *J. Pharm. Sci.*, 74, 399, 1985. With permission.)

TABLE 2
In Vitro Evaluation of Polymer Bioadhesion to Rabbit Stomach Tissue Usin Modified Surface Tensiometer[a]

Test Material	Weight for detachment (mg)[b]	Forc (dyn
Polyacrylic acid (divinyl glycol)	855(54)	106
Polyacrylic acid (divinylbenzene)	876(57)	108
Polyacrylic acid (2,5-dimethyl 1,5-hexadlene)	864(56)	106
Polymethacrylic acid (divinylbenzene)	306(45)	38
Poly(2-hydroxyethyl methacrylate)	30(8)	3
Amberlite 200 resin beads	0	
Gelatin microcapsules[c]	0	

[a]   All studies used 4 mg of 30/40 mesh cut material.
[b]   Mean (SEM).
[c]   Crosslinked with formaldehyde.

Different crosslinking agents did not seem to have a significant effect on bioadhesive strength. However, there was a reduction in bioadhesive strength upon substitution of a methyl group on the PAA backbone. This reduction in bioadhesion is hypothesized to be due to an increase in hydrophobicity, which would result in a decrease in hydration of the polymer network.[70] Such a decrease in hydration would result in a decrease in the flexibility and mobility of the segment chains. Thus, the monomeric unit of a bioadhesive polymer plays an important role in bioadhesion, more so than the crosslinking agent. This, of course, may be a direct result of the relative structural contributions, since the crosslinking agent is a very small part of the total polymer network.

Any structural modification that increases interfacial interaction or interpenetration will increase the chances of a successful bioadhesive polymeric structure. Thermodynamically, it was shown that the work of detachment is proportional to the degree of interaction between the adhesive and substrate networks.[72] Moreover, the diffusion coefficient decreases with increasing relative amounts of crosslinking.[73]

As described earlier, the presence of negative groups promotes better bioadhesion. This was further supported by the observed increase in bioadhesive strength of hydrocolloids possessing carboxyl groups, such as acrylic acid, over those with neutral groups like 2-hydroxyethyl methacrylate.[70]

Another bioadhesive mechanism that is a function of charge or ionization is hydrogen bonding. This mechanism gained relevance when the adhesive strength of crosslinked PAA, pKa = 4.5, was examined as a function of the pH of the media (Figure 5).[74]

The pKa of PAA was found to depend on the degree of neutralization. It is likely that crosslinked PAA may have maximum bioadhesion at a pH < 4, where the majority of carboxyl groups are nonionized and available for formation of hydrogen bonds.[74]

Therefore, knowing the pKa of the basic bioadhesive polymer, the bioadhesive strength can be affected by manipulation of the degree of ionization of the charged moieties with respect to the targeted tissue pH.

It is clear that water plays an important role in bioadhesion. Bioadhesion of a polymer to a tissue surface can be conceptualized as a dynamic equilibrium of formation and breaking of interactive bonds between the adhesive and the substrate tissue through the presence of water.[75] A bioadhesive polymer must be able to broach the weak aqueous boundary layer of the substrate tissue. Once this occurs, the polymer must possess the appropriate functional groups, and general physical and structural attributes that will allow for good interpenetration and interaction with tissue and/or mucosal structural components, resulting in adhesion. This dynamic equilibrium of bond formation and bond breaking, in the presence of water, allows stress relaxation of the interface.[75] This conceptualization can be extended to the adhesion of plastics and ice to moist surfaces, barnacles to underwater structures, and plaque to teeth.[75]

It follows that the amount of water in the interactive interface is important. This is evidenced by the decrease in adhesive strength of a bioadhesive polymer when insufficient water is present to hydrate the bioadhesive fully. Insufficient hydration of a bioadhesive polymer results in not all of the adhesive sites or functional groups being liberated or exposed for interaction. Moreover, insufficient hydration would result in a decrease of bioadhesive polymer chain mobility, thereby decreasing the degree or extent of interpenetration.

The dynamic equilibrium of adhesion with respect to water is indeed an equilibrium, and thereby is dependent not only on too little water present, but on too much water present as well. Too much water present at the interface can result in excessive swelling which, in turn, results in an overextension of the available interactive hydrogen bonds and other adhesive forces between the polymer and the substrate.[76] In the case of water-insoluble polymers, the three-dimensional network in an aqueous medium is maintained by covalent crosslinks formed during polymerization. Excessive water may result in a decrease of adhesive strength for water-insoluble, but swellable, bioadhesive polymers. In swellable pol-

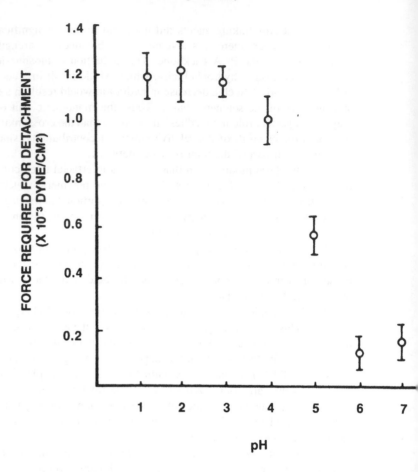

FIGURE 5.   Effect of pH on *in vitro* bioadhesion of crosslinked polyacrylic acid to rabbit stom‑
tissue.

ymers, the force of retraction of the stretched network structure depends on the d
extent of crosslinking. The degree of swelling at equilibrium has been found tc
with increasing degrees of crosslinking.[77]

Swelling, which is a direct manifestation of the degree of hydration, affects the
concentration of polymer solutions. This directly influences chain-segment mo
therefore the diffusion coefficient of the liquid polymer.[78] The swelling time
hydration is important to the polymer's bioadhesiveness. The faster a polymer hyc
faster the initiation of diffusion, formation of adhesive interactions, and increase
glement or interpenetration at the interface.

Hydration and the resulting chain-segment liberation and mobility are particula
to bioadhesion. However, interpenetration, entanglement, and resultant adhesive in
are also a function of applied pressure. The effect of applied pressure is illustrated
6[79] and 7.[71] The tensile and shear stress increases to plateau values with increasir
force. The increase in applied pressure results in a corresponding increase in cor
i.e., mechanical entanglement and interpenetration, which also allows for an i
adhesive interactions. If the applied pressure is increased, the molecular contact
number of adhesive interactions or degree of possible entanglement reaches a n
This would correspond to the maximum adhesive strength for that particular poly

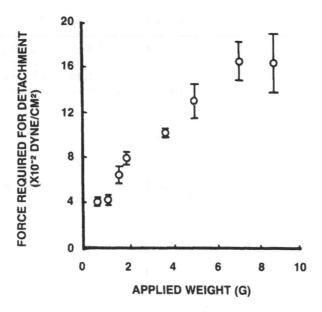

FIGURE 6. Effect of applied weight on mucin-mucin tensile stress using pH 1.2 USP simulated gastric fluid. (From Park, H. and Robinson, J. R., *J. Controlled Release*, 2, 47, 1985. With permission.)

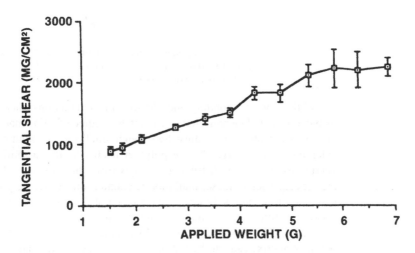

FIGURE 7. Effect of applied weight on mucin-mucin shear stress using pH 2 isotonic phosphate buffer. (From Leung, S. H. S. and Robinson, J. R., *J. Controlled Release*, 12, 187, 1990. With permission.)

V. GENERAL MOLECULAR CHARACTERISTICS

Hydrophilicity is an important component for bioadhesive polymers. Particularly since hydrophilic functional groups like carboxyl, hydroxyl, amide, and sulfate groups have the ability to form hydrogen bonds. As mentioned earlier, hydrogen bonding plays a significant role in bioadhesion, and has a correlation with the degree of hydration. Park and Robinson[79] found that the degree of hydration of crosslinked polyacrylic acid with carboxyl groups can be controlled by adjusting the pH of the medium (Figure 8).[79]

The buffer systems were dilute hydrochloric acid (pH 1.2), 0.1M phosphate buffer (pH 2.0, 3.0, 4.0, 6.0, and 7.0) and 0.1M acetate buffer (pH 5.0). Ionic strength was controlled in all buffers with NaCl and temperature was kept at 37°C. Each point is the mean to two measurements.

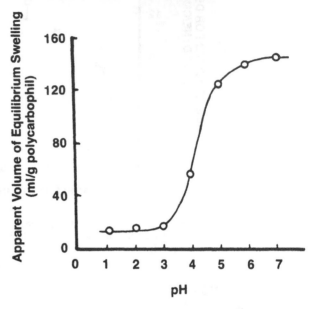

FIGURE 8.   Apparent volume of equilibrium swelling of polycarbophil at various pHs. (From Park, H. and Robinson, J. R., *J. Controlled Release, 2,* 47, 1985. With permission.)

With hydrogen bonding and electrostatic interactions playing such a predomir in bioadhesion, Donnan effects cannot be neglected. For macromolecular solutio electrically neutral, there must be enough small ions in solution to interact with a macromolecular charges.[80] The polymer itself acts like a semi-permeable membra venting the randomly distributed charges from diffusing into the bulk solution. Th the concentration of these small mobile counter ions inside the polymer matrix will b than that of the bulk solution. The presence of this ion concentration differential es a swelling force or swelling pressure due to a net osmotic pressure differential ac interface.[77] This osmotic pressure differential is the driving force for solvent to e polymer matrix, causing hydration to form a more dilute and flexible network sys

The counter ions also serve to reduce swelling or expansion of the polymer prior to hydration. For anionic and cationic polymers, e.g., polyacrylic acid and p the charged groups within the polymer structure can establish an electrostatic re which would tend to expand the polymer network. At a given pH, the electrostatic r can be reduced by the presence of small mobile counter ions.

Another important physical characteristic of bioadhesive polymers is molecular Studies by Chen and Cyr[81] suggested that bioadhesive strength increased as the m weight of the polymer increased above 100,000. Polyethylene glycols, with a m weight of 20,000, did not demonstrate adhesiveness, whereas Polyvox WSR 35 molecular weight of 200,000, demonstrated improved adhesiveness, and Polyvox W with a molecular weight up to 4 million, showed excellent adhesive properties.[81]

It is clear that chain length and molecular weight are important factors in bioa

It is likely that a critical bioadhesive chain length exists for a given bioadhesive interface that results in optimum interpenetration or entanglement of the polymer with the substrate.[82]

As we have seen, interpenetration and entanglement seem to be very important to good bioadhesion. Since bioadhesive polymers are able to hydrate and swell, this should lead to increases in general molecular flexibility and mobility of the polymer chains. The ability of the polymer chains to interpenetrate can be approximated by their ability to diffuse. This suggests that chain-sgement mobility can be related to polymer viscosities as well as their diffusion coefficients. The diffusion coefficient of the solute polymer increases with the degree of swelling of the polymer network, and decreases with increasing solute size.[83] The experimental diffusion coefficient, D, demonstrates an Arrhenius type temperature dependence within a restricted temperature range.[82]

$$D = D_0 \exp(-E/RT) \tag{10}$$

where D_0 is a constant and is independent of temperature over a given temperature range, and E is the experimental activation energy for diffusion or mobility of polymer chains. Therefore, it can be seen that the higher the chain-segment mobility at a given temperature, the greater the interpenetration.

Viscosity is also a measure of intermolecular chain flexibility and mobility. A bioadhesive polymer's viscosity depends on polymer-solvent, interaction, flexibility, degree of ionization, concentration of the polymer, and the pH.[84] The viscosity of most polymers does not have a single value, but varies with the shearing force.[85] The relationship between shear force per unit area, b_s, and the velocity gradient of flow, $\Delta V/\Delta Y$, is:[85]

$$b_S = \eta \, \Delta V/\Delta Y \tag{11}$$

where η is the coefficient of viscosity, or "viscosity", of the polymer system. This may also be written as

$$b_S = \eta \, dv/dy \tag{12}$$

Systems that follow equation 12 are known as Newtonian, as shown in Figure 9. Generally, solutions of low molecular weight are Newtonian, whereas solutions of macromolecules are non-Newtonian. This is a direct consequence of the polymers' ability to entangle with one another.

Viscosity is dependent on molecular weight.[85] Branched polymers tend to have lower viscosities since their backbone structures are shorter than linear polymers of the same molecular weight, and they are more compact structurally.

Polymer viscosity is affected by the degree of entanglement of the polymer chains. Polymers that reside in a "good" solvent find that polymer-solvent interactions are favored over polymer chain interactions. In "poor" solvent conditions, polymer chain interaction forces would be favored over polymer-solvent interactions, and the polymer would remain in a compact interdependent network, as shown in Figure 10. The polymer chain is more extended in a good solvent system, and thus the intrinsic viscosity of the polymer would be higher.

Most bioadhesive polymers are solvated in aqueous media, and owe their expanding networks to hydration and subsequent swelling. The hydration of macromolecules involves three types of water:[86] tightly bound water, which is believed to be hydrogen bound; loosely bound water, which differs from bulk water in enthalpy; and bulk water.

The rate and extent of water uptake by a bioadhesive polymer depends on the type and number of hydrophilic groups in the polymer structure, the pH of the media, and the ionic

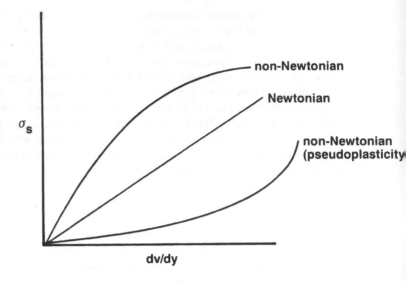

FIGURE 9.   Differentiation between Newtonian and non-Newtonian behavior.

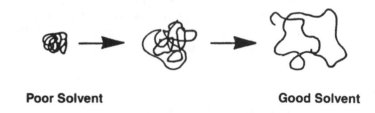

Poor Solvent   **Good Solvent**

FIGURE 10.   Schematic representation of dissolution/swelling of polymer in good and poor solvents.

strength of the aqueous environment. The amount of water sorbed, the degree of decreases, as shown in Figure 11, as the percent of charged groups (acrylic acid) and the percent of uncharged groups (methyl methacrylate) increases.[71]

Different degrees of adhesive properties can be seen with different degrees of Systems can exhibit maximum adhesion at an optimum degree of hydration.[81] This that depends on the polymer. Some will exhibit adhesiveness at a low degree of and lose adhesiveness as the water content is increased. The loss in adhesiveness to be due to the formation of a slippery, nonadhesive mucilage when excess water at or near the interface, the general mechanism of which was described earlier.[8]

Leung and Robinson[71] synthesized a series of 0.2% crosslinked acrylic a methacrylate copolymers. Bioadhesive studies of these crosslinked copolymers ducted at pH 2; the results of these studies are shown in Figure 12. When comp Figure 11, one can find similarities in both curves. As the percent of acrylic acid the amount of absorbed water, i.e., the degree of hydration, and the tensile stress in a similar fashion.

Figure 13 shows a correlation between degree of hydration and tensile stres copolymers.[71] The highest bioadhesion was found with a copolymer of the highest or greatest expanded network.

The contribution of the expanded nature of the mucus network was also stu a divalent ion, calcium; a monovalent ion, sodium; and a chelating agent, ED shear stress of the mucin-mucin interaction was studied using a dual tensiomete

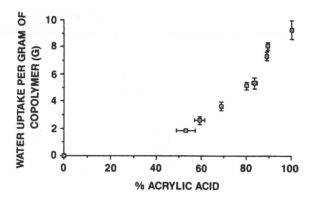

FIGURE 11. Hydration of copolymers with different percent of acrylic acid. (From Leung, S. H. S. and Robinson, J. R., *J. Controlled Release*, 12, 187, 1990. With permission.)

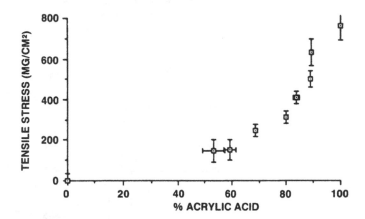

FIGURE 12. Correlation of tensile stress with percent of acrylic acid. (From Leung, S. H. S. and Robinson, J. R., *J. Controlled Release*, 12, 187, 1990. With permission.)

(Figure 14).[71] It was found that the addition of EDTA results in the highest mucin-mucin shear stress, followed by sodium chloride, and calcium chloride with the lowest. Addition of calcium caused precipitation of mucin and decreased openness of the mucin network. This resulted in a decrease in interpenetration and entanglement at the interface with a resultant reduction of bioadhesive strength. The addition of EDTA-chelated calcium in the mucus layer increased the openness of the network by exposing more of the charged groups and thus promoting internal electrical repulsion. This allows the process of interpenetration of entanglement to be enhanced, with a concomitant increase in the strength of bioadhesion.

In a bioadhesive system, after contact is established, the expanded networks of the bioadhesive polymer and mucus tend to maximize mechanical interpenetration and entanglement, and adhesive interactions, e.g., van der Waals' bonds, hydrophobic interactions, and hydrogen bonding.

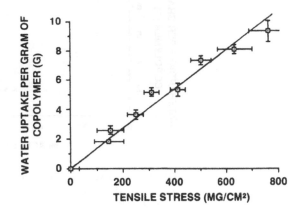

FIGURE 13.   Correlation of tensile stress with water uptake. (From Leung, S. H. S. and Robinson, J. R., *J. Controlled Release*, 12, 187, 1990. With permission.)

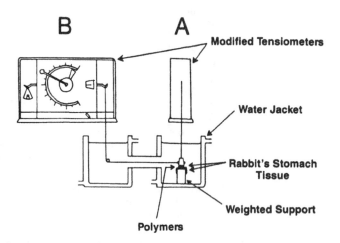

FIGURE 14.   Dual tensiometer. (From Leung, S. H. S. and Robinson, J. R., *J. Controlled Release*, 12, 187, 1990. With permission.)

VI. METHODS OF MEASURING BIOADHESION

Specialized techniques have been developed for measuring bioadhesion to va ological surfaces.

The majority of these methods are based on determination of the shear stress c stress of the bioadhesive system.[81,87,88] The tensile strength between water-soluble p and mucus was measured by Smart et al.,[82] using the Wilhelmy plate method (Fig The plates were coated by dipping them into a 1% solution of the test polymer ar drying at 60°C to a constant weight. The polymer-coated glass plate was then imm homogenized mucus samples. The adhesive force was measured after 7 min of con shortest time necessary to achieve a measurable degree of bioadhesion. This is be the need for polymer hydration and the subsequent expansion of the polymer netw

As mentioned earlier, Park and Robinson studied the bioadhesive strength of a

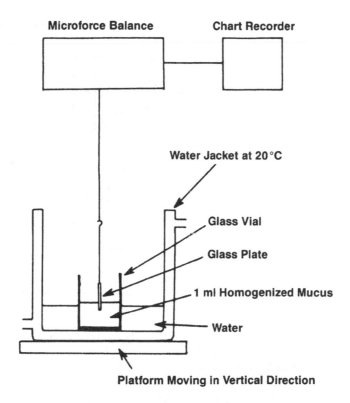

FIGURE 15. The *in vitro* mucoadhesion apparatus. (From Bremecker, K. D., et al., *J. Pharm. Sci.*, 73, 548, 1984. With permission.)

of polymers in different ionization states, using a fluorescent probe technique.[67] Polymers were added to the surface of pyrene-labeled lipid bilayers of cultured human conjunctival epithelial cells. The binding of a polymer to the bilayer compressed the bilayer, causing a change in fluorescence. A large value of fluorescence change indicated a strong binding potential.

The charge densities of both water-soluble and insoluble anionic bioadhesive polymers have been measured by potentiometric titration[74] and an acridine orange binding technique.[89] Acridine orange showed a one-to-one binding with either sulfate or carboxyl groups.[90,91]

The tensile stress of mucin-mucin and polymer-mucin interactions were determined using a modified tensiometer,[70,71] and is shown in Figure 16.[70] The tensile strength was determined by measuring the force of detachment of the polymer mucus interface. Both tensile and shear stresses are measurable in bioadhesive systems. A dual tensiometer apparatus may be used to measure the shear stress in bioadhesion (Figure 14).[71] Measuring both shear and tensile stress can provide a clearer understanding of the forces involved in the *in vivo* situation.

Mikos and Peppas,[92] and Peppas and Buri[54] utilized a thin channel filled with artificial mucus gel or natural mucus to measure both the static and dynamic bioadhesiveness of polymer particles. The polymeric particles were preswollen in a mucin solution. Pictures of the motion of the particles were taken, their velocities determined, and the hydrodynamic force necessary for particle detachment calculated. Motion of the polymeric particles was generated by a controlled air flow.

Bioadhesion has been studied as a function of gastrointestinal transit in rats.[70] A capsule containing the test bioadhesive polymer or the control, nonadhesive beads was surgically inserted into the rat stomach with subsequent sacrifices at various time intervals, post-surgery. The number and location of the polymer-coated beads were noted upon necropsy.

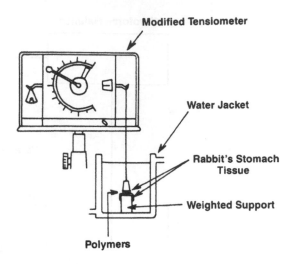

FIGURE 16.   A modified surface tensiometer for an *in vitro* evaluation of bioadhesion. (From Ch'ng, H. S., et al., *J. Pharm. Sci.*, 74, 399, 1985. With permission.)

In drug delivery systems the amount of sequestered drug present may infl bioadhesive strength of the systems. The determination of the adhesive ability of the bioadhesive dosage form is necessary. Ishida et al.[95] developed a test apparatus the adhesiveness of tablets (Figure 17) and ointments (Figure 18).

The tendency of tablets and capsules to adhere to the esophagus was exami isolated swine esophagi (Figure 19). These are but a few of the numerous a determining *in vivo* bioadhesiveness for drug delivery systems.

VII. DRUG DELIVERY

Bioadhesive polymers can be used as platforms for delivery of drugs locally ically. Use of bioadhesive drug delivery systems can result in maximal and effi absorption with a concomitant improvement in therapy and/or a decrease in extran load in the body. External targeted tissues are basically any mucosal epithelial tissue the eye, mouth, gastrointestinal tract, nasal regions, rectum, urinary tract, and vagin examination of some of these routes follows.

A. ORAL

The short gastrointestinal tract transit time in humans results in frequent dosin to maintain an effective therapeutic blood level. This, in turn, may introduce pa pliance problems as well as peak and trough blood drug levels. Application of muc dosage forms which can be designed to localize in specific areas of the gastrointes may increase transit time of the dosage form and permit once-daily dosing, alon possibility of exploitation of site-specific absorption windows.

Polycarbophil (crosslinked PAA) has been used in an albumin bead form develop a sustained release dosage form for chlorothiazide.[96] The presence of poly was shown to have no effect on the release rate of chlorothiazide. The formul shown to double the bioavailability of chlorothiazide and prolong the gastrointesti time in rats.[96] The mucoadhesive binds the dosage form to the mucus/epithelial su increases the transit time. When this study was repeated in dogs and humans, t

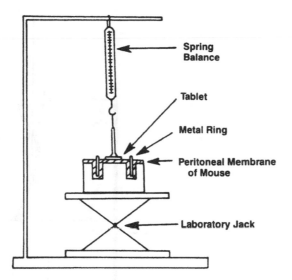

FIGURE 17. Schematic illustration of a stickiness test apparatus. (From Ishida, M., et al., *Chem. Pharm. Bull.*, 29, 810, 1981. With permission.)

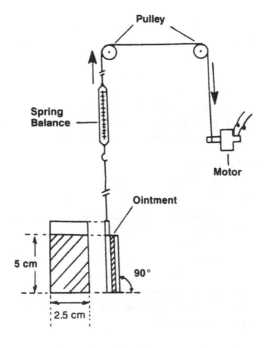

FIGURE 18. Schematic illustration of the shearing stickiness test apparatus. (From Ishida, M., et al., *Chem. Pharm. Bull.*, 31, 1010, 1983. With permission.)

were less dramatic, due to soluble mucin in the stomachs of the test subjects that binds the mucoadhesive before it can attach to the wall of the stomach.

B. BUCCAL

The buccal area has a very significant potential for mucoadhesive drug delivery because

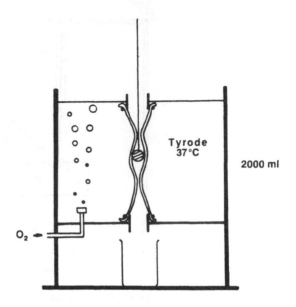

FIGURE 19.   Schematic illustration of the organ bath for isolated esophageal preparations. (From Marvola, M., et al., *J.
Pharm. Sci.*, 71, 975, 1982. With permission.)

of the abundant blood supply in the buccal area. Moreover, buccal delivery provides
for delivery of acid labile drugs. Other advantages of oral mucosal delivery[97] are

1. It bypasses hepatic first-pass metabolism.
2. It has excellent accessibility, and can be applied, localized, and removed ea
3. It can be made unidirectional, to insure only buccal tissue absorption.
4. It prevents the buildup of diffusion-limiting mucus.
5. The buccal tissue is generally more permeable than the skin.

C. OCULAR

A significant problem with ocular drug delivery is the low bioavailability du
corneal drug loss via drainage, tear turnover, nonproductive absorption, and protein
Other pharmaceutical dosage forms have not solved the problem of bioavailability
of short residence time and/or poor dissolution.

The bioadhesive polymer polycarbophil was used as a platform for ocular de
progesterone.[98] It was shown that polycarbophil has good bioadhesion to the con
mucus/epithelial surface, although the bioadhesive strength is approximately one fo
of the gastric mucus/epithelial surface. Bioavailability studies in rabbits showed
mucoadhesive formulation had an "area under the curve" 4.2 times greater than
suspension preparation.[98]

D. NASAL

The nasal mucosa provides a potentially excellent route for systemic drug deliv
area of the human nasal mucosa[99] is about 150 cm^2 and, together with its dense
network, provides an extraordinary absorptive surface.

A new powder dosage form consisting of freeze-dried insulin and carbopol-
developed.[100] This bioadhesive nasal dosage form demonstrated that absorption o
via the nasal route was possible. Results on beagle dogs showed that the absor
insulin from the nasal mucosa was fastest in the preparation with crystalline cellul

was sustained in the preparation with sodium carbopol. The sustained release effect seemed to increase with carbopol concentration.

E. RECTAL

Bioadhesive dosage forms for delivery of antipyrine and theophylline have been developed.[101] The dosage form is cylindrical in shape, and consists of hydroxyethyl methacrylate (HEMA) crosslinked with ethylene glycol dimethacrylate. This dosage form gave a rapid increase in plasma concentration of theophylline for the first 4 to 5 hr, and then an almost constant release thereafter. Similar results were observed *in vivo* with antipyrine.

F. VAGINAL

Generally, most vaginal therapeutic drugs are delivered by means of creams, foams, suppositories, gels, or tablets. Williams[102] designed a soluble hydroxypropyl cellulose cartridge impregnated with drug for vaginal drug delivery. During vaginal residence, moisture from the vaginal wall and the cervical gland slowly dissolves the polymer cartridge. Thus, the medicament can be released over an extended period of time. Furthermore, hydroxypropyl cellulose converts to a high viscosity gel upon hydration and provides a soothing effect on the vaginal wall.

VIII. SUMMARY

There is great promise for bioadhesive polymers as platforms for local and systemic drug delivery. Polymers being considered for a drug delivery role must not only be assessed for specific bioadhesive properties, but also for drug loading and delivery characteristics as well. The bioadhesive polymer may only be part of a drug delivery system. This system may include other polymers designed for controlled drug delivery, such as matrix diffusion. Moreover, specificity to a particular adhesion site may be desired. This would require not only an understanding of the bioadhesive polymer, but also a more complete understanding of the morphology, chemistry, and physiology of the target tissue, specific mucus, and the biological environment present at the desired delivery site.

Mucus certainly plays an intricate role in bioadhesion. It may indeed be the primary site of bioadhesive interaction with substrate tissues. This continuous network of glycoproteinaceous material that coats most of the body orifices carries a substantial negative charge due to the presence of sialic acid and sulfonic acid residues. It is this predominance of negative charges in the mucin network that is most likely responsible for a great deal of the bioadhesive interaction seen to date, particularly with charged bioadhesive polymers.

The bioadhesive process can be conceptualized as the establishment of intimate contact, by diffusion or network expansion, of the polymer chains, with subsequent interpenetration. This process may be further enhanced by viscoelastic deformation between the bioadhesive and substrate tissue through applied force or pressure. This is followed by formation of secondary bonds, e.g., electrostatic and hydrophobic interactions, hydrogen bonding, and van der Waals' intermolecular interactions. It follows that the more compatible the two surfaces, the better the adhesive interaction potential will be. This applies to both charged and neutral bioadhesive polymers.

In addition, the expanded nature of both the mucin and polymer networks permits mutual interpenetration. Interpenetration/interdiffusion of mucin and adhesives results in an increase in contact area and establishment of physical entanglement of the two different macromolecules. Physical entanglement will strengthen the network in the interfacial area, whereas an increase in contact area will result in an increase in formation of secondary bonds. There are a number of factors that may affect interpenetration: chain-segment mobility, chain entanglement, crosslinking density of both networks, equilibrum swelling, porosity, additives, and compatibility of the adhesive and mucin.

There are, of course, many factors to be considered with respect to the bi substrate, mucin. A lot remains to be elucidated concerning mucin, including its pl properties, turnover rate, flow, various ionic and concentration gradients within network, mucin organization at various tissue sites in the body, and its role in ulti absorption. This remains a difficult and challenging task, since attempts to obtain m measurements or observations, to date, have generally been done *in vitro*. It is n clear if any artifact or perturbations have been introduced that are not present *in* more is learned and discovered about the natural properties of mucin, a better und of the structure-activity relationships of bioadhesive polymers and various mucins will

This evolution, as such, coincides with, and compliments, the ever-growin vancing pool of knowledge that embodies controlled and targetted drug delivery.

REFERENCES

1. **Manley, R. S., Ed.,** *Adhesion in Biological Systems,* Academic Press, New York, 1970.
2. **Gross, L. and Hoffman, R.,** Medical and biological adhesives, in I. Skeist, Ed., *Handbook c* 2nd ed., Van Nostrand-Reinhold, New York, 1977, 818.
3. **Wright, P. S.,** Composition and properties of soft lining materials for acrylic dentures, *J. D* 1981.
4. **Ducheyne, P., van der Perre, G., and Aubert, A. E., Eds.,** *Biomaterials and Biomechani* Amsterdam, 1984.
5. **Refojo, M. F., Dohlman, C. H., and Koliopoulos, J.,** *Surv. Ophthalmol.,* 15, 217, 1971.
6. **Wang, P. Y.,** Surgical adhesives and coatings, in C. D. Ray, Ed., *Medical Engineering,* Year B Publishers, Chicago, 1974, 1123.
7. **Vezin, W. R. and Florence, A. T.,** *In vitro* heterogeneous degradation of poly (*n*-alkyl α-cya *J. Biomed Mater. Res.,* 14, 93, 1980.
8. **Mugin, C., Cogalniceanu, D., Leibovici, M., and Negulescu, I.,** On the medical use of esters: toxicity of pure *n*-butyl-α-cyanoacrylate, *J. Polym. Sci. Symp.,* 66, 189, 1979.
9. **Harper, M. C. and Ralston, M. J.,** Isobutyl 2-cyanoacrylate as an osseous adhesive in osteochondral fractures, *J. Biomed. Mater. Res.,* 17, 167, 1983.
10. **Leonard, F., Kulkarui, R. K., Nelson, J., and Brandes, G. J.,** Tissue adhesives and he including compounds: the alkyl cyanocryltes, *J. Biomed. Mater. Res.,* 1, 3, 1967.
11. **Meyer, G., Muster, D., Schmitt, D., Jung, P., and Jaeger, J. H.,** Bone bonding through b present status. *Biomat. Med. Dev. Art. Org.,* 7, 55, 1979.
12. **Park, J. B.,** Acrylic bone cement: *In vitro* and *in vivo* property-structure relationship — a selec *Ann. Biomed. Eng.,* 2, 297, 1983.
13. **Schachter, H. and Williams, D.,** *Biosynthesis of mucus glycoproteins, Adv. Exp. Med. B.* 1982.
14. **Ginsburg, V. and Neufeld, E. F.,** Complex heterosaccharides of animals, *Annu. Rev. Bioche* 1969.
15. **Kornfeld, R. and Kornfeld, S.,** Comparative aspects of glycoprotein structure, *Ann. Rev. B* 217, 1976.
16. **Forstner, J. F.,** Intestinal mucins in health and disease, *Digestion,* 17, 234, 1978.
17. **Pigman, W.,** *The glycoconjugates,* Vol. 1, Horowitz, M. I. and Pigman, W., Eds., Academic York, 1977.
18. **Allen, A. and Garner, A.,** Progress report: mucus and bicarbonate secretion in the stoma possible role in mucosal protection, *Gut,* 21, 249, 1980.
19. **Silverberg, A. and Meyer, F. A.,** Structure and function of mucus, in *Mucus in Health and Advances in Experimental Medicine and Biology,* Vol. 144, Chantler, E. N., Edler, J. B., and Eds., Plenum Press, New York, 1982, 53.
20. **Chantler, E. N., Elder, J. B., and Elstein, M., Eds.,** *Mucus in Health and Disease.* II. *Experimental Medicine and Biology,* Vol. 144, Plenum Press, New York, 1982, 53.
21. **Carlstedt, I. and Sheehan, J. K.,** Macromolecular properties and polymeric structure of m proteins, in *Mucus and Mucosa,* Ciba Foundation Symposium, Nugent, J. and O'Connor, M., E London, 1984, 157.

22. **Pigman, W. and Gottschalk, A.,** *Glycoprotein,* Vol. 2, Elsevier, Amsterdam, 1966.
23. **Gibbons, R. A.,** Mucus of the mammalian genital tract, *Br. Med. Bull.,* 34, 43, 1978.
24. **Phelps, C. F.,** Biosynthesis of mucus glycoprotein, *Br. Med. Bull.,* 34, 43, 1978.
25. **Schwartz, R. T. and Datema, R.,** Inhibition of lipid-dependent glycosylation, in Horowitz, M. I., Ed., *The Glycoconjugates,* Vol. 3, Academic Press, New York, 1982, 47.
26. **Meyer, F. A., Eliezer, N., Silverberg, A., Vered, J., Sharon, N., and Sade, J.,** Biochemical basis for the transport function of epithelial mucus, *Bull. Physiol. Path. Resp.,* 9, 259, 1973.
27. **Scawen, M. and Allen, A.,** The action of proteolytic enzymes on the glycoprotein from pig gastric mucin, *Biochem. J.,* 163, 363, 1977.
28. **Mantle, M. and Allen, A.,** Isolation and characterization of the native glycoprotein from pig small intestinal mucus, *Biochem. J.,* 195, 267, 1981.
29. **Souheng, W.,** *Polymer Interface and Adhesion,* Marcel Dekker, New York, 1982.
30. **Good, R. J.,** Definition of adhesion, *Adhesion,* 8, 1, 1976.
31. **Pritchard, W. H.,** The role of hydrogen bonding in adhesion, *Aspects Adhes.,* 6, 11, 1971.
32. **Gledhill, R. A., Kinloch, A. J., and Shaw, S. J.,** Effect of relative humidity on the wettability of steel surface, *J. Adhes.,* 9, 81, 1977.
33. **Leclerq, B., Satton, M., Baszkin, A., and TER-Minassian-saraga, L.,** Surface modification of corona treated poly (ethylene terephthalate) film: adsorption and wettability studies, *Polymer,* 18, 675, 1977.
34. **Darjaguin, B. V. and Smilga, V. P.,** *Adhesion: Fundamentals and Practice,* McLaren, London, 1969.
35. **Derjaguin, B. V., Toporov, Y. P., Mueler, V. M., and Aleinikova, I. N.,** On the relationship between the electrostatic and molecular component of the adhesion of elastic particles to a solid surface, *J. Colloid Interface Sci.,* 58, 528, 1977.
36. **Kammer, H. W.,** Adhesion between polymers, *Aeta Polym.,* 34, 112, 1983.
37. **Lake, G. J. and Thomas, A. G.,** The strength of highly elastic materials, *Proc. R. Soc. London Ser. A,* 300, 108, 1967.
38. **Ahagon, A. and Gent, A. N.,** Threshold fracture energies for elastomer, *J. Polym. Sci. Polym. Phys. Ed.,* 13, 1903, 1975.
39. **Ahagon, A. and Gent, A. N.,** Effect of interfacial bonding on the strength of adhesion, *J. Polym. Sci. Polym. Phys. Ed.,* 13, 1285, 1975.
40. **Gent, A. N. and Tobias, R. H.,** Effect of interfacial bonding on the strength of adhesion of elastomers. III. Interlinking by molecular entanglements, *J. Polym. Sci. Polym. Phys. Ed.,* 22, 1483, 1984.
41. **Kinloch, A. J.,** The science of adhesion. I. Surface and interfacial aspects, *J. Mater. Sci.,* 15, 2141, 1989.
42. **Huntsberger, J. R.,** Mechanisms of adhesions, *J. Paint Technol.,* 39, 199, 1967.
43. **Good, R. J.,** Surface free energy of solids and liquids: thermodynamics, molecular forces and structure, *J. Colloid Interface Sci.,* 59, 398, 1977.
44. **Tabor, D.,** Surface forces and surface interactions, *J. Colloid Interface Sci.,* 71, 350, 1979.
45. **Norde, W. and Lyklema, J.,** Thermodynamics of proteins adsorption, *J. Colloid Interface Sci.,* 71, 350, 1979.
46. **Norde, W. and Lyklema, J.,** The adsorption of human plasma albumin and bovine pancreas ribonuclease at negatively changed polystyrene surface. II. Hydrogen ion titrations, *J. Colloid Interface Sci.,* 66, 266, 1978.
47. **Norde, W. and Lyklema, J.,** The absorption of human plasma albumin and bovine pancrease ribonuclease at negatively charged polystyrene surface. IV. The charge distribution in the absorbed state, *J. Colloid Interface Sci.,* 66, 295, 1978.
48. **Anand, J. N.,** Interfacial contact and bonding in autoadhesion. III. Parallel plate attraction, *J. Adhes.,* 1, 31, 1969.
49. **Hiemenz, P. C.,** *Principles of Colloid and Surface Chemistry,* Hiemenz, P. C., Ed., Marcel Dekker, New York, 1977.
50. **Schultz, J., Tsutsumi, K., and Donnet, J. B.,** Surface properties of high energy solids, *J. Colloid Interface Sci.,* 59, 277, 1977.
51. **Owens, D. and Wendt, R. C.,** Estimation of the surface free energy of polymers, *J. Appl. Polym. Sci.,* 13, 1740, 1969.
52. **Kaelbe, D. H. and Uy, K. C.,** Reinterpretation of organic liquid — PTFE surface interactions, *J. Adhes.,* 2, 50, 1970.
53. **Kaelbe, D. H. and Moacanin, J.,** A surface energy analysis of bioadhesion, *Polymer,* 18, 475, 1977.
54. **Peppas, N. A. and Buri, P. A.,** Surface, interfacial and molecular aspects of polymer bioadhesion on soft tissues, *J. Controlled Release,* 2, 257, 1985.
55. **Van Wachem, P. B., Beugeling, T., Feizen, J., Bantjes, A., Detmers, J. P., and van Aken, W. G.,** Interaction of cultural human endothelial cells with polymeric surfaces of different wettabilities, *Biomaterials,* 6, 403, 1985.

124   *Polymers for Controlled Drug Delivery*

56. **Schonhorn, H. and Hansen, R. H.,** A new technique for preparing low surface energy pol adhesive bonding, *J. Polym. Sci.,* 54, 203, 1966.
57. **Helfand, E. and Tagami, Y.,** Theory of the interface between immiscible polymers, *Polym. Lett* 1971.
58. **Helfand, E. and Tagami, Y.,** Theory of the interface between immiscible polymers, *J. Chem. I* 3592, 1972.
59. **Helfand, E. and Tagami, Y.,** Theory of the interface between immiscible polymers, *J. Chem. I* 1812, 1972.
60. **Voyutskii, S. S.,** *Autoadhesion and Adhesion of High Polymers,* John Wiley & Sons/Interscie York, 1963.
61. **Campion, R. P.,** The influence of structure of autoadhesion (self-tack) and other forms of diff polymers, *J. Adhes.,* 7, 1, 1974.
62. **Reinhart, C. T. and Peppas, N. A.,** Solute diffusion in swollen membranes. II. Influence of cr on diffusive properties, *J. Membrane Sci.,* 18, 227, 1984.
63. **Peppas, C. T. and Lustig, S. R.,** The rate of crosslinks, entanglements and relaxations of the olecular carrier in the difusional release of biologically active materials: Conceptual and sealing rela *Ann. N.Y. Acad. Sci.,* 44, 26, 1984.
64. **Gilmore, P. T., Falabella, R., and Laurence, R. L.,** Polymer/polymer diffusion, *Macromole* 880, 1980.
65. **Leung, S. H. S. and Robinson, J. R.,** The contribution of anionic polymer structural featur coadhesion, *J. Controlled Release,* in press.
66. **Park, K., Ch'ng, H. S., and Robinson, J. R.,** Alternative approaches to oral controlled drug bioadhesives and *in situ* systems, in *Recent Advances in Drug Delivery Systems,* Anderson, J. M. S. W., Eds., Plenum Press, New York, 1984, 163.
67. **Park, K. and Robinson, J. R.,** Bioadhesive polymers as platforms for oral-controlled drug method to study bioadhesion, *Int. J. Pharm.,* 19, 107, 1984.
68. **Katchalsky, A., Damon, D., and Nevo, A.,** Interactions of basic polyelectrolytes with the red t II. Agglutination of red blood cells by polymeric bases, *Biochim. Biophys. Acta,* 33, 120, 195S
69. **Quinton, P. M. and Philpott, C. W.,** A role for anionic sites in epithelial architecture, *J. Cell* 787, 1973.
70. **Ch'ng, H. S., Park, H., Kelly, P., and Robinson, J. R.,** Bioadhesive polymers as platform controlled drug delivery. II. Synthesis and evaluation of some swelling, water-insoluble bioadh ymers, *J. Pharm. Sci.,* 74, 399, 1985.
71. **Leung, S. H. S. and Robinson, J. R.,** The contribution of anionic polymer structural featur coadhesion, *J. Controlled Release,* 12, 187, 1990.
72. **Bhowmick, A. K. and Gent, A. N.,** Effect of interfacial bonding on the self-adhesion of SBR and *Rubber Chem. Technol.,* 57, 216, 1984.
73. **Barrer, R. M., Barrie, J. A., and Wong, P. S. L.,** The diffusion and solution of gases in hig linked copolymers, *Polymers,* 9, 609, 1968.
74. **Park, H.,** On the Mechanism of Bioadhesion, Ph.D. thesis, University of Wisconsin, Madison
75. **Plueddemann, E. P.,** Adhesion through silane coupling agents, *J. Adhes.,* 2, 184, 1970.
76. **Chen, J. L. and Cyr, G. N.,** Compositions producing adhesion through hydration, in *Adhesive System,* Manly, R. S., Ed., Academic Press, New York, 1970, chap. 10.
77. **Flory, P. J.,** *Principle of Polymer Chemistry,* Cornell University Press, Ithaca, NY, 1953, 541
78. **Gent, A. N. and Tobias, R. H.,** Diffusion and equilibrium swelling of macromolecular networl linear homologs, *J. Polym. Sci.,* 20, 2317, 1982.
79. **Park, H. and Robinson, J. R.,** Physico-chemical properties of water insoluble polymers im mucin/epithelial adhesion, *J. Controlled Release,* 2, 47, 1985.
80. **Tanford, C.,** Thermodynamics, in *Physical Chemistry of Macromolecules,* Tanford, C., Ed., J & Sons, New York, 1961, chap. 4.
81. **Chen, J. L. and Cyr, G. N.,** Compositions producing adhesion through hydration, in *Adhesive System,* Manly, R. S., Ed., Academic Press, New York, 1970, chap. 10.
82. **Smart, J. O., Kellaway, I. W., and Worthington, H. E. C.,** An *in vitro* investigation of mucos materials for use in controlled drug delivery, *J. Pharm. Pharmacol.,* 36, 295, 1984.
83. **Peppas, N. A. and Reinhart, C. T.,** Solute diffusion in swollen membranes, I. A new theory, *Sci.,* 15, 275, 1983.
84. **Florence, A. T. and Atwood, D.,** Polymeric system, in *Physicochemical Principles of Phar* ed., Chapman and Hall, New York, 1982, chap. 8.
85. **Hiemenz, P. C.,** The viscous state, in *Polymer Chemistry,* Hiemenz, P. S., Ed., Marcel Del York, 1984, chap. 2.
86. **Wallace, D.,** The role of hydrophobic bonding in collagen fibril formation: a quantitative mod lymers, 24, 1705, 1985.

87. **Anderson, G. P., Bennet, S. J., and DeVries, K. L.,** *Analysis and Testing of Adhesive Bonds,* Academic Press, New York, 1977.
88. **Reich, S., Levy, M., Meshores, A., Blumental, M., Yalon, M., Sheets, J. W., and Goldberg, E. P.,** Interocular-lens-endothelial interface: adhesive force measurements, *J. Biomed. Mater. Res.,* 18, 737, 1984.
89. **Leung, S. H. S.,** The Determination of Change Density for Water-Soluble and Water Insoluble Anionic Bioadhesives, M.S. thesis, University of Wisconsin, Madison, 1985.
90. **Cundall, R. B., Phillips, G. O., and Rowlands, D. P.,** A spectrofluorimetric procedure for the assay of carrageenan, *Analyst,* 98, 857, 1973.
91. **Diakuin, G. P., Edwards, H. E., Wedlock, O. J., Allen, J. L., and Phillips, G. O.,** The relationship between counterion activity coefficient and the anticoagulant activity of heparin, *Macromolecules,* 11, 1110, 1978.
92. **Mikos, A. B. and Peppas, N. A.,** Comparison of experimental techniques for the bioadhesive forces of polymeric materials with soft tissues, in Proc. 13th Int. Symp. Controlled Release of Bioactive Mater., Choudry, I. A. and Thies, C., Eds., Controlled Release Society, Inc., Lincolnshire, Ill., 1986, 97.
93. **Morris, E. R. and Rees, D. A.,** Principles of biopolymer gelation: Possible models for mucus gel structure, *Br. Med. Bull.,* 34, 49, 1978.
94. **Clamp, J. R., Allen, A., Gibbons, R. A., and Roberts, G. P.,** Chemical aspects of mucus, *Br. Med. Bull.,* 34, 25, 1978.
95. **Ishida, M., Nambu, N., and Nagai, T.,** Ointment-type mucosal dosage form of carbopol containing prednisolone for treatment of aphtha, *Chem. Pharm. Bull.,* 31, 1010, 1983.
96. **Longer, M. A., Ch'ng, H. S., and Robinson, J. R.,** Bioadhesive polymers as platforms for oral controlled drug delivery. III. Oral delivery of chlorothiazide using a bioadhesive polymer, *J. Pharm. Sci.,* 74, 406, 1985.
97. **Veillard, M. M., Longer, M. A., Martens, T. M., and Robinson, J. R.,** Preliminary studies of oral mucosal delivery of peptide drugs, submitted.
98. **Hui, H. W. and Robinson, J. R.,** Ocular delivery of progesterone using a bioadhesive polymer, *Int. J. Pharm.,* 26, 203, 1985.
99. **Nagai, T. and Machida, Y.,** Advances in drug delivery. Mucosal adhesive dosage forms, *Pharma Int. Engl. Ed.,* August, 196, 1985.
100. **Nagai, T., Nishimoto, Y., Nambu, N., Suzuki, Y., and Sekine, K.,** Powder dosage form of insulin for nasal administration, *J. Controlled Release,* 1, 15, 1984.
101. **deLeede, L. G. J., deBoer, A. G., Portzger, E., Feijer, J., and Breimer, D. D.,** Rate-controlled rectal drug delivery in man with a hydrogel preparation, *J. Controlled Release,* 4, 17, 1986.
102. **Williams, B. L.,** Soluble Medicated Hydroxypropyl Cellulose Cartridge, U.S. Patent 4,317,447, 1982.
103. **Eirich, F. R.,** The conformational states of macromolecules absorbed at solid-liquid interface, *J. Colloid Interface Sci.,* 58, 423, 1977.

Chapter 7

SYNTHETIC BIODEGRADABLE POLYMER DRUG DELIVERY SYSTEMS

Kam W. Leong

TABLE OF CONTENTS

I. INTRODUCTION

The use of biodegradable polymers for biomedical applications has dramatically i▮ in recent years.[1-4] As temporary scaffolds, these materials have been explored as ▮ many other applications, biodegradable orthopedic prostheses, guides for nerve reger▮ vascular grafts, and drug carriers, the last of which is the theme of this book. While ▮ researchers in the past tended to just adapt what is available commercially, more a▮ polymer scientists are teaming with life scientists to custom-design the polymeric bior▮ for specific applications. The number of synthetic biodegradable polymers being ▮ for controlled-release applications has been growing rapidly. Since there have been ▮ and thorough reviews on this topic just recently,[5-9] we would like to focus on on▮ developments.

As a starting point, Figure 1 provides a schematic of biodegradation types as char▮ by Heller.[78] In the simple case, the drug solute is physically dispersed in the matri▮ released as the polymer biodegrades. It must be noted that biodegradation taken in t▮ does not necessarily mean a reduction of the molecular weight of the polymer, as exe▮ by the change of the side chains which lead to solubilization. The disintegration of th▮ can also be effected by stress, fatigue, or absorption of biological fluid.[10-14] Besid▮ physically dispersed in the matrix, the drug can also be chemically linked to e▮ backbone or the side chain of the polymer.

In other parts of the book, the different major mechanisms of drug release, ▮ diffusion, chemical, and swelling-controlled, have been discussed in detail. When▮ with a biodegradable system, it is common for nonpractitioners to presume that th▮ gradation of the drug-carrier or the cleavage of the polymer-drug bond is the only i▮ factor in the release kinetics. In reality, it is rare that matrix degradation consiti▮ sole controlling mechanism. Diffusion always plays an important role. If the dru▮ drophilic and the drug loading level is high, swelling of the matrix may also be a ▮ affecting the drug release. In predicting the release from a biodegradable system, c▮ therefore be aware of the interplay of these three mechanisms.

The major hurdle in developing new biodegradable polymers is in proving the ▮ of the degradation products. In that sense, the drug-carrier is treated like a drug its▮ mathematical models which help describe and predict the release kinetics are less▮ than those for the non-biodegradable systems because of the complexity of the ▮ mechanisms. On the other hand, in addition to eliminating the necessity of remc▮ biodegradable system has several potential advantages in comparison to non-biode▮ systems:

1. *The release rate is less dependent on the drug properties*. Since the matrix deg▮ plays a role in controlling the release, the release rate is more amenable to manipu▮ parameters such as drug loading level and geometry. Whereas drug solutes might be▮ in some diffusion-controlled systems, if below a threshold drug loading level, a c▮ release can always be expected in a biodegradable system.

2. *The release rate may be more steady with time*. In a diffusion-controlled sy▮ release rate typically declines with time. Only with elaborate fabrication design, ▮ nonuniform drug distribution or limiting the release to special geometries, can this▮ in concentration gradient be compensated for a zero-order release. On the other ▮ biodegradable system may yield constant release even with a simple monolithic ▮ somehow the matrix degradation can compensate for this decline, perhaps with an ▮ of drug permeability. In the idealized case where the matrix undergoes constant ▮ degradation, and drug diffusion is minimal, the release rate will also be consta▮ surface area of the device remains unchanged during the course of the release. H▮ one must be aware that this means the release can also be erratic if the matrix deg▮

Type IA

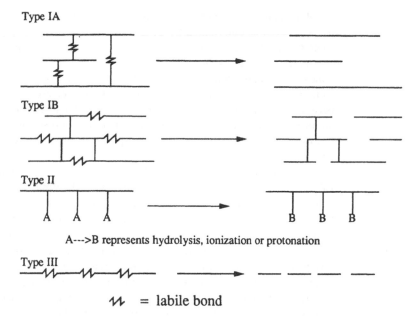

Type IB

Type II

A--->B represents hydrolysis, ionization or protonation

Type III

↯ = labile bond

FIGURE 1. Schematic diagrams of different biodegradation mechanisms.[78]

is unpredictable. For instance, there is the danger of dose dumping if the matrix suddenly disintegrates.

3. *Biodegradable systems may be more suitable to the delivery of unstable drugs.* This point is of particular importance in the light of the advances in molecular biology and genetic engineering which lead to many potent bio-macromolecules. For a non-biodegradable matrix, the steps leading to release are water diffusion into the matrix, dissolution of the drug solutes, and out-diffusion of the solute. The mean residence time of drug particles existing in solution state is therefore longer for a non-biodegradable than for a biodegradable matrix, since a long passage through the channels for a biodegradable matrix may not be required. It is conceivable that a fraction of the drug is decomposed inside the non-biodegradable matrix before it can be released. Some of them would aggregate and reprecipitate, clogging the channels for diffusion.

Given these potential advantages, it is not surprising that an increasing number of researchers have joined in the effort of designing new biodegradable systems, as evidenced by the vigorous activities in the literature. We shall cover those recent developments below.

II. POLYESTER

A. POLY(LACTIDE-GLYCOLIDE) COPOLYMERS

The copolymers of lactic and glycolic acids (PLGA) remain a popular choice as the biodegradable drug-carrier. In an attempt to avoid the use of catalysts, a study used bulk polycondensation techniques to obtain low molecular weight PLGA (Mn = 1600 to 3300).[15] The *in vitro* degradation rate is highest at a composition of 30/70 mole % LA/GA. This value is similar to the one found with the higher molecular weight of PLGA (Mn = 25,000 to 40,000) obtained by ionic polymerization using catalysts. It is also found that the period of complete degradation varies linearly with the molecular weight within this range. Release of lutenizing hormone-releasing hormone agonist into rats produces near constant serum levels for the first 10 weeks, and then continues at a declining rate for another 4 weeks.

In examining the effect of gamma-sterilization on the stability and degradation of the

copolymers in microsphere form, it is found that sterilization decreases the molecu
by 30 to 40% as determined by gel permeation chromatography.[16] The polymer
catastrophic disintegration when the molecular weight is approximately 25,000
storage at room temperature the molecular weight of these gamma-irradiated sa
clines, up to approximately 40% of their original value in 9 months. This decline of
weight caused by sterilization in turn affects the release profile. For example, t
period of cisplatin was reduced from 60 to 8 d. An earlier study reported that the c
parameter of the release kinetics is the cisplatin drug distribution in the microsphe
in turn is affected by drug loading, the presence of extra cisplatin in the dispersi
and the molecular weight of the polymer.[17]

Microspheres made of PLA, PLGA, and poly(ε-caprolactone-co-L-lactic ac
LA) have been used to deliver L-methadone subdermally for the maintenance
addicts.[18] Degradation of the PLA and PLGA microspheres is believed to be ca
the basic drug. Although each type of microsphere yields distinct and non-zero-or
profiles, a combination of these types provides a 1-week constant release needed
methadone maintenance therapy (Figure 2). Using prednisolone-21 as a model dru
group studied the effect of matrix characteristics of microspheres on release.[19] T
spheres obtained by the solvent extraction-precipitation or the freeze-drying techn
different porosities, which in turn yield distinct release profiles. To overcome
vantage of non zero-order of release from microspheres, a hollow fiber of PLA
the drug suspended in oil was developed.[20,21] The device is small enough to be i
a syringe, and it is removable in case of an emergency. The *in vitro* release of levo
shows a near constant release rate of over 320 d. The researchers also find tha
sterilization decreases the molecular weight of the polymer, lowering the Mw to
of its original value, as well as chemically modifying the drug. Release from the
sample is no longer zero-order. The inclusion of castor oil in the design of th
system might be a concern of biocompatibility, but the animal studies conclud
hollow fiber evokes only a moderate foreign body reaction. The absence of for
giant cells and lymphoid elements is suggested to indicate the inertness of the d
reason for the near zero-order release kinetics observed in this study is offered.
that the slow dissolution rate of the drug contributes to this phenomenon.

B. POLYLACTIDE AND COPOLYMERS

A delayed-release delivery system for water-soluble macromolecules was
based on polylactide.[22] By coating a macromolecule, such as a protein, with PLA o
molecular weight and thickness, various delay periods can be obtained. Such
system is expected to be useful in delivering vaccines which require occasion
shots.

To retain the desirable feature of having the polymer break down into non-toxi
in the body, cyclo(glycine-DL-lactic acid) (1) can be copolymerized with DL-dil
by ring-opening techniques as shown in Equation 1.[23]

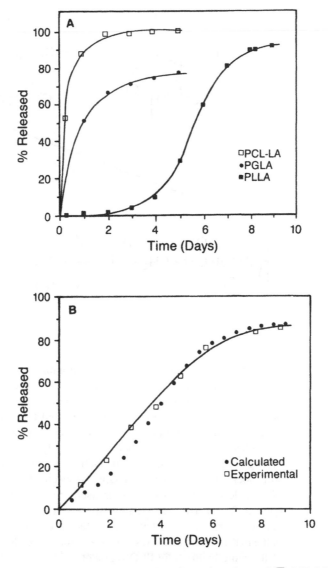

FIGURE 2.   (a) *In vitro* release of L-methadone from microspheres of (□) PCL-LA, 50-212 μm, (●) PGLA, 106-212 μm; and (■) PLLA, 106-212 μm. Reservoir: 0.04 *M* phosphate buffer, pH 7.4. (b) *In vitro* release of L-methadone from combinations of different micros-pheres, and comparison with rates calculated from individual components: 11:48:41 mixture of PCL-LA (85% LA), PCL-LA (95% LA), and PLLA microspheres. (From Cha, Y. and Pitt, C. G., A one week subdermal delivery system for L-methadone based on biodegradable microcapsules, *J. Controlled Release*, 7, 69, 1988. With permission.)

1   **2**

x = Mole Fraction of Mono

The glycine renders PLA more hydrophilic and accelerates the degradation. Si PLGA systems, the degradation mechanism of these glycine/PLA copolymers is drolysis, and is autocatalyzed by the generated carboxylic end groups. Tissue bio bility in rats suggests a macrophage-mediated foreign body reaction. The tissue re dependent on the degradation rate, and hence is more severe with higher glycine The other new PLA copolymers involve polyethylene oxides (PEO). The aim is t biodegradable copolyesters, with lactic acid and PEO representing the crystalline soft blocks of the segmented chains, respectively.[24,25] A two-phase matrix is obse PEO molecular weight of 6000 is used; below that PEO chain length, no soft se noticed. The *in vitro* degradation studies of these copolymers indicate that the deg rate increases with pH, but is not affected by carboxylic ester hydrolase. The cry of the matrices also increases as degradation proceeds, probably due to the selective e of the more hydrophilic PEO segments.

C. MISCELLANEOUS

An approach of simply using a compressed admixture of a water-soluble poly a biodegradable polymer as drug-carrier was presented.[26] When acetylated poly(vinyl (PVA) and polycaprolactone are used, a sustained release of the model drug methyl is observed. The release can be controlled by the ratio of the soluble/biodegradah ponents as well as by the degree of acetylation of PVA. It is concluded that one can the drug with an insoluble component, not necessarily a bioerodible polymer, to sustained release. Using insulin therapy of diabetic rats as an example, the autho that normoglycemia can be achieved in rats treated with implants composed of ins cholesterol. Presumably, this will work only if the insoluble component is comp and most importantly if the drug is highly insoluble in buffer. The dissolution of then becomes the rate-determining step to effect sustained release.

Other polyesters designed with the goal of producing natural or nontoxic bre products include the hydroxybutyrate-hydroxyvalerate copolymers,[27,28] and the on on aspartic acid and different aliphatic diols.[29] Presumably these polyesters will be suitable for drug delivery and offer alternatives to the PLGA matrices. A series of poly(alkylene tartrates) and their copolymers with polyurethanes have also been evaluated as drug carriers.[30]

III. POLYAMIDE

Polyglutamates with various ester contents, and with chemically or enzymatically degradable bonds, have been evaluated as drug-carriers.[31] These poly[(tert-butyloxycarbonylmethyl) glutamates] are obtained by partial esterification of poly(glutamic acid) with tert-butyl bromoacetate (Equation 2).

$$(NH\text{-}CH\text{-}CO)_n$$

$$\begin{array}{l} CH_2 \\ CH_2 \\ C=O \\ OH \end{array} \quad + \text{Br-CH}_2\text{-COO-C(CH}_3)_3 \longrightarrow$$

Polyglutamic acid   *Tert*-butyl bromoacetate

$$(NH\text{-}CH\text{-}CO)_x\text{-}(NH\text{-}CH\text{-}CO)_y$$

$$\begin{array}{ll} CH_2 & CH_2 \\ CH_2 & CH_2 \\ C=O & C=O \\ O & OH \\ CH_2 \\ C=O \\ O \\ CH_3\text{-C-CH}_3 \\ CH_3 \end{array} \tag{2}$$

These polymers are amorphous and extrudable at low temperatures. The degradation proceeds by cleavage of the tert-butanol side chain, leading to a soluble polymer, followed by cleavage of the backbone by leucine aminopeptidase. The hydrophobicity of the polymer can be increased by the ester content. Good tissue biocompatibility is reported for the progesterone-impregnated polymers in rat implantation studies.

Other biodegradable nonpeptidic polyamides are obtained by the ring-opening polymerization of 2,2'-bis[5(4H)-oxazolones] with dinucleophiles, such as diamines (Equation 3).[32]

$$\left(\begin{array}{c} O \;\; R_2 \quad\quad O \quad\quad O \;\; R_2 \quad\quad O \\ \| \;\; | \quad\quad \| \quad\quad \| \;\; | \quad\quad \| \\ C\text{-}C(CH_3)\text{-}NH\text{-}C\text{-}R_1\text{-}CNH\text{-}C(CH_3)\text{-}CNH\text{-}R_3\text{-}NH \end{array}\right)_n \tag{3}$$

Release of amaranth as a marker from one of these polymers shows a near zero-ord
The fact that the polymer erosion lags behind the drug release is used to suggest t
swelling, and not erosion, is the controlling release mechanism. The release per
short, under 20 h. Subsequent studies incorporate an acid anhydride into the matri
the pH of the bulk in order to slow down the polymer dissolution. The release
extended this way, and the release mechanism becomes dominantly surface-er
trolled.

Polymers composed of amino acids as monomers have also been proposed
carriers. However, the side chains of the amino acids are used, resulting in a
linkage that is not peptidic. For instance, 4-hydroxy-L-proline can be polymeri
polyester when the secondary amine is protected.[33]

IV. POLYANHYDRIDE

A. SYNTHESIS

Research on polyanhydride drug-carriers has continued at a strong pace i
several years. Significant progress has been made in synthesis, structural ider
stability determination, and potential and clinical applications. A minor drawb
polyanhydrides synthesized in the past has been the relatively low molecular weig
studies show that by optimizing the melt-polycondensation conditions such as p
purity, reaction time and temperature, and removal of the condensation by-pi
intrinsic viscosity as high as 1.16 dL/g could be obtained.[34] To facilitate the
interchange in the polymerization, coordination catalysts have been used to er
nucleophilicity of the carbonyl carbon. In the synthesis of the copolyanhy
bis(carboxyphenoxy)propane and sebacic acid (CPP-SA), significantly higher
weights in shorter times are achieved by using cadmium acetate, earth metal o
zinc-etherate as catalysts. The average molecular weights range from 141,000 t
with catalysts, compared to 116,800 without catalysts. The catalysts are also fc
effective in improving the molecular weights of other polyanhydrides.

With the intention of preparing the polymer in an even milder reaction co
single-step, one-pot synthesis in which a dicarboxylic acid monomer can be directly
into the polyanhydride at room temperature has been reported. Limited success i
with the use of organophosphorus compounds as dehydrative coupling agents.[3]
vantage of the use of these coupling agents is the difficulty in isolating and pu
final products without evoking hydrolytic decomposition. To circumvent this diffic
work-up, as well as to improve the molecular weight, a one-step polymerization u
chloride, phosgene, or diphosgene as coupling agents was developed.[36] The study
ways to remove the acid acceptor-hydrochloride salt from the polymerization r
either using an insoluble acid acceptor (e.g., crosslinked polyamides, inorganic
using solvents that dissolve exclusively either the polymer or the salt. In eithe
by-product or the precipitating polymer is isolated by simple filtration. For insta
yields and reasonable molecular weights were obtained for poly(sebacic acid) (P
the reaction of sebacoyl chloride and sebacic acid is conducted in DMF or tolu
crosslinked poly(4-vinylpyridine) (PVP) or triethylamine (TEA).

In improving the physical properties of the polyanhydrides, these studies si
enhance their attractiveness in controlled release applications.

B. NEW STRUCTURES

New types of polyanhydrides with the general structure of $+OOC-C_6H_4-O+CF$
(x = 1-10), have been reported.[37] These polymers are characterized by a uniform d
of aliphatic and aromatic residues in the backbone. This uniformity is advantag

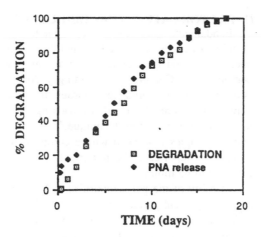

FIGURE 3. *In vitro* release of *p*-nitroaniline from poly(carboxyphenoxyvaleric acid) (5 weight %). (From Domb, A and Langer, R., Polyanhydrides: stability and novel composition, *Makromol. Chem. Macromol. Symp.*, 19, 189, 1988. With permission.)

random copolyanhydrides of aromatic and aliphatic diacids because in those random co-polymers, the more hyrolytically sensitive aliphatic blocks would lead to a nonuniform degradation profile. The new aliphatic-aromatic homopolymers remove this undesirable feature. A linear *in vitro* degradation profile is indeed observed for these polymers. The degradation rate is dependent on the length of the aliphatic moiety in the diacid monomer. The release of a model drug *p*-nitroaniline from compression-molded discs of poly(carboxyphenoxyvaleric acid) also correlates with the matrix degradation (Figure 3). An unsaturated polyanhydride with fumaric acid in the backbone as a comonomer has also been synthesized.

Other new polyanhydrides are conceived by including amino acids or short peptides into the backbone (Equation 4).[38,39]

$$\text{(4)}$$

The amino acids are incorporated via hydrolytically labile anhydride bonds at the carboxylic acid terminal, and imide bonds at the amine terminal. It is postulated that the breakdown products of these poly(anhydride-co-imides) have the chance of being nontoxic. The structure is speculated to circumvent the limitations of poly(α-amino acid), which include antigenicity and vulnerability to enzymatic attack.

C. FACTORS AFFECTING DEGRADATION

Fundamental studies to elucidate the parameters which control the degradation ▌
of polyanhydrides have been carried out using NMR, X-ray diffraction, scanning
microscopy, and differential scanning calorimetry.[40,41] Fabrication is shown to b▌
portant factor. Compression molding yields a porous structure. Film casting of cr▌
polyanhydrides also produces a porous structure, but casting of semi-crystalline or an▌
polyanhydrides results in a dense packing. Such dense packing is also seen in micr▌
made by the hot-melting technique.[42] Surface erosion or a clear eroding zone is ▌
only in samples fabricated with a compact morphology. The solubility of the deg▌
products is reported to be important. Presumably, in a well-stirred and perfect s▌
role should be minimized.

Stability of the polyanhydrides in both the solution and solid state has been s▌
Aliphatic polyanhydrides are found to self-depolymerize under anhydrous conditio▌
solid state. For instance, the molecular weight of PSA declines from 130,000 to ▌
mately 80,000 in 60 d. The self-depolymerization mainly affects the high molecula▌
fraction. The Mn is hence affected to a lesser extent than Mw. In contrast, aroma▌
anhydrides such as poly[bis(*p*-carboxyphenoxy)methane anhydride] and poly[bis(*p*▌
yphenoxy)hexane anhydride] show no signs of depolymerization over a 12-mont▌
when stored anhydrously at room temperature. The stability of polyanhydrides in ▌
has also been studied. Except for the aromatic polyanhydrides, which remain st▌
depolymerization rate is higher than that in the solid state, as shown in Figure ▌
depolymerization rate is found to follow a first-order kinetics, and increases with ▌
perature and polarity of the solvent. Finally, the depolymerized products can be ▌
merized to yield the original polymer, which suggests that inter- or intramolecular a▌
interchange took place in the depolymerization.

D. MICROSPHERES

To broaden the use of the polyanhydrides as drug-carriers, two microenca▌
formulations have been reported. The first technique[42] consists of dispersing the d▌
ecules in the molten polymer. The mixture is then suspended in either silicon or ▌
that is heated at 5° C above the melting temperature of the polymer. While bein▌
the suspension is gradually cooled for the solidification of the microspheres. After ▌
with petroleum ether, free-flowing powder can be formed. With this hot-melting te▌
microparticles of spherical shape and different diameters, as controlled by the agita▌
can be obtained. Release of acid orange, *p*-nitroaniline, and insulin have been studie▌
correlation between the release and matrix degradation profiles are observed for ▌
two drugs. To avoid the use of high temperatures in melting the polymer, as req▌
the hot-melt techniques, a solvent extraction or removal process has been develo▌
The technique involves dropwise addition of a drug-containing polyanhydride solu▌
an oil phase undergoing vigorous agitation. As the organic solvent diffuses into the o▌
the droplets become more and more concentrated, and nucleation takes place. Dru▌
microspheres are thus produced.

E. BIOCOMPATIBILITY AND *IN VIVO* STUDIES

To prepare for clinical trials, extensive safety evaluations have been conducte▌
CPP-SA 20:80 copolyanhydride. Studies suggest that the copolymer is biocompatib▌
neural tissue.[46-48] When implanted in the frontal lobe of the rabbit brain, these poly▌
not induce any behavioral changes or neurological deficits suggestive of toxicity. The▌
also survive to their date of sacrifice. In comparison to Gelfoam™, another biode▌
polymer that has been clinically used in the brain, the polyanhydrides produce no si▌
differences in terms of histological response. Similar studies have been conducte▌
brain of Sprague-Dawley rats, in which the tissue reaction to poly(CPP-SA) 2(▌

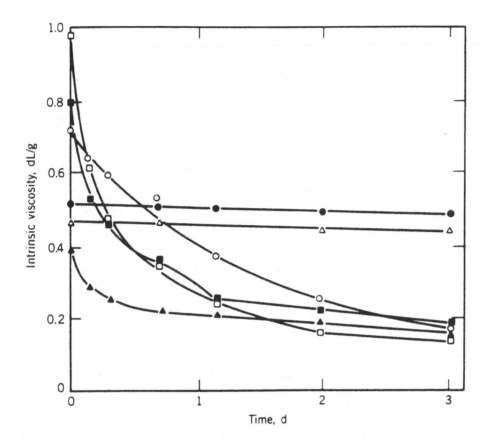

FIGURE 4. Solution of depolymerization of polyanhydrides in chloroform (10 mg/ml) stored under nitrogen at 37°C. ☐, Poly(SA); ■, poly(CPP-SA) 20:80; ○, poly(CPP-SA) 50:50; ●, poly[bis(carboxyphenoxy)hexane anhydride]; ▲, poly(phenylenedipropionic anhydride); △, poly[bis(carboxyphenoxy)methane anhydride]. (From Domb, A. and Langer, R., Solid state and solution stability of poly(anhydrides) and poly(esters), *Macromolecules*, 22, 2117, 1989.)

compared to Surgicel™ (an oxidized regenerated cellulose) and Gelfoam. Results similar to that of the rabbit studies are obtained. The polymer evokes a well localized inflammatory reaction comparable to that of Surgicel, which disappears as the polymer degrades over 5 weeks.

The purpose of these studies is to establish the safety of the polymer in neurological applications, particularly in the treatment of glioblastoma multiforme. The proposed approach is to line the surgical cavity, created by the removal of the tumor, by the drug-loaded implant. The anti-cancer drug studied is bischloronitrosourea (BCNU). In the preclinical studies, the distribution of the drug delivered by poly(CPP-SA) 20:80 in the rabbit brain was studied using autoradiographic techniques.[49,50] While the drug is almost completely cleared from the brain in 3 d when given by direct injection, over 10% of the brain is still exposed to measurable BCNU concentration at 21 days post-implantation, when delivered from the polyanhydride implant. It is further estimated that in 3 d after implantation, a BCNU concentration of 6.5 mM is achieved at the implant-brain interface, declining to approximately 200 μM at 1 cm from the implant. This represents a much improved AUC over conventional intravenous administration. This delivery system is being tested in Phase III human clinical trials.

The same polyanhydride (CPP-SA) 20:80 has also been used to deliver the angiogenesis inhibitor of a combination of heparin and cortisone acetate for the inhibition of 9L glios-

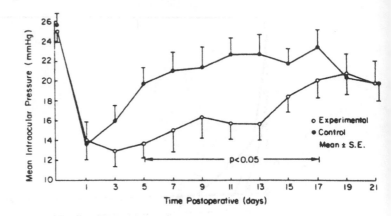

FIGURE 5.   Postoperative intraocular pressures over time. Statistically significant lower pressures occurred in experimental eyes between postoperative days 5 through 17. (From Lee, D. A., et al., The use of biodegradable polymers and 5-fluorouracil in glaucoma filtration surgery, *Invest. Ophthal. Vis. Sci.*, 29, 1692, 1988.)

arcoma.[51] It is postulated that the glioblastoma multiforme, being highly vascular a
as a focal lesion intracranially, would respond well to the localized release of an
inhibitors. Using a model of 9L gliosarcoma in the flank of Fischer rats, it is s
the localized release significantly inhibits the tumor growth. At day 14 the tum
of experimental animals is 195 mm³ vs. 919 mm³ for the controls. Presumably, this
to treatment of malignant gliomas has the potential of bypassing the blood-bra
thereby allowing the use of a greater variety of therapeutic agents and reducing th
toxic effects. To improve the drug bioavailability to the brain, a similar approach
taken in the delivery of bethanechol for Alzheimer's disease.[52] Rats with memo
produced by lesion in the brain is used as a model. Using a radial maze test, it
that experimental rats receiving the bethanechol polyanhydride implant display
improvement within 10 d of implantation.

To improve the success of glaucoma filtration surgery for patients with po
prognoses, the antimetabolite 5-fluorouracil is embedded in poly(CPP-SA) 20:80 f
into the eye.[53,54] The primary cause of filtration surgery failure is the blockage by
of the opening which drains the fluid from the eye. It is hoped that the localized and
release to the sclerostomy site would inhibit fibroblast proliferation and subsequen
The drug-loaded implant is placed over the sclera adjacent to the sclerostomy
subconjunctival space. The results show that intraocular pressures (IOP) are lo
experimental subjects' eyes during the 5th through 17th postoperative days (Figu
favorable result is due to the longer duration of the filtration blebs in the ex
subjects' eyes, when compared to control subjects' eyes. It is strongly suspecte
onset of bleb failure coincides with the exhaustion of the drug. Work is in progres
the delivery system by extending the release period and exploring other antif
agents in altering the wound healing process.

In the form of microspheres formulated by both the hot-melt and the solver
technique, the polymer has been used to deliver insulin into diabetic Sprague Dawle
A 200 mg dose of 5% loaded microspheres gives a 3 d effective decrease in uri
and 1 d of normoglycemia, while a 100 mg of 10% loaded microspheres e
normoglycemia period to 2 d. In comparison, the insulin-loaded slabs are able t
blood glucose control for at least 7 d, although there is a one-day delay in both
blood glucose responses.

Delivery of polypeptides has been a topic of great interest, and polyanhyd been used for the sustained release of bovine somatotropin, horseradish peroxidase, alkaline phosphatase, β-galactosidase, and chondrogenic-stimulating proteins.[55,56]

V. POLY(PHOSPHOESTER)

The use of poly(phosphoesters) as a pendant drug delivery system has been implicated by Penczek in the early 1980s.[57,58] Recent studies look at the linkage of pharmacologically active amines on aliphatic polyphosphonates.[59,60] The linkage is achieved through the Atherton-Todd reaction, in which the poly(dialkyl phosphonate) is converted to the poly(dialkyl phosphoramidate) by amines in the presence of carbon tetrachloride and a base. Benzocaine and phenethylamine have been coupled to the poly(propylene phosphonate) and poly(3,6,9-trioxaundecamethylene phosphonate) by this reaction. Another study examines the coupling of model drugs with different groups to an aliphatic poly(phosphoester).[61] As shown in Equation 5, the polymer is synthesized by an anionic polymerization of 2-hydro-2-oxo-1,3,2-oxaphosphorinane **1**. After the chlorination of **2**, the model compounds of benzoic acid, aniline, thiophenol, and p-nitrophenol are linked to the polymer via dehydrochlorination.

(5)

An anticancer drug 5-fluorouracil (5-FU) has also been linked to the polymer via trimethylsilyl derivatization. These model drugs are all freely water-soluble compounds, which in a diffusion-controlled release system would be depleted extremely rapidly. Shown in

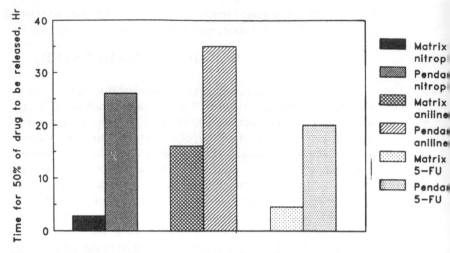

FIGURE 6.   Comparison of *in vitro* release of model drugs from poly(phosphate esters) as either a ▮ pendant delivery system.

Figure 6 is the comparison of the release of nitrophenol, aniline, and 5-FU from a b▮ A/ethoxy (BPA/EOP) matrix and from the pendant system. The time it takes 50▮ drug to be released from the polymer-drug conjugate is significantly longer, sho▮ the pendant system is indeed capable of prolonging the release of hydrophilic drugs a phosphate ester or phosphoroamide bond.

The evaluation of the poly(phosphoesters) as matrix drug delivery systems ▮ conducted on a bisphenol A backbone with different side chains: ethoxy (BPA/EO (BPA/EP), phenoxy (BPA/POP), phenyl (BPA/PP).[62-64] As expected, the BPA/PF siderably more stable than the BPA/EOP. Implantation studies conducted in rabbit▮ that the degradation is faster *in vivo*. The weight loss for BPA/EOP at 11 weeks i▮ *vivo* versus 7.8% *in vitro*. The discrepancy suggests that either the poly(phospho vulnerable to enzymatic attack, or the breakdown products of the polymers are mor▮ in the physiological fluid. Although the mass loss of these polymers slows down first few weeks, there is clear evidence of backbone cleavage as analyzed by GPC, su▮ of a homogeneous degradation mechanism. The swelling of the polymers decrea▮ the hydrophobicity of the side chains: ethoxy > ethyl > phenoxy > phenyl. At l average water uptake of the polymers in that order is 61.3%, 18.5%, 16.6%, an▮ respectively.

Shown in Figure 7 is the *in vitro* release of cortisone acetate from the four matrices.[64] This shows that a variation of the side chain does alter the drug release The release is faster from the carriers with the aliphatic than the aromatic side cha▮ relative constant and sustained release observed is probably due to the low water s of the drug. For more hydrophilic drugs, the release more typically decreases w▮ From the same carrier BPA/EOP, the release rate increases with the water solubili▮ drug (Figure 8). The linear profiles observed for some of the hydrophilic drugs are int▮ As observed by SEM, the carrier becomes significantly more porous during the c release. It is speculated that in those cases the release is controlled by a combir▮ drug diffusion, matrix swelling, and matrix degradation.

VI. POLY(PHOSPHAZENE)

Poly(phosphazenes) were first explored as drug-carriers in 1983 to deliver nap▮ Previous studies suggest that the degradation products of the polymer consists of a▮

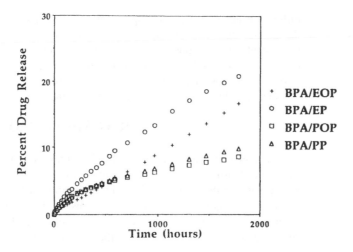

FIGURE 7. *In vitro* release of cortisone acetate from four different poly(phosphoesters) with bisphenol-A backbone but with different side chains (10 wt% drug loading).

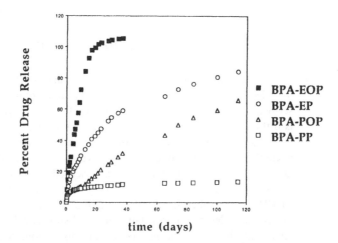

FIGURE 8. *In vitro* release of drugs with different water solubilities from a poly(phosphate ester) with a bisphenol-A backbone and an ethoxy side chain (10 wt% drug loading).

phosphate, and the side-group substituent.[66] It appears that these polymers would be attractive candidates for a pendant delivery system. A recent study looks at the controlled release applications using imidazole and methylphenoxy side chains. As monolithic devices, the hydrolytic instability of the polymer is imparted by the imidazole group.[67] Through variation of the imidazole content, the initial biodegradation rate can be altered. Since the degradation rate declines with time as the imidazole content decreases, it would be interesting to see if the degradation would completely stop as the imidazole side groups are depleted. Release of *p*-nitroaniline, even at low loading level, indicates a square root of time relationship, suggesting that the matix functions essentially as a diffusion-controlled delivery system. This is further corroborated by release studies of bovine serum albumin, which show signs of the protein being trapped in the matrix. Supposedly, the chemical structure of the side chains can be further modified to render the release truly matrix-degradation controlled. A

different usage of the polyphosphazene is for microencapsulation formulation.[68]
the manner alginate microcapsules are formed when a solution containing ionic ph
is sprayed into an aqueous solution of calcium chloride, the complexation be
polyelectrolyte and the metal salt leads to microcapsule formation. BSA and β-gal
have been encapsulated this way with high efficiency. Coating the microspheres
L-lysine and chitosan further sustains the release for the proteins.

VII. POLY(IMINOCARBONATE)

Another new candidate in the biodegradable polymer field is poly(iminocar
The general structure as shown in Equation 6 is produced by a reaction between
a dicyanate. In the initial studies a hydroquinone or bisphenol-A backbone was u
polymers biodegrade *in vitro*. Release of Eosin Y from both polymers appears to be
controlled, while release of *p*-nitroaniline from poly(BPA iminocarbonate) is m
sustained. Recent studies focus on the polymerization of other structures, such a
dipeptide derivatives.[70]

$$HO-R-OH + NCO-R-OCN \longrightarrow \left(R-O-\overset{\overset{NH}{\|}}{C}-O \right)_n$$

VIII. POLY(ORTHO ESTER)

The use of a crosslinked poly(ortho ester) to release 5-fluorouracil and LHF
intended for glaucoma filtration surgery and contraception, respectively, has
scribed.[71] To achieve a sustained release of 5-FU, a hydrophilic drug, from a mat
is difficult. However, this study shows that by manipulation of the poly(ortho e
position, a sustained release of over 1 month can be attained. The crosslinking d
a readily erodible component, 9,10-dihydroxystearic acid, in the polymer controls
kinetics. A near-constant release is observed in some cases as a result of the
permeation rate caused by the cleavage of the crosslinking bonds (Figure 9).
LHRH on the other hand follows a biphasic profile. The initial release corre
diffusional release, and the latter to the hydrolytic liberation of the protein tha
chemically bound to the matrix during fabrication. Studies focusing on the ero
acteristics of catalyzed poly(ortho ester) matrices,[72] and the effect of crosslinkin
incorporation on the polymer degradation behavior, have also been reported.[73]

IX. RESPONSIVE SYSTEMS

Although controlled release represents a significant improvement over the co
mode of drug administration, it is still not the ideal delivery system. The idea
system would be one which responds to physiological needs. Increasing attenti
being paid to these self-regulated or triggered delivery systems. A poly(ortho est
is designed with a tertiary amine function to render the degradation of the poly(o
more sensitive to pH changes.[74] The responsive release system thus consists of i
glucose oxidase embedded in this polymer. As glucose diffuses into this matrix,
acid is produced as a result of the enzyme-substrate reaction. This lowers the
microenvironment, which accelerates the degradation of the polymer, and in tu
a higher release of insulin. A different approach to release narcotic antagonists
by opiates, involves a more elaborate design. As shown in Figure 10, the naltrexo

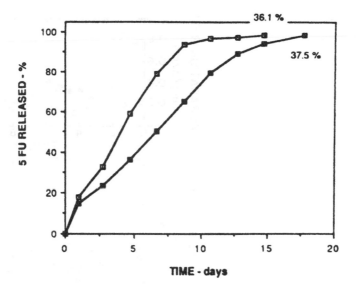

FIGURE 9. Cumulative release of 5-fluorouracyl from a crosslinked poly(ortho ester) prepared from a 15/85 mole ratio of triethylene glycol and 1,2-propylene glycol in the prepolymer,
crosslinked with 1,2,6 hexanetriol and containing varying amounts of copolymerized 9,10-
dihydroxystearic acid (DHSA). Discs 1.2*6.4 mm in a pH 7.4 buffer at 37° C. Numbers
indicate weight loss. Device contains 10 wt% (5 mg) 5-fluorouracyl (□) 0.005 mol DHSA,
(■) 0.001 mol DHSA. (From Heller, H., et al., Use of poly(ortho esters) for the controlled
release of 5-fluorouracil and a LHRH analogue, *J. Controlled Release*, 6, 217, 1987. With
permission.)

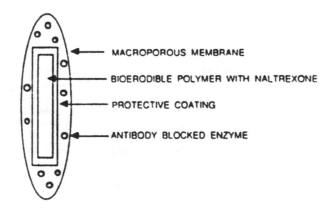

FIGURE 10.   Schematic representation of triggered drug delivery device. (From Heller, J., Chemically self-regulated drug delivery systems, *J. Controlled Release*, 8, 111, 1988. With permission.)

ded in the poly(ortho ester) is released only in response to external opiates. According to
this scheme, the opiate diffuses into the device and activates the enzyme, which can remove
the protective hydrogel coating. This leads to the contact of the alkaline labile poly(ortho
ester) with physiological pH, thereby initiating the matrix erosion and naltrexone release
process. Another design is based on reversible antibody binding to haptens attached to the
surface of permeable or biodegradable polymers.[75] Hydroxylated polyester-urethanes are
being studied as the coating membrane to which morphine can be grafted. To take advantage
of the fact that hydrolysis of carboxylic and phosphate esters and amides is greatly enhanced

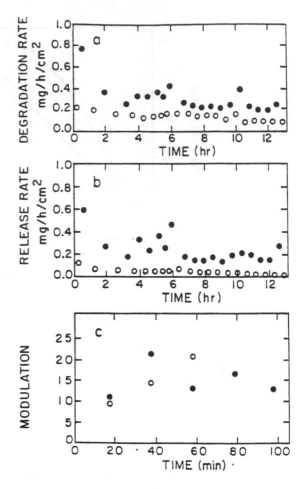

FIGURE 11.   Effect of ultrasound on polymer degradation and drug release. The repeated ultrasound exposure durations were 15 min for the on period (●), the intervals between these exposures in which the samples were not exposed to ultrasound were 15 min to 1.5 h (○). (a) Degradation rate of poly[bis-(*p*-carboxyphenoxy methane] (PCPM) vs. time; (b) Release rate of *p*-nitroaniline (PNA) from PCPM 10 wt % drug loading) vs time; (c) Modulation vs. time of PNA release from polylactic acid (10 wt% loading) (●), and from polyglycolic acid (10 wt% loading) (○). (Modulation is defined as the ratio of degradation or release rates during ultrasound exposure to the mean of the rates during the time intervals before and after that exposure). (From Kost, J., et al., Ultrasound-enhanced polymer degradation and release of incorporated substances, *Proc. Natl. Acad. Sci. U.S.A.*, 86, 7663, 1989. With permission.)

by transition metals, a delivery system of metal chelating agents responsive to m
has been proposed.

A more mechanical approach to an externally controllable delivery system is **t**
the use of ultrasonic energy.[76,77] As the ultrasonic energy accelerates the degradati
polymeric matrix, that in turn leads to an enhanced drug release. Success is clea
onstrated *in vitro* with polylactide, polyglycolide, and the polyanhydrides based c
carboxyphenoxy) alkanes (Figure 11). The extent of release rate enhancement is pro
to the intensity of the ultrasonic energy. An increase as high as 20 times has been o
Success *in vivo* is less dramatic but still observable in testing the subcutaneous de
p-aminohippurate in Sprague-Dawley rats. During the *in vivo* experiment, the u
applicator head was applied for 20 min to the catheterized rats' skin above the in
a pulsed mode (50% duty cycle, at a frequency of 20kHz, and a power of 5W,

pronounced effect is observed 15 to 30 min after the ultrasound application. The drug concentration in the urine rises from a base level of approximately 40 to 180 μg/ml. The delay is presumably due to the time it takes for the drug to be released from the polymer, equilibrated with plasma, and removed by the kidney. It appears that there are no histopathological differences between the normal skin and the skin which has been exposed to irradiation for 1 h.

X. CONCLUSION

Compared to natural biodegradable drug delivery systems, synthetic systems enjoy the tremendous advantage of versatility. Through creative polymer chemistry, the synthetic systems can be custom designed to meet specific needs. The toxicology of the breakdown products and tissue biocompatibility of the polymers are the major issues in deciding the success of the devices. When intended as a long-term delivery system, the cytotoxicity of the degradation products may be less of a problem because of the slow degradation rate and hence the low dose. Any acute inflammatory response to the implant may also have the chance of being resolved as the polymer disappears. However, other potential side effects such as carcinogenicity and teratogenicity are difficult to address and evaluate. Nevertheless, with the tremendous potential advantages, research in this area is still rewarded with a high benefit to risk ratio.

It is unlikely that a single biodegradable system will satisfy the requirements of all controlled release applications. Although it may not be immediately apparent, each system possesses distinct advantages and disadvantages. It is safe to say that all current biodegradable drug-carriers possess varying degrees of imperfection, be it weak mechanical strength, unfavorable degradation characteristics, toxicity, synthetic complexity, or fabrication difficulty. Continued improvement over existing systems, as well as exploration of new ones, should therefore be encouraged. There are ample opportunities for polymer chemists to express their creativity in this field, and the challenges will certainly be gratifying.

ACKNOWLEDGMENT

The support of the Whitaker Foundation to this work is gratefully acknowledged.

REFERENCES

1. **Langer, R. and Wise, D., Eds.,** Medical Applications of Controlled Release, Vol. I & II, CRC Press, Boca Raton, FL, 1986.
2. **Hanker, J. S. and Giammara, B. L., Eds.,** Biomedical Materials and Devices, Materials Research Society Sympo. Proc., Vol. 110, Materials Research Society, 1989.
3. **de Putter, C., de Lange, G. L., de Groot, K., and Lee, A. J. C.,** Implant materials in biofunction, *Advances in Biomaterials,* Vol. 8, 1987.
4. **Gebelein, C. G.,** *Advances in Biomedical Polymers,* Plenum Press, New York, 1987.
5. **St. Pierre, T. and Chiellini, E.,** Biodegradability of synthetic polymers used for medical and pharmaceutical applications: Part 1. Principles of hydrolysis mechanisms, *J. Bioactive and Compatible Poly.,* 1, 467, 1986.
6. **St. Pierre, T. and Chiellini, E.,** Biodegradability of synthetic polymers used for medical and pharmaceutical applications: Part 2. Backbone hydrolysis, *J. Bioactive and Compatible Polym.,* 2, 4, 1987.
7. **St. Pierre, T. and Chiellini, E.,** Biodegradability of synthetic polymers used for medical and pharmaceutical applications: Part 3. Pendant group hydrolysis and general conclusions, *J. Bioactive and Compatible Polym.,* 2, 238, 1987.
8. **Linhardt, R.,** Biodegradable Polymers for Controlled Release of Drugs, Springer Verlag, 1988.

9. **Rosen, H., Kohn, J., Leong, K., and Langer, R.,** Bioerodible polymers for controlled rele in, *Controlled Release Systems: Fabrication Technology,* Vol. 2, Hsieh, D., Ed., CRC Press, FL, 1988.

10. **Dolezel, B., Adamirova, L., Naprstek, Z., and Vondracek, P.,** *In vivo* degradation of Change of mechanical properties in polyethylene pacemaker lead insulations during long-term in the human body, *Biomaterials,* 10, 96, 1989.

11. **Dolezel, B., Adamirova, L., Vondracek, P. and Naprstek, Z.,** *In vivo* degradation of Change of mechanical properties and crosslink density of silicone rubber pacemaker lead insul long-term implantation in the human body, *Biomaterials,* 10, 387, 1989.

12. **Smith, R., Oliver, C., and Williams, D. F.,** The enzymatic degradation of polymers *in vitr Mat. Res.,* 21, 991, 1987.

13. **Huang, S. J.,** Biodegradable polymers, in *Encyclopedia of Polymer Science and Technolo ed.,* Mark, H., Bikales, N. M., Overberger, C. G., and Menges, G., Ed., John Wiley & So

14. **Szycher, M.,** Biostability of polyurethane elastomers: a critical review, *J. Biomaterials A 1988.

15. **Asano, M., Fukuzaki, H., Yosihida, M., Kumakura, M., Mashimo, T., Yuasa, H., In manaka, H., and Suzuki, K.,** *In vivo* characteristics of low molecular weight copoly(L-lactic acid) formulations with controlled release of luteinizing hormone-releasing hormone agonist, . *Release,* 9, 111, 1989.

16. **Spenlehauer, G., Vert, M., Benoit, J. P., and Boddaert, A.,** *In vitro* and *in vivo* degradatio lactide/glycolide) type microspheres made by solvent evaporation method, *Biomaterials,* 10,

17. **Spenlehauer, G., Vert, M., Benoit, J. P., Chabot, F., and Veillard, M.,** Biodegrada microspheres prepared by the solvent evaporation method: morphology and release characteri: *trolled Release,* 7, 217, 1988.

18. **Cha, Y. and Pitt, C. G.,** A one week subdermal delivery system for L-methadone based on b microcapsules, *J. Controlled Release,* 7, 69, 1988.

19. **Redmon, M., Hickey, A. J., and DeLuca, P.,** Prednisolone-21-acetate poly(glycolic acid) r influence of matrix characteristics on release, *J. Controlled Resl.,* 9, 99, 1989.

20. **Schakenraad, J. M., Oosterbaan, J. A., Nieuwenhuis, P., Molenaar, I., Olijslager, J., I Ednink, M. J. D., and Feijen, J.,** Biodegradable hollow fibers for the controlled relea *Biomaterials,* 9, 116, 1988.

21. **Eenink, M. J. D., Feijen, J., Olijslager, J., Albers, J. H. M., Rieke, J. C., and Greid** Biodegradable hollow fibers for the controlled release of hormones, *J. Controlled Rel.,* 6, 2:

22. **Marcotte, N., Polk, A., and Goosen, T.,** Programmed drugs: delayed-release of albumin fro pellets, *Polym. Prep,* 30, 476, 1989.

23. **Schakenraad, J. M., Nieuwenhuis, P., Molenaar, I., Helder, J., Dijkstra, P. J., and I** *vivo* and *in vitro* degradation of glycine/DL-lactic acid copolymers, *J. Biomed. Mat. Res.,* 23,

24. **Younes, H. and Cohn, D.,** Morphological study of biodegradable PEO/PLA block copolymer *Mat. Res.,* 21, 1301, 1987.

25. **Cohn, D. and Younes, H.,** Compositional and structural analysis of PELA biodegradable bloc degrading under *in vitro* conditions, *Biomaterial,* 10, 466, 1989.

26. **Wang, P. Y.,** Compressed poly(vinyl alcohol)-polycaprolactone admixture as a model to eva implants for sustained drug delivery, *J. Biomed. Mat. Res.,* 23, 91, 1989.

27. **Holland, S. J., Jolly, A. M., Yasin, M., Tighe, B. J.,** Polymers for biodegradable medica Hydroxybutyrate-hydroxyvalerate copolymers: hydrolytic degradation studies, *Biomaterials,* 8

28. **Holland, S. J., Jolly, A. M., Yasin, M., Tighe, B. J.,** Polymers for biodegradable medical Hydroxybutyrate-hydroxyvalerate copolymers: accelerated degradation of blends with polysacc *materials,* 10, 400, 1989.

29. **Pramanick, D. and Ray, T. T.,** Synthesis and biodegradation of polymers derived from *Biomaterials,* 8, 325, 1987.

30. **DiBenedetto, L. J. and Huang, S. J.,** Biodegradable hydroxylated polymers as controlled re *Poly. Preprint,* 30, 453, 1989.

31. **Lescure, F., Gurny, R., Doelker, E., Pelaprat, M. L., Bichon, D., and Anderson, J** histopathological response to a new biodegradable polypeptidic polymer for implantable c system, *J. Biomed. Mat. Res.,* 23, 1299, 1989.

32. **Harris, F. and Eury, R.,** Synthesis and evaluation of bioerodible non-peptide polyamides amino acid residues, *Poly. Preprint,* 30, 449, 1989.

33. **Kohn, J. and Langer, R.,** Polymerization reactions involving the side chains of α-L-amino *Chem. Soc.,* 109, 817, 1987.

34. **Domb, A. and Langer, R.,** Polyanhydrides. I. Preparation of high molecular weight polya *Poly. Sci.,* 25, 3373, 1987.

35. **Leong, K. W., Simonte, V., and Langer, R.,** Synthesis of polyanhydrides: melt-polycondensation, dehydrochlorination, and dehydrative coupling, *Macromolecules*, 20, 705, 1987.
36. **Domb, A., Ron, E., and Langer, R.,** Polyanhydrides. II. One step polymerization using phosgene or diphosgene as coupling agents, *Macromolecules*, 21, 1925, 1988.
37. **Domb, A., and Langer, R.,** Polyanhydrides: stability and novel composition, *Makromol. Chem. Macromol. Symp.*, 19, 189, 1988.
38. **Staubli, A., Mathiowitz, E., and Langer, R.,** Correlation Between Structural Characteristics and Material Properties of Poly(anhydride co-imides), 2nd Topical Conf. Emerging Technol. in Mater. AICHE Annu. Meet, San Francisco, 1989, 53.
39. **Staubli, A., Ron, E., and Langer, R.,** Synthesis and characterization of poly(imide-co-anhydrides), *Polym. Prepr.*, 30, 451, 1989.
40. **Mathiowitz, E., Ron, E., Mathiowitz, G., and Langer, R.,** Surface morphology of bioerodible poly(anhydrides), *Polym. Prepr.*, 30, 460, 1989.
41. **Ron, E., Mathiowitz, E., Mathiowitz, G., and Langer, R.,** A novel computerized approach to predict degradation rates of new biodegradable copolymers, *Polym. Prepr.*, 30, 462, 1989.
42. **Mathiowitz, E. and Langer, R.,** Polyanhydride microspheres as drug-carriers. I. Hot-melt microencapsulation, *J. Controlled Release*, 5, 13, 1987.
43. **Domb, A., and Langer, R.,** Solid state and solution stability of poly(anhydrides) and poly(esters), *Macromolecules*, 22, 2117, 1989.
44. **Bindschaedler, C., Leong, K., Mathiowitz, E., and Langer, R.,** Polyanhydride microsphere formulation by solvent extraction, *J. Pharm. Sci.*, 77, 696, 1988.
45. **Mathiowitz, E., Saltzman, W. M., Domb, A., Dor, Ph., and Langer, R.,** Polyanhydride microspheres as drug carriers. II. Microencapsulation by solvent removal, *J. Appl. Poly. Sci.*, 35, 755, 1988.
46. **Tamargo, R. J., Epstein, J. I., Reinhard, C. S., Chasin, M., and Brem, H.,** Brain biocompatibility of a biodegradable controlled-release polymer in rats, *J. Biomed. Mat. Res.*, 23, 253, 1989.
47. **Brem, H. Tamargo, R. J., Pinn, M., and Chasin, M.,** Biocompatibility of a BCNU-Loaded Biodegradable Polymer: A Toxicity Study in Primates, Abstr. Annu. Meet. Am. Assoc. Neurological Surgeons, 1988, 381.
48. **Brem, H., Kader, A., Epstein, J. I., Tamargo, R., Domb, A., Langer, R., and Leong, K.,** Biocompatibility of bioerodible controlled release polymers in the rabbit brain, *Selective Cancer Therapeutics*, 5, 55, 1989.
49. **Grossman, S. A., Reinhard, C. S., Brem, H., Brundrette, R., Chasin, M., Tamargo, R., and Colvin, O. M.,** The intracerebral delivery of BCNU with surgically implanted biodegradable polymers: a quantitative autoradiographic study, *Proc. Am. Soc. Clin. Oncology*, 7, 84, 1988.
50. **Brem, H., Ahn, H., Tamargo, R. J., Pinn, M., and Chasin, M.,** A Biodegradable Polymer for Intracranial Drug Delivery: A Radiological Study, Abstr. Annu. Meet. Am. Assoc. Neurological Surgeons, 1988, 399.
51. **Tamargo, R. J., Leong, K. W., and Brem, H.,** Growth inhibition of a gliosarcoma by the local sustained release of heparin and cortisone acetate, *J. Neuro-oncology*, in press.
52. **Howard, M. A., Gross, A., Grady, M. S., Langer, R., Mathiowitz, E., Winn, H. R., and Mayberg, M. R.,** Intracerebral drug delivery in rats reverses lesion-induced memory deficits, *J. Neurosurg.*, 71, 105, 1989.
53. **Lee, D. A., Leong, K. W., Panek, W. C., Eng., C. T., and Glasgow, B.,** The use of bioerodible polymers and 5-fluorouracil in glaucoma filtration surgery, *Invest. Ophth. Vis. Sci.*, 29, 1692, 1988.
54. **Lee, D. A., Flores, R. A., Anderson, P. J., Leong, K. W., Teekhasaenee, C., de Kater, A. W., and Herzmark, E.,** Glaucoma filtration surgery in rabbits using bioerodible polymers and 5-fluorouracil, *Ophthalmology*, 94, 1523, 1987.
55. **Chasin, M., Domb, A., Ron, E., Mathiowitz, E., Leong, K. W., Laurencin, C., Brem, H., Grossman, S., Langer, R.,** Polyanhydrides as drug delivery systems, in *Biodegradable Polymers as Drug Delivery Systems*, Langer, R. and Chasin, M., Eds., Marcel Dekker, New York, in press.
56. **Lucas, P. A., Laurencin, C., Syftestad, G. T., Domb, A., Goldber, V. M., Caplan, A. I., and Langer, R.,** Ectopic induction of cartilage and bone by water-soluble proteins from bovine bone using a polyanhydride delivery vehicle, *J. Controlled Rel.*, in press.
57. **Penczek, S., Lapienis, G., and Klosinski, P.,** Synthetic analogues of phosphorus containing biopolymers, *Pure Appl. Chem.*, 56, 1309, 1984.
58. **Pretula, J., Kaluzynski, K., and Penczek, S.,** Synthesis of poly(alkylene phosphates) with nitrogen containing bases in the side chains. I. N- and C-substituted imidazoles, *Macromolecules*, 19, 1797, 1986.
59. **Derouet, D., Piatti, T., Brosse, J. C.,** Synthese de polyesters phosphoriques supports de molecules actives. II. Etude de monomeres du type phosphorodichloridate de *O*-alkyle (OU *O*-acryle) ave les diols, a,w-lineaires non aromatiques, *Eur. Polym. J.*, 23, 657, 1987.
60. **Brosse, J. C., Derouet, D., Fontaine, L., and Chairatanathavorn, S.,** Fixation of pharamocologically active amines on polyphosphonates, *Makromol. Chem.*, 190, 2339, 1989.

61. **Li, N. H., Richards, M., Brandt, K., and Leong, K. W.,** Poly(phosphate esters) as drug-carr *Preprint,* 30, 454, 1989.
62. **Richards, M., Dahiyat, B. I., Arm, D. M., Lin, S., Leong, K. W.,** Interfacial polyconden characterization of polyphosphates and polyphosphonates, *J. Polym. Sci.,* in press.
63. **Richards, M., Dahiyat, B. I., Arm, D. M., Brown, P. R., and Leong, K. W.,** Evaluatio phosphates and polyphosphonates as degradable biomaterials, *J. Biomed. Mat. Res.,* submitted.
64. **Dahiyat, B. I., Richards, M. and Leong, K. W.,** Poly(phosphoesters) as controlled release m *Controlled Release,* submitted.
65. **Grolleman, C. W. J., deVisser, A. C., Wolke, J. G. C., van der Goot, H., and Timmer** Studies on a bioerodible drug carrier system based on polyphosphazene, *J. Controlled Releas* 1986.
66. **Allcock, H. R., Fuller, T. J., and Matsumura, K.,** Hydrolysis pathways for aminophosphazer *Chem.,* 21, 515, 1982.
67. **Laurencin, C. T., Koh, H. J., Neenan, T. X., Allcock, H. R., and Langer, R.,** Control using a new bioerodible polyphosphazene matrix system, *J. Biomed. Mat. Res.,* 21, 1231, 198
68. **Cohen, S., Chung, W., Ramachandran, B., Chow, M., Kwon, S., Allcock, H., and La** Novel polyphosphazene for drug delivery applications, 2nd Topical Conf. Emerging Techno AICHE Annual Meeting, San Francisco, 1989, 49.
69. **Kohn, J. and Langer, R.,** Poly(iminocarbonates) as potential biomaterials, *Biomaterials,* 7, 1
70. **Li, C. and Kohn, J.,** Synthesis of poly(iminocarbonates): degradable polymers with potential a as disposable plastics and as biomaterials, *Macromolecules,* 22, 2033, 1989.
71. **Heller, H., Ng, S. Y., Penhale, D. W., Fritzinger, B. K., Sanders, L. M., Burns, R. A. M. G., and Bhosale, S. S.,** Use of poly(ortho esters) for the controlled release of 5-fluorou LHRH analogue, *J. Controlled Release,* 6, 217, 1987.
72. **Nguyen, T. H., Higuchi, T., and Himmelstein, K. J.,** Erosion characteristics of catalyzed ester) matrices, *J. Controlled Release,* 5, 1, 1987.
73. **Chow, A. W., Hamlin, R. D., Heller, J.,** Cure behaviour of neat and drug-loaded poly(o bioerodible implants, *J. Controlled Release,* 9, 123, 1989.
74. **Heller, J.,** Chemically self-regulated drug delivery systems, *J. Controlled Release,* 8, 111, 19%
75. **Pitt, C. G., Gu, Z. W., Hendren, R. W., Thompson, J., and Wani, M. C.,** Triggered dru systems, *J. Controlled Release,* 2, 363, 1985.
76. **Kost, J., Leong, K. W., and Langer, R.,** Ultrasonically controlled polymeric drug therapy, *Chem.,* Macromol. Symp., 19, 275, 1988.
77. **Kost, J., Leong, K. W., and Langer, R.,** Ultrasound-enhanced polymer degradation and incorporated substances, *Proc. Natl. Acad. Sci. U.S.A.,* 86, 7663, 1989.

Chapter 8

COLLAGEN-BASED DRUG DELIVERY DEVICES

Mou-ying Fu Lu and Curt Thies

TABLE OF CONTENTS

I. INTRODUCTION

Much attention and publicity for the past 10 to 20 years has been focus development of synthetic polymers for drug delivery devices, particularly devices from synthetic polymers that degrade under *in vivo* conditions.[1-5] The possible co of natural polymers to this field have received far less publicity, even though th contains many reports that demonstrate that they have a role to play.

Figure 1 contains generalized repeat units for three broad classes of natural proteins, polysaccharides, and polyesters derived from β-hydroxyacids. Each cla many polymers that are viable candidates for drug delivery applications.[6] They are r diverse in terms of source, composition, molecular structure, size, and prope diversity exists because natural polymers are synthesized enzymatically. Althoug and Ulbrich[7] correctly note that synthetic polymers offer certain advantages ove occurring polymers, the technologies currently used to prepare synthetic poiym cannot create the elegant molecular structures and unique properties that characte natural polymers. This is a prime reason for considering the latter. Insight into the as drug carriers will develop as they are used, and this may lead to the creation o synthetic polymers for such applications.

Biodegradability by enzymatic attack and biological activity are two desirable that natural polymers may possess. Fabrication of drug delivery devices from ma will undergo controlled degradation in a biological environment by enzymatic most desirable property, particularly when the products of such degradative pro components of the normal metabolic process of the body. The ability of so polymers to show bioactivity offers interesting possibilities that are being explore degree, but warrant further study. In such cases, the carrier becomes an active in the therapeutic process. Although antigenicity, a form of bioactivity possessed polymers like proteins, can be a very dangerous property, it has not been a maje to date.

The recent medical literature contains a number of references to several applications for collagen-based drug delivery devices. Accordingly, it is appropriat the nature of such applications. It is relevant to point out first that the collagen a complex family of proteins. They are the most common proteins of connective form a major part of the organic matrix of bones.[8] Although 11 types of collagen recognized and characterized to varying degrees, Miller and Gay[9] are confident types will be identified in the future.

Collagens used to fabricate drug delivery devices have been derived from a different sources including fresh human placenta, rat tail tendon, and calfskin. Th Corporation, Palo Alto, CA, is a commercial source of collagen.

The potential value of collagen for medical and surgical applications has be for some time. Chrapil et al.[10] outlined many uses. They summarized the favorable of collagen, as well as the general technology associated with preparing collagen Such products exist in many forms, including solutions, gels, flour, fibers, sp tubing. Their 1973 list of medical and surgical applications of collagen is long, an the use of collagen as a drug delivery system; however, the latter was discus context of using the ability of collagen to interact in solution with various substanc forming complexes that show prolonged drug delivery when injected.[10]

II. DRUG DELIVERY DEVICES

Since most current promising drug delivery applications of collagen involve lagen-based implants or ocular inserts, this survey is concerned primarily with types of applications.

FIGURE 1

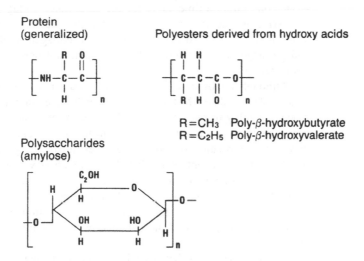

Protein
(generalized)

Polyesters derived from hydroxy acids

$R=CH_3$ Poly-β-hydroxybutyrate
$R=C_2H_5$ Poly-β-hydroxyvalerate

Polysaccharides
(amylose)

FIGURE 1. Generalized structures for protein, polyesters, and polysaccharides.

A. IMPLANTS FOR ANTIBIOTIC THERAPY

A number of studies have examined how well collagen functions as a carrier for antibiotics, designed to prevent infection after bone surgery. Firsov, et al.[11] studied the *in vitro* and *in vivo* performance of spongy collagen lamellae implants loaded with 25 w/w% gentamicin. The implants contained 5 mg gentamicin; their dimensions were unspecified. Crosslinked and uncrosslinked implants were evaluated, but the crosslinking agent and degree of crosslinking were not specified. *In vitro* and *in vivo* gentamicin release profiles were constructed by using a bioassay protocol involving *Bacillus subtilis* ATCC 6633.

The release rates of genatmicin from crosslinked lamellae into water and into pH 7.35 phosphate buffer of 0.29 ionic strength (temperature unspecified) were similar. Approximately 50 to 60% of the gentamicin payload was released in 30 d. Gentamicin release from the uncrosslinked lamellae occurred more rapidly in phosphate buffer than in water. In both media, 60 to 70% of the gentamicin payload was released within 1 h.

In vivo studies were carried out by making small incisions in the backs of 200 to 250 g Wistar rats, inserting the implant, and then pushing the implant approximately 1 cm away from the incision before it was sutured. The number of animals per test was not specified.

Gentamicin blood levels of animals that received either uncrosslinked or crosslinked implants fell to 0.1 µg/ml within 8 h after injection. The gentamicin content of tissue surrounding the crosslinked implants was assayed and found to reach 210 µg/g tissue within 1 h after implantation. It declined in 6 h to 5.2 + 1.9 µg/g tissue, and remained at this concentration for 14 d. The tissue concentration then declined slowly to 1 µg/g tissue at 30 d. The uncrosslinked sample gave a gentamicin concentration of 365 µg/g tissue at 1 h after implantation. The gentamicin concentration declined to 1.2 + 0.3 µg/g tissue 6 h after implantation and remained there for 7 d. It then declined steadily and reached 0.1 µg/g tissue at 14 d.

With both the crosslinked and uncrosslinked implants, the gentamicin content of tissue surrounding the implants immediately after implantation (the most probable time period for development of infections) was many times higher than that found if the gentamicin was given systemically.[11] The essentially constant gentamicin tissue concentration of 5.9 + 1.9 µg/g tissue, maintained by the crosslinked collagen implant for 14 d, is higher than the MIC

of gentamicin for most pathogens causing wound and surgical infections. The area ι
tissue concentration-time curve for the crosslinked collagen implant was superior t
a poly(methyl methacrylate) implant, but this was not true for the uncrosslinked
Thus, it was concluded that the crosslinked collagen implant is capable of provid
and prolonged concentrations of gentamicin, and possibly other antibiotics, at th
implantation.

Although Firsov et al.[11] consistently indicated that their collagen implants w
degradable, no direct histological, weight loss, or radiotracer data demonstrating
biodegradability or rate of biodegradation were presented. They did note that the pι
period of relatively constant gentamicin tissue concentration observed with their
was due to formation of fibrous capsules surrounding the implants. This implie
histological assessment of implant biodegradation was made. Sorg et al.[12] also
briefly on the behavior of implanted drug-loaded sponges and sheets as carriers for anι
antiseptics, and labile drugs like blood-clotting factors. They formed their devic
bovine tendon collagen. Sterilization by γ-irradiation or ethylene oxide did not
haemostyptic properties of the collagen or destroy the potency of aminoglycoside
on the device.

In vivo behavior of their $10 \times 10 \times 0.5$ cm collagen sponges coated with aminoς
(4 to 7 mg/kg body weight) and loaded with 120 mg gentamicin or 240 mg netilm
determined by implanting them in rabbits at the site of a severe bone infection. The
was induced by implantation of an intramedullary rod and *Staphylococcus aureus*,
before the collagen sponge was implanted. Scintigraphic and histological examina
vealed remission of osteomyelitis within 8 weeks after the sponge was implan
aminoglycoside serum levels were low, but comparatively high levels were foun
cortical bone even 28 d after the onset of therapy. Complete collagen resorption was ι
within 6 weeks after implantation. Results of the *in vivo* study in rabbits prompted thι
to initiate a controlled clinical study. As of 1988, over 200 patients suffering froι
post-traumatic or hematogenic bone infections or septic loosening of prostheses ι
treated. With these patients, no collagen-derived side effects have been detected, ι
noglycoside concentration in the serum and urine have been far below toxic concer
The haemostyptic effects of collagen are regarded as beneficial in reducing bleed
bone.

B. IMPLANTS AS PROTEIN CARRIERS

A number of workers have studied the performance of collagen-based delivery
loaded with proteins. For example, Deatherage and Miller[13] studied the *in vivo* beh
a collagenous implant loaded with bone induction factors. They fabricated their disι
cm diameter and 0.4 cm thickness by compacting a mixture of 90 mg Type I collε
60 mg of factors active in cartilage and bone induction, extracted from the long
Sprague-Dawley rats. One such disc was implanted subcutaneously in each of 2
breeder rats. A control disc, free of bone extract components, was also implanted
rat. One animal was sacrificed on each of 21 d after implantation and the two imι
each animal were subjected to gross and histological examination.

The implants elicited minimal immunologic response. By day 21, endochond
fication of the established hyaline cartilage model had occurred in the implant loaι
bone extract. The cartilage-bone structure formed had essentially the same dimer
the original implant. This observation suggests that a sufficient amount of bonι
components, needed to cause formation of bony tissue, is retained within the collager
at least long enough to cause formation of such tissue. In contrast, by day 21 thι
implant, free of bone extract, did not promote osteogenesiι. It was encapsulated,
further cellular activity appeared at the periphery of the implant or within the impι

Deatherage and Miller[13] felt that their implant system meets many criteria of an ideal delivery system. The disc implants were readily prepared and had sufficient strength to withstand the handling steps that occurred during implantation. No chemical crosslinking was used. Since the implant essentially dictates the size and shape of bony tissue produced, they believe a particular desired contour can be anticipated and achieved.

Muthukumaran et al.[14] studied the dose dependence of bone induction by a demineralized collagen bone matrix (DBM) and an osteogenin-enriched fraction in the presence/absence of inactive collagenous bone matrix (ICBM). This was done by preparing a variety of small pellets from various combinations of these components. Dimensions of the pellets were unspecified; most had a total mass of 25.5 to 26.5 mg. All implants also contained 0.5 mg chondroitun 6 sulfate; several contained 1 mg Type I collagen isolated from rat tail tendon. All pellets evaluated were implanted subcutaneously in male Long-Evans rats (two implants per animal).

It was concluded that at least 10 mg DBM was required for bone induction. A dose-dependent increase in bone induction, as measured by alkaline phosphatase activity and calcium content, occurred as the amount of DBM increased from 10 to 25 mg.

Lucas et al.[15] studied ectopic induction of cartilage and bone by water-soluble proteins extracted from bovine bone with 4 M guanidine hydrochloride. The crude protein extract was used, since it contained the factors needed to support the entire osteogenic cascade. The extract was incorporated in Type I collagen pellets by dialyzing an aqueous solution of both components against ethanol. The pellets were dehydrated, implanted in the dorsal thigh of 5- to 7-week-old CBA/J mice, and subjected to histological examination at 9, 16, and 25 d after implantation. The weight of collagen associated with the weight of water-soluble protein varied from below 1:1 to 25:1. The minimum protein weight per pellet was 2 mg. Total weight of each pellet evaluated was not clearly specified, but implants with a 1:1 or 2:1 w/w collagen/protein ratio contained 20 mg of water-soluble proteins. Thus, they had a total weight of 40 and 60 mg, respectively. Total pellet volume was approximately 1 mm³; pellet dimensions were not specified.

All implants with collagen:protein ratios ranging from 1:1 to 25:1 induced cartilage and bone formation, while collagen:protein ratios below 1:1 did not. The crude water-soluble protein extract implanted alone caused no signs of cartilage or bone formation. The same was true for collagen pellets loaded with bovine serum albumin. Only the combination of water-soluble protein extract and Type I collagen in pellet form induced cartilage and bone formation.

Soluble bone matrix-derived protein factors which regulate specific cellular processes must interact with local target cell populations for a sufficient period of time in order to initiate a biological response.[15] The Type I collagen pellet loaded with water-soluble protein extract accomplished this. Consistency of results obtained with the implants was checked by making three separate preparations of such pellets from extracts of different bovine bones. Out of 17 such implants, 13 contained some cartilage and bone 9 d after implantation, to give a 76% positive response.

Since the purpose of this study was to design a delivery vehicle for osteogenesis, the authors used a crude protein extract that would contain the inductive protein and support the entire osteogenic cascade process. Future studies will stress improving the consistency of performance of the device and increasing the size of the osteogenic response that it creates. It was suggested that the device makes possible further studies with purified proteins. Such studies may lead to identification of which protein(s), if any, support the entire osteogenic cascade, and if other individual, purified, soluble bioactive factors in combination can initiate or optimally sustain the osteogenic cascade.

Lucas et al.[15] noted that the Type I collagen they used is a homogeneous substance. It acts as a noninflammatory, biodegradable substrate that promotes cell attachment. They also

stressed that their dehydrated collagen delivery vehicle could be applicable to th
of a number of bioactive factors that act upon local cell populations. Suggested
applications include delivery to orthotopic sites of purified, soluble bioactive(s) is
bone induction, and delivery of bioactive factors like TGF-β, FGF, and PDGF
upon local cell populations in wound healing or angiogenesis.[15]

Significantly, all observations reported by Lucas et al.[15] were derived from h
observations of *in vivo* implants. The rate of water-soluble protein release from th
was not defined either under *in vitro* or *in vivo* conditions. This is an importan
remains to be done.

Weiner et al.[16] incorporated human growth hormone in plurilamellar vesicles
immobilized the vesicles in a collagen gel. They used two collagens: rat tail collage
by acid digestion, and bovine dermal collagen isolated by acid and pepsin diges
vesicle/collagen gels were formed at 37°C and then administered to rats by a sin
muscular or subcutaneous injection. Vesicles loaded with [^{125} I]-labelled growth
immobilized in a 0.3% collagen gel, gave a sustained level of [^{125} I] label at the
site for over 14 d. At 14 d, approximately 20% of the initially injected label re
the injection site. When the hormone-loaded vesicles were injected alone, only 16.
label remained at the injection site 3 d after injection.

Rosenblatt et al.[17] have modeled the diffusional release rates of proteins from
matrices. Their model assumed that diffusion of proteins was hindered when the
of the confining collagen matrix approached the size of the entrapped protein. *In vi*
behavior of two proteins of different size, chymotrypsinogen and fibrinogen, we
test predictions of their model.

The matrices from which diffusion occurred were fabricated from a fibrilla
sample or sample of succinylated collagen.[17] Each fibrillar collagen matrix conta
mg of radio-labeled protein and 35 mg fibrillar collagen (0.17 w/w percent activ
succinylated collagen matrix contained 0.1 mg of radio-labelled protein and 38
nylated collagen (0.3 w/w % actives). These gel-like mixtures were converted in
in the bottom of the test tube by centrifugation, and evaluated without an int
isolation and drying step. Protein elution from the pellets was measured under
ditions by layering 2 ml of buffer on the test pellets and changing this buffer pe
Succinylated pellets were studied at room temperature; fibrillar collagen pellets we
at 37°C.

The release data obtained were complex, and indicated that protein release
collagen pellets involved several mechanisms. In the case of chymotrypsinogen
in the fibrillar collagen implant, approximately 25% appeared to be bound to th
The rest appeared to be released by a free-diffusion mechanism. Release of fib
large protein, was slightly hindered by the fibrillar collagen matrix. The succinylate
pellet, a non-fibrillar matrix, had a significant retardation effect on chymotrypsi
fibrinogen release. These observations led to the conclusion that diffusional relea
proteins from collagen matrices can be controlled. However, it also was noted that
binding-debinding interactions with the collagen matrix can alter predicted releas
can changes in matrix morphology caused by fragmentation of the matrix and/o
cells.

C. IMPLANTS FOR ENHANCED WOUND HEALING

The ability of collagen implants loaded with a glycosaminoglycan to enhar
healing has been studied by several groups. McPherson et al.[18] evaluated the in
heparin on the wound healing response to *in vivo* collagen implants. They were
with the development of biomaterials that could promote the healing of chronic, r
wounds like decubitus, venous stasis, and diabetic ulcers. Materials for such ap

should provide a transient latticework or scaffold for fibroplasia and neovascularization of wound beds, while simultaneously providing a support for epidermal cell migration, proliferation, and differentiation. Their implants were formed by injecting 0.5 to 1.0 ml of sterile fibrillar collagen suspension, with or without heparin, into the supracascapular region of Sprague-Dawley rats (8 to 10 weeks old). The same collagen suspension (0.1 ml), with or without heparin, was also injected into guinea pig dermal wounds. The injected suspensions contained 18 to 30 mg collagen per ml. The heparin content was 10, 50, or 300 μg/ml suspension or 0.3 to 20 μg heparin per mg collagen. Thus, on a dry weight basis the implants contained from 0.03 to 2 wt% heparin.

Increasing heparin concentrations in the injected collagen suspension had a positive dose-response effect on fibroblast invasion into the collagen implants injected in the rat subcutis. The same concentrations of chondroitin sulfate or hyaluronate had no positive effect on cell invasion. Heparin-containing implants had a more distinct fibrillar organization than implants free of heparin, and this may have provided a better environment for cell invasion.[18]

Radiolabel experiments made[18] with [³H] collagen and [³⁵S] heparin showed that approximately 65% of the heparin injected in the rat subcutis had migrated from the implantation site in 2 d. The remaining heparin was eliminated from this site at a much slower rate. Approximately 10% remained there 28 d after implantation. Approximately 55% of the collagen injected to this location had disappeared 28 d after implantation. The presence of heparin in the implant did not affect the rate of collagen disappearance as measured by loss of [³H] at the injection site.

The heparin-free and heparin-loaded implants caused similar rates of guinea pig dermal wound closure. Approximately 50% of the [³H] collagen injected had disappeared from the implant site 5 d after injection; 98% had disappeared after 28 d. The presence of heparin had no effect on rate of collagen disappearance; however, histological examination showed that the collagen/heparin implants had a more porous appearance. This was associated with more penetration of developing granulation tissue into the implant relative to that observed with heparin-free implants. Laser Doppler flowmetry suggested that heparin-containing implants were more vascular than control wounds or wounds treated with collagen-free of heparin.[18]

McPherson et al.[18] believe that perhaps the most important result of their studies is the convincing evidence that fibrillar collagen gels, with or without heparin, can effectively support the wound healing response. Collagen-based implants support neovascularization, fibroplasia, and epidermal regeneration. They do not interfere with the long-term course of wound repair because they are resorbable. For these reasons they feel that collagen-based matrices are ideal candidates for the delivery of certain chemotactic, mitogenic, and differentiative factors to promote the healing of soft and hard tissue defects.

Docherty et al.[19] studied the movement of choroid fibroblasts through three-dimensional Type I collagen matrices. They noted that the movement of cells through extracellular matrices is intrinsic to many tissue processes such as wound healing, tumour metastasis, differentiation, and ovulation. Their gels were formed in clear tissue-culture plastic multi-wells (35 mm diameter). The cells were subsequently seeded on these gels. They found that increasing the collagen concentration in the matrix from 1 to 2.5 mg/ml increased cell invasiveness. Collagen concentrations above 3.5 mg/ml were too high to allow cell invasion; concentrations below 0.5 mg/ml gave unstable gels. These observations were similar to those of Schor et al.[20]

Fibroblast invasion was facilitated by incorporating hyaluronate or chondroitin sulfate, two glycosaminoglycans, into the collagen gel. Hyaluronate was significantly more effective, although its concentration in the collagen matrix (0.5 to 2.0 mg/ml gel) had a major effect on cell invasion. It caused maximum cell invasion when its concentration in a matrix, formed from 1.5 mg collagen/ml, was 1 mg/ml. Higher or lower concentrations markedly reduced

invasion relative to that observed at the optimum concentration. A combination of hya
and chondroitin sulfate promoted cell movement in a synergistic manner. Addition c
component, fibronectin, caused a further increase in invasion, even though fibronec
had no effect.

The enhanced fibroblast invasion caused by glycosaminoglycans appeared to •
with more dense packing of collagen fibrils within the collagen gels, since increased
concentration of glycosaminoglycan-free gels caused the same effect. Results of s
electron microscopy assays of fixed collagen gels, with and without glycosamino
were interpreted as suggesting that the glycosaminoglycans caused changes in the
of fibrils in the gels, and this accounted in part for the observed differences in th
fibroblast invasion. That is, physical properties of the matrix influence movement
into the matrix. However, it was noted that factors other than gel stability and fibril
may be important for enhanced migration caused by the glycosaminoglycans.

Docherty et al.[19] attempted to study how heparin affected choroid fibroblast inv
collagen gels, but found that heparin had such an adverse effect on gel stability that
measurement of cell invasion was not possible. They noted that Guidry and Grinnel
that heparin inhibits polymerization of collagen gels.

Although McPherson et al.[18] stated that neither chondroitin sulfate nor hya
enhanced fibroblast invasion of their *in vivo* collagen implants, Docherty et al.[19] fc
both glycosaminoglycans enhanced *in vitro* fibroblast invasion of their gels. In th
case, the glycosaminoglycan concentrations used were 0.01 to 0.3 mg/ml, lower
0.5 to 2.0 mg/ml concentrations used by Docherty et al.[19] The implants of McPh
al.[18] were also formed *in situ* by injection. It would be of value to define what dif
in experimental conditions affected the differences in cell invasion behavior obse
these two groups of workers.

D. OCULAR INSERTS

The concept of using collagen inserts to provide prolonged delivery of drugs tc
has been studied for some time. Initial studies focused upon fabrication of drug-loade
cut from drug-loaded collagen film, prepared by evaporating to dryness an aqueous
of drug and collagen. In some cases the film was chemically crosslinked. In other
was not. Succinylated collagen also was used.[22] More recent work has concentra
formation of drug-free inserts that are immersed in an aqueous drug solution (or sus
immediately before placement in the eye.

Rubin et al.[23] described preliminary *in vitro* and *in vivo* results obtained with a pi
nitrate-loaded collagen strip insert (0.32 cm² surface area and 0.46 mm thicknes
strip contained 12.8 mg pilocarpine and 4.2 mg collagen, so the pilocarpine nitrate
was 75 wt%. *In vitro* release of pilocarpine nitrate from the inserts into stirred
solution at 37°C was complete in 20 min. Strip inserts placed in the inferior forni
right eye of five rabbits caused pupillary constriction within 7 min, and it lasted
inserts dissolved in 25 min and caused no inflammation in the eye. There also
detectable long-term effects (up to 30 d) of placing the inserts in the rabbit eye.
or not strip inserts were moistened before insertion into a rabbit's eye was not spe

Vasantha et al.[24] prepared pilocarpine nitrate-loaded collagen film by a protoc
ogous to that of Rubin et al.[23] Circular disc inserts were die cut from the film
diameter of 1.5 cm or a surface area of 7.07 cm². One set of discs evaluated
chemically treated; a second set was treated with 1% glutaraldehyde at pH 7.4 fc
after film formation had been completed. In both cases, the discs initially contain
pilocarpine nitrate. The weight of collagen associated with this weight of pilocarpir
was not specified. Furthermore, all films were washed for 1 h (presumably in wate
they were evaluated *in vitro*. This was done in order to remove adsorbed and loosel
pilocarpine nitrate.

As the amount of pilocarpine nitrate and collagen carried by a disc at the time it was evaluated was not specified, it is difficult to accurately compare performance of the Vasantha et al.[24] discs with the strips of Rubin et al.[23] Nevertheless, the former released pilocarpine nitrate over a much longer period under *in vitro* conditions. Discs not treated with glutaraldehyde released 350 μg pilocarpine nitrate during the first 4 h of immersion in 37°C physiological pH 7.4 phosphate buffer. The rate of release during this period declined to a steady-state value of 140 μg/d and remained at this rate for 5 d. Discs treated with glutaraldehyde released less pilocarpine nitrate (265 μg) during the first 4 h of immersion in the same buffer, and had a lower (120 μg/d) steady-state release rate that was maintained for 7 d. A series of discs of varying thickness, but constant drug content, also showed an initial rapid rate of drug release that declined quickly to a steady-state value lasting 4 d. The steady-state release rate measured increased in direct proportion to disc thickness. It is reasonable to suggest that the much longer release times reported by Vanantha et al.[24] are due to a much lower initial pilocarpine nitrate content. They did not report results of *in vivo* studies.

Bloomfield et al.[22] prepared a slow pulse delivery system from oval-shaped discs of soluble succinylated collagen. Each disc weighted 10 mg and carried 1.1 mg of ^{14}C-labeled gentamicin sulfate. The performance of these inserts in the eye of New Zealand rabbits was compared with that of three other routes of administration: drop, ointment, and injection. The collagen disc gave a higher gentamicin concentration in the tear film than the other routes of administration, even 2 h after the experiment began. Gentamicin tear film concentration peaked approximately 0.6 h after the insert was placed in the eye, and decreased rapidly thereafter. The insert was completely dissolved 6 h after placement in the eye. Sclera and cornea tissue gentamicin concentration measured 1 and 3 h after initiation of treatment were highest with the collagen insert. At these times it consistently gave a sclera concentration higher than the corneal concentration. It was concluded that a modest improvement in pulse delivery leads to substantially enhanced drug uptake, and a soluble collagen insert is a practical way to achieve this.

Beginning in 1988, several articles that characterize the performance of collagen shields soaked in different drug solutions have appeared in the ophthalmic literature. The collagen shield was originally developed by Svyatoslav Fyodorov as a corneal bandage for use after radial keratotomy, in keratorefractive procedures, and for corneal abrasions.[25] The concept was to use the collagen shield to maximize corneal healing by supplying the injured cornea with "building blocks" required in the healing process. However, it was recognized that this device could also serve as a way to deliver drugs to the eye.

BioCor,™ the commerically available collagen shield studied by most workers since 1988, is sold by Bausch and Lomb Pharmaceutical, Clearwater, FL. It is fabricated from porcine scleral collagen, has a diameter of 14.5 mm, base curve of 9.0 mm, and thickness of 0.0127 to 0.0170 mm. The rate at which is dissolves in the eye can be varied (12, 24, and 72 h) by varying the degree of UV-induced crosslinking. As the shields dissolve, they provide a layer of biologically compatible collagen solution that seems to lubricate the surface of the eye, minimize rubbing of the lids on the cornea, and foster epithelial healing.[26]

Thus far, no single protocol has been followed for loading drug-free collagen shields with drug(s). Many workers soak then in an aqueous drug solution at 25°C immediately before use, but some add the drug to the shield in drop form after the shield is in place in the eye. A drug-soaked shield may be used alone or in combination with eye drops applied after the shield has been in place in the eye for a finite time. All of these protocols have yielded improved therapeutic benefits.

The drug used in conjunction with a collagen shield is often a water-soluble antibiotic like gentamicin sulfate, vancomycin, or tobramycin, but dexamethasone and prednisolone-21-acetate, two topical steroids, have also been evaluated. When a collagen shield is immersed in a drug solution, drug uptake by the shield is rapid. It appears that a soak time of

TABLE 1
Effect of Soak Solution Drug Concentration and
Drug Combinations on Collagen Shield Six-Hour
Release Data

Soak solution drug conc (mg/ml)		Wt of drug released at 6 hours *in vitro* (μg)	
Gentamicin	Vancomycin	Gentamicin	Vancomycin
40	—	419 + 25	—
40	25	460 + 10	—
40	50	691 + 58	—
—	50	—	2291 + 101
40	25	—	1373 + 31
40	50	—	2321 + 186

5 to 10 min is adequate for loading a shield. For example, Hobden et al.[27] essentially the same amount of tobramycin (800 to 890 g) was taken up by a shi soaks of 10, 30, 60, and 120 min in a 4% tobramycin solution. Unterman et a that 12 shields soaked 5 min in a 40 mg/ml tobramycin solution contained an a 829 ± 48 μg tobraymcin, while 12 shields soaked 5 min in a 200 mg/ml solution 5525 ± 736 μg tobramycin. Phinny et al.[29] reported that the minimum time to impregnate a collagen shield with gentamicin sulfate and vancomycin remains to t but a limited number of trials revealed that collagen shields receiving a 5-min so to be as effective as samples soaked 2 h. In their study they used a 2-hr soak i be sure that the shields were fully loaded. Most workers use soak times of 5 to

The amount of drug taken up by a collagen shield and the rate at which it is a function of the drug being loaded into the shield and the concentration of c loading solution. As mentioned above, Unterman et al.[28] found that increasing the t concentration by a factor of 5 (from 40 to 200 mg/ml) increased shield uptake of t by a factor of more than 6. The presence of a second drug in the soak solution individual drug uptake. For example, Table 1 contains concentrations of soak solt by Phinney et al.,[29] and the amount of drug released into saline after 6 h by shie with genatmicin, vancomycin, and combinations of these drugs. The amount of released at 6 h increased as the concentration of vancomycin increased from 0 ml. It appears that the amount of vancomycin in the shield is not affected signif the presence of gentamicin in the system. Although these data are limited, the that drug type, soak concentration, and combinations of drug can affect drug u collagen shield, and hence must be regarded as experimental parameters that mu trolled carefully and well-defined.

Unterman et al.[28] found that tobramycin-loaded shields rapidly release their t payload under *in vivo* conditions. Shields loaded by a 5-min soak in a 40-mg tc ml solution contained only 16.8% of their initial tobramycin content after 1 h in eye, while shields loaded by soaking in a 200 mg/ml solution contained 4.1% of tobramycin content after 1 h.

Several *in vivo* studies carried out with New Zealand rabbits have establis combined collagen shield/drug regimen increases drug penetration into the cornea a humor. For example, Sawusch et al.[30] compared the effectiveness of applying t to rabbit eyes in six sequential one-drop doses given every 30 min with and collagen shield in place. The mean tobramycin concentration in the aqueous hum with a collagen shield, 30 min after the last dose, was 6.48 ± 3.18 μg/ml, without a shield had a mean concentration below 0.16 μg/ml at this time. Rab

which stromal keratitis was induced were also subjected to tobramycin treatment (one drop per 30 min for 12 h) with and without a collagen shield in place. Treated eyes with a collagen shield had a mean ± SD bacterial colony forming unit count of 49.4 ± 55.4/ml, and 313 + 258.3/ml without a shield.

Hobden et al.[27] soaked collagen shields in a 4% tobramycin solution and found that they were as effective in treating experimental *Pseudomonas keratitis* in rabbit eyes over a 4-h test period as the 4% tobramycin solution administered topically with no shield in place. However, the amount of drug used to load the shield was only approximately 5% of that applied topically without a shield.

Unterman et al.[28] found that shields loaded by soaking in 40 or 200 mg tobramycin/ml solutions gave a tobramycin concentration in the cornea or aqueous humor that exceeds the mean antibiotic inhibitory concentration for most strains of *Pseudomonas* for 8 h.

Phinney et al.[29] found that collagen shields soaked 2 h in gentamicin, vancomycin, or a combination of these drugs gave tear, cornea, and aqueous humor levels that were at least comparable, if not higher, after 6 h than those obtained with frequent drop therapy for this period. They concluded from their data that the collagen shield is an attractive modality for drug delivery, although additional studies will be necessary to further define the role that collagen shields can play in bacterial ulcer management.

The use of collagen shields in conjunction with topical steroids has been evaluated *in vivo*. Sawusch et al.[25] examined the penetration of a 1% prednisolone-21-acetate solution into the cornea and aqueous humor of rabbit eyes with and without a collagen shield in place. In one series of experiments, 12-h shields were soaked for 15 min in the drug solution before they were placed in the eyes. In a second series of experiments, a drop of drug solution was administered to each collagen shield after it was placed dry in the eyes. Prednisolone penetration into the cornea and aqueous humor at 30 and 120 min after placement of either type shield in the eyes was higher than that observed when no collagen shield was present. Shields loaded with prednisolone 15 min before insertion in the eyes gave a higher prednisolone concentration than shields to which prednisolone was added after the shield was placed in the eye.

Hwang et al.[31] studied the increase in dexamethasone penetration in the cornea, aqueous, iris, and vitreous of rabbit eyes at six time-intervals during treatment with and without collagen shields. Four protocols were compared:

- Protocol 1: No shield; one topical drop of 0.1% dexamethasone.
- Protocol 2: No shield; one-hourly topical drop of 0.1% dexamethasone for 6 h.
- Protocol 3: 24-h shield soaked 15 min in 0.1% dexamethasone.
- Protocol 4: 24-h shield soaked 15 min in 0.1% dexamethasone plus one-hourly topical drop of 0.1% dexamethasone for 6 h.

The shield that was simply soaked with dexamethasone (Protocol 3) gave peak and cumulative drug concentrations equivalent or superior to those recorded when 6-hourly topical drops were administered (Protocol 2). However, drug-soaked shields plus 6-hourly drops (Protocol 4) gave dexamethasone concentrations 2 to 4 times above that observed with hourly drops (Protocol 2).

Poland et al.[32] recently summarized the performance of tobramycin-soaked shields in 47 patients who had some form of ocular surgery, and 13 patients with nonsurgical epithelial healing problems. In all cases, there were no detrimental effects on the ocular surface caused by the combined use of a collagen shield and tobramycin. Significantly, the oxygen permeability of the collagen shield was initially about twice as high as that of a hydrophilic contact lens, and this permeability increased exponentially as the degradation process progressed. They concluded that collagen shields appear to promote improved healing in patients with postsurgical and acute epithelial defects, as well as provide adequate antibiotic pro against infection in these vulnerable eyes.

III. SUMMARY

In the past 2 years, a number of studies have demonstrated that drug delivery fabricated from collagen offer much promise. Many potential applications of such have not been fully explored. However, results obtained to date suggest that full exp is warranted and undoubtedly will occur.

REFERENCES

1. **Wood, D. A.,** Biodegradable drug delivery systems, *Int. J. Pharm.*, 7, 1, 1980.
2. **Heller, J.,** Biodegradable polymers in controlled drug delivery, *Crit. Rev. Ther. Drug Carri* 39, 1984.
3. **Juni, K. and Nakano, M.,** Poly(hydroxy acids) in drug delivery, *Crit. Rev. Ther. Drug Carri* 209, 1987.
4. **Thies, C.,** Biodegradable polymers for parenteral administration, *Int. J. Pharm. Technol. Pro* 2, 25, 1981.
5. **Holland, S. J., Tighe, B. J., and Gould, P. L.,** Polymers for biodegradable medical devic potential of polyesters as controlled macromolecular release systems, *J. Controlled Release*, 4,
6. **Graham, N. B. and Wood, D. A.,** Polymeric inserts and implants for the controlled release *Macromolecular Biomaterials*, Hastings, G. W. and Ducheyne, P., Eds., CRC Press, Boca 1984, chap. 8.
7. **Kopecek, J. and Ulbrich, K.,** Biodegradation of biomedical polymers, *Prog. Polym. Sci.*, 9,
8. **Johns, P.,** Chemical constitution of gelatin, in *The Science and Technology of Gelatin*, Ward, Courts, A., Eds., Academic Press, New York, 1977, chap. 2.
9. **Miller, E. J. and Gay, S.,** The collagens: an overview and update, *Methods Enzymol.*, 144,
10. **Chrapil, M., Kronenthal, R. L., and Van Winkle, W.,** Medical and surgical applications o in *International Review of Connective Tissue Research*, Vol. 6, Hall, D. A. and Jackson, D Academic Press, New York, 1973, 1.
11. **Firsov, A. A., Nazarov, A. D., and Fomina, I. P.,** Biodegradable implants containing genta release and pharmacokinetics, *Drug Dev. Ind. Pharm.*, 13, 1651, 1987.
12. **Stemberger, A., Sorg, K. H., Ascherl, R., Scherer, M. A., Ergardt, W., Machka, K., I R., Lechner, F., Blmel, G., and Schlemmer, H.,** Investigations on collagen as a resorbable d *Polym. Mater. Sci. Eng.*, 59, 817, 1988.
13. **Deatherage, J. R. and Miller, E. J.,** Packaging and delivery of bone induction factors in a implant, *Collagen Rel. Res.*, 7, 225, 1987.
14. **Muthukumaran, N., Ma, S., and Reddi, A. H.,** Dose-dependence of and threshold for op induction by collagenous bone matrix and osteogenin-enriched fraction, *Collagen Rel. Res.*, 8,
15. **Lucas, P. A. Syftestad, G. T., Goldberg, V. M., and Caplan, A. I.,** Ectopic induction of c bone by water-soluble proteins from bovine bone using a collagenous delivery vehicle, *J. Biom Res. Appl. Biomater.*, 23, 23, 1989.
16. **Weiner, A. L., Carpenter-Green, S. S., Soehngen, E. C., Lenk, R. P., and Popescu, M. C., collagen gel matrix: a novel sustained drug delivery system, *J. Pharm. Sci.*, 74, 922, 1985.
17. **Rosenblatt, J., Rhee, W., and Wallace, D.,** The effect of collagen fiber size distribution on rate of proteins from collagen matrices by diffusion, *J. Controlled Release*, 9, 195, 1989.
18. **McPherson, J. M., Ledger, P. W., Ksander, G., Sawamura, S. J., Conti, A., Kincaid, S. D., and Clark, R. A. F.,** The influence of heparin on the wound healing response to collage *in vivo*, *Collagen Rel. Res.*, 1, 83, 1988.
19. **Docherty, R., Forrester, J. V., Lackie, J. M., and Gregory, D. W.,** Glycosaminoglycans f movement of fibroblasts through three-dimensional collagen matrices, *J. Cell Sci.*, 92, 263, 1
20. **Schor, S. L., Schor, A. M., and Bazill, G. W.,** The effects of fibronectin on the migratio foreskin fibroblasts and Syrian hamster melanoma cells into three-dimensional gels of native coll *J. Cell Sci.*, 48, 310, 1981.

21. **Guidry, C. and Grinnell, F.**, Heparin modulates the organisation of hydrated collagen gels and inhibits gel contraction by fibroblasts, *J. Cell Biol.*, 104, 731, 1987.
22. **Bloomfield, S. E., Miyata, T., Dunn, M. W., Bueser, N., Stenzel, K. H., and Rubin, A. L.**, Soluble gentamicin ophthalmic inserts as a drug delivery system, *Arch. Ophthalmol.*, 96, 885, 1978.
23. **Rubin, A. L., Stenzel, K. H., Miyata, T., White, M. J., and Dunn, M.**, Collagen as a vehicle for drug delivery, *J. Clin. Pharmacol.*, 13, 309, 1973.
24. **Vasantha, R., Sehgal, P. K., and Rao, K. P.**, Collagen ophthalmic inserts for pilocarpine drug delivery system, *Int. J. Pharm.*, 47, 95, 1988.
25. **Sawusch, M. R., O'Brien, T. P., and Updegraff, B. S.**, Collagen corneal shields enhance penetration of topical prednisolone acetate, *J. Cataract Refract. Surg.*, 15, 625, 1989.
26. **Kaufman, H. E.**, Collagen shield symposium, *J. Cataract Refract. Surg.*, 14, 487, 1988.
27. **Hobden, J. A., Reidy, J. J., O'Callaghan, R. J., Hill, J. M., Insler, M. S., and Rootman, D. S.**, Treatment of experimental pseudomonas keratitis using collagen shields containing tobramycin, *Arch. Ophthalmol.*, 106, 1605, 1988.
28. **Unterman, S. R., Rootman, D. S., Hill, J. M., Parelman, J. J., Thompson, H. W., and Kaufman, H. E.**, Collagen shield drug delivery: therapeutic concentrations of tobramycin in the rabbit cornea and aqueous humor, *J. Cataract Refract. Surg.*, 14, 500, 1988.
29. **Phinney, R. B., Schwartz, S. D., Lee, D. A., and Mondino, B. J.**, Collagen-shield delivery of gentamicin and vancomycin, *Arch. Ophthalmol.*, 106, 1599, 1988.
30. **Sawusch, M. R., O'Brien, T. P., Dick, J. D., and Gottsch, J. D.**, Use of collagen corneal shields in the treatment of bacterial keratitis, *Am. J. Ophthalmol.*, 106, 279, 1988.
31. **Hwang, D. G., Stern, W. H., Hwang, P. H., and MacGowan-Smith, L. A.**, Collagen shield enhancement of topical dexamethasone penetration, *Arch. Ophthalmol.*, 107, 1375, 1989.
32. **Poland, D. E. and Kaufman, H. E.**, Clinical uses of collagen shields, *J. Cataract. Refract. Surg.*, 14, 489, 1988.

Chapter 9

ACRYLIC LATEX SYSTEMS

Kevin M. Scholsky, Peter J. Tarcha, and Ann Hsu

TABLE OF CONTENTS

I. INTRODUCTION

The need for devices capable of administering drugs in a controlled manne
established.[1,2] Encompassed within a wide range of available drug delivery de
polymer particles in the colloidal size range. These colloidal devices include nanoc
liposomes,[4] and latex particles,[5] and have been reviewed by several different i
tors.[6,7,8] Ideally, a colloidal delivery system would transport a drug to the target site
producing an excessive immune response, release it at a controlled rate, and then bi
to nontoxic by-products capable of being metabolized or eliminated. Obviously,
all these requirements presents a difficult task. This chapter will discuss the me
preparing and characterizing acrylic latex delivery devices, as well as their advant
limitations.

In a broad sense, a colloid can be defined as a suspension of finely divided pa
a continuous phase, that are approximately 5 to 1000 Å in diameter. Due to their si
particles are difficult to filter, and do not settle out readily. A polymer colloid re
similar dispersion of polymeric particles. If the continuous phase is water, the
colloid is a conventional latex.[9] Most latexes belong to the lyophobic classification
they are synthesized using hydrophobic monomers. This is in contrast to lyophilic
which are solutions of hydrophilic polymers such as polyvinyl alcohol or methyl c
or suspensions of gel nanoparticles such as crosslinked poly(acrylamide) latexes.[10]

Due to their small size, latex particles exhibit enormous surface-to-volume ra
example, 1 ml of a latex containing 0.10 g of polymer and an average particle dia
800 nm, contains 3.56×10^{11} particles, representing a total surface area of 7.15
A^2 or 71.5 m[2].[11] Thus, the properties of latex particles are determined largely by thei
characteristics.

II. SYNTHESIS OF ACRYLIC LATEXES

A. CONVENTIONAL EMULSION POLYMERIZATION

Latex particles are prepared by the process commonly called emulsion polyme
but more correctly called latex polymerization. A typical recipe requires monome
persing medium (usually water, which can contain surfactants), and an initiator.
of polymerization usually starts in the continuous phase. Harkins was the first to
mechanism of latex particle formation.[12] A more quantitative description was later
Smith and Ewart.[13] According to these theories, latex particles are formed whe
soluble oligoradicals formed in the continuous phase during initiation, are cap
monomer-swollen micelles. Polymerization then continues, as additional monomer
into the swollen micelles from surrounding emulsified monomer droplets.

As latex particles continue to form by nucleation, and the total surface are
dispersed phase increases, additional surfactant and surface-active oligoradicals are
from the surrounding medium. This mechanism ultimately prevents formation of
ticles, as the quality of available surfactant falls below the critical micelle conce
and all newly formed oligoradicals are captured by existing particles. Fitch et al.[14,15]
a particle nucleation mechanism for surfactant-free solutions. In these systems, wate
oligoradicals, which have reached a critical chain length, homogeneously nucleate
primary polymer particles, which then combine to form larger particles. These
electrostatically self-stabilized by charged end-groups derived from the initiator,
swollen by monomer diffusing from the emulsion droplets, and continue to grow
case where nonionic stabilizers are used, stabilization is achieved by a steric mech
In view of the fact that polymerization inside the coexisting monomer emulsion dr
practically nonexistant, the term "emulsion polymerization" is somewhat a misno

TABLE 1

Experimental Conditions for Latex Synthesis

Latex no.	Reaction temp (°C)	H_2O (g)	Principal monomer (g)	Crosslinking monomer (g)	Redox initiator			Surfactant[e] (g)
					$NaHSO_3$ (g)	$K_2S_2O_8$ (g)	FAS[d] (g)	
1	30	150	4.00SA[a,f]	—	0.2500	0.5000	0.0030	0.2000
2	30	150	1.45SA[a,g]	0.145 EDA[c,g]	0.1200	0.2500	0.0020	0.2000
3	45	300	2.90SA[a,f]	0.290 EDA[c,f]	0.2400	0.5000	0.0040	0.4000
4	65	120	0.75 CA-PA[b,h]	0.120 EDA[c,h]	0.1200	0.2500	0.0020	0.5000

[a] Salicyl acrylate; [b]Chloramphenicol acrylate; [c]Ethylene diacrylate; [d]Ferrous ammonium sulfate ($\cdot 9H_2O$); [e]Sodium dodecyl sulfonate; [f]Monomer dissolved in 40 ml of acetone before addition; [g]Monomer dissolved in 20 ml of acetone before addition; [h]Monomer dissolved in 30 ml of acetone before addition

From Schlosky, K. and Fitch, R. M., Controlled release of pendant bioactive materials from acrylic polymer colloids, *J. Controlled Release*, 3, 87, 1986. With permission.

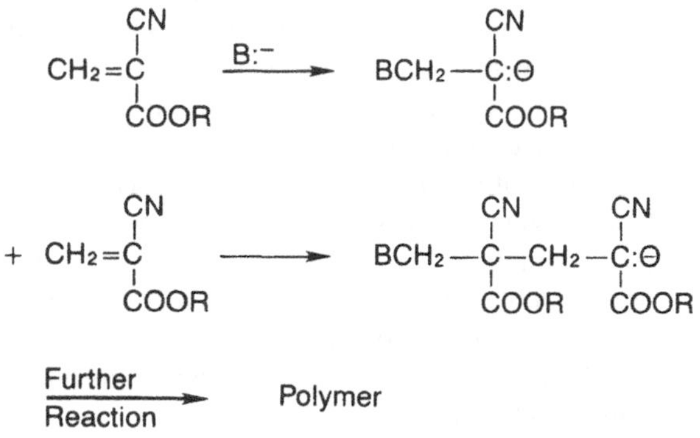

FIGURE 1. Mechanism of anionic polymerization of cyanoacrylate.

A typical latex polymerization procedure uses a stirred (100 to 300 rpm) vessel which is purged free of oxygen and maintained under an inert atmosphere. The flask is charged with deoxygenated distilled water, which may contain a surfactant and one or more components of an initiator system. Monomer(s) are added either in bulk or dropwise after the polymerization has begun. The reaction can be initiated by adding the complementary components of a redox initiator system, or by heating if a thermal initiator is used. Table I shows some experimental conditions for latex polymerizations of salicyl acrylate and chloramphenicol acrylate for use in controlled release systems.[5]

There has been considerable interest in the use of polycyanoacrylates as possible biodegradable drug carriers. Their synthesis is fairly straightforward, and the mechanism is presumed to be an anionic polymerization, when performed under slightly acidic to neutral conditions in water (Figure 1). The stabilizing effect of the electron-withdrawing cyano and ester moieties permits a weak Lewis base such as water to serve as the initiator for the anionic polymerization reaction. Adjustment of the pH to basic greatly accelerates the polymerization.[17] Typically a 0.01 N hydrochloric acid solution is used initially as the continuous phase, to which a nonionic stabilizer such as polysorbate 20, dissolved at 0.5 wt%, is added. The cyanoacrylate monomer is then added with stirring at room temperature, and allowed to react for several hours. Subsequently, the pH is raised to 7.0 by addition of

base and the reaction is allowed to continue for several additional hours, during w
a polymer colloid is formed. Detailed synthetic methods can be found in the w
Egakey and Speiser,[18] Couvreur et al.,[19] and others.

Methods for forming nanocapsules have been described in the work of Al Khou
et al.[20] Their procedure involves the injection through a fine tube of an oil phase,
an oil such as Miglyol (a coconut oil), ethanol, isobutylcyanoacrylate, and dr
magnetically stirred aqueous phase, containing a nonionic surfactant. During thi
the nanocapsules are formed immediately. Their method provides a means of enc
lipophilic drugs into a cyanoacrylate-based carrier.

B. NONAQUEOUS DISPERSIONS AND INVERSE PHASE LATEX POLYMERIZATION

Polymer colloids can also be prepared as nonaqueous dispersions (NADs).[21]
persions differ from conventional latexes in that an organic solvent is used as the
phase, and a nonionic surfactant is used in place of a typical ionic surfactant. Poly
proceeds via homogeneous nucleation, and the resulting particles are stabilized
mechanism.[16] Aqueous latexes can be prepared from their nonaqueous dispersion cc
by serum replacement methods such as centrifugation and washing, or by dialysis
the latter method requires that the dialysis membrane not be attacked by the solven
dialysis units should prove useful in this regard.

The technique of inverse phase latex polymerization is used to produce late
composed of normally water-soluble polymers. The monomers, which may inclu
linking agent, are dissolved in water, and this aqueous solution is dispersed into
phase with the aid of a nonionic surfactant. The reaction is then initiated using wa
or oil-soluble free-radical initiators, and polymerization occurs either inside the w
droplet or homogeneously in the oil phase. The resulting latex usually exhibits a
broader particle size distribution than is typically produced by conventional latex
ization methods.

Birrenbach and Speiser[22] have prepared latexes comprised of copolymers of
and *N,N'*-methylenebisacrylamide using such a technique. Sjoholm and Edman[2]
polyacrylamide latexes for *in vivo* studies by the procedure of Ekman and Sjoho
method employs an aqueous phase initiator and produces a polydisperse latex with
particle diameter of 0.2 to 0.3 μm. Polyacrylamide latexes can also be polyme
oil-soluble initiators such as azobisisobutylnitrile. A typical method, derived from
of Visioli,[25] was found to work well in our experience, and can be seen schem
Figure 2. This method has been used to produce a poly(*N*-vinyl pyrrolidinone) l

El Samaligy et al.[27] synthesized water-containing nanocapsules by first emulsif
into a (4:1) cyclohexane-chloroform mixture containing 5% Arlacel A. A separa
of the same organic solvent, containing a measured amount of cyanoacrylate, was
to the emulsified system and was stirred with a magnetic stirrer. This technique
means of encapsulating water-soluble drugs.

C. PSEUDO-LATEXES

Another category of polymer colloid is the so-called pseudo-latex, develope
derhoff et al.[28] These dispersions are prepared by first dissolving polymers in
solvent which is then emulsified in a continuous, aqueous phase. The organic
then stripped off, leaving a solvent-free, aqueous polymeric dispersion. Alterna
polymer can be dissolved in water and emulsified in an organic, continuous pha
technique allows for the preparation of a wide variety of polymer colloids which are
of being formed by conventional emulsion polymerization techniques. For exampl
has prepared cellulose acetate hydrogen phthalate pseudo-latexes by such a me

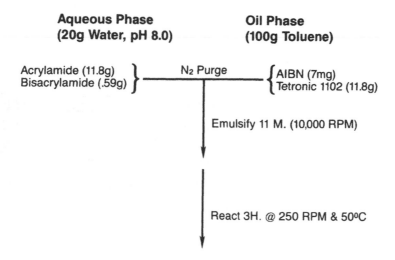

Aqueous Phase
(20g Water, pH 8.0)

Oil Phase
(100g Toluene)

Acrylamide (11.8g)
Bisacrylamide (.59g)

N₂ Purge

AIBN (7mg)
Tetronic 1102 (11.8g)

Emulsify 11 M. (10,000 RPM)

React 3H. @ 250 RPM & 50ºC

FIGURE 2.   Inverse emulsion polymerization.

particles were used to administer pilocarpine HCl into the lachrimal fluid of the eye as a possible treatment for glaucoma. Gurny et al.[30] have also used this method to prepare biodegradable latexes comprised of poly-*d,l*-lactic acid.

III. LATEX PURIFICATION AND CHARACTERIZATION

After synthesis, latex particles typically need to be purified to remove unreacted monomer, surfactant, initiator fragments, and soluble oligomeric ions. This can be done using dialysis, ion-exchange, centrifugation and washing, ultrafiltration, or a combination of the above.

A. DIALYSIS
Hollow-fiber dialysis can be performed by circulating the latex outside the hollow fiber bundle, while passing distilled water inside the fibers in a countercurrent direction as seen in Figure 3. Dialysis is quite effective at removing the bulk of electrolyte impurities, with the capability of removing up to 95% within several hours.[31] The extent of purification can be determined by measuring the conductivity of the dialysis effluent, which decreases as the latex is purified. Dialysis has been used for the quantitative removal of electrolytes and surfactants from poly(butylcyanoacrylate) nanoparticles.[18]

B. ION EXCHANGE
To remove trace levels of impurities often present in a latex, it is customary to follow dialysis by treatment with ion-exchange resins. This can be done using a mixed bed of resins such as Dowex 50W-X4 (cation) and Dowex 1-X4 (anion) exchange resin in their hydrogen and hydroxyl counterion forms, respectively. Ion exchange is performed by shaking a mixture of the latex and resins for at least 1 h, using a fivefold excess of resin based on the expected amount of electrolyte present. An exhaustive cleaning procedure is used to purify the resins prior to use,[32] since unconditioned resins contain fragments of uncrosslinked polyelectrolyte, which are leachable and can contaminate the latex. After ion exchange, the purified latex can be freed from the resin by passing it through prewashed glass wool.

C. CENTRIFUGATION
Centrifugation followed by washing is a rather labor-intensive method for purifying latexes. By this method, the particles are sedimented under the influence of a centrifugal

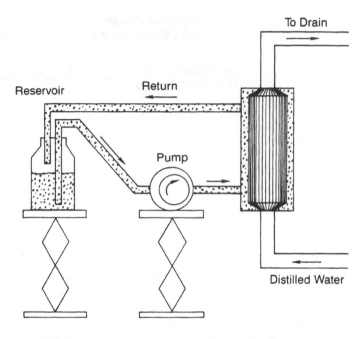

FIGURE 3.   Schematic of continuous dialysis of latex suspensions.

field, the strength of which is chosen based on particle size. Typical values in the la
range from 5,000 to 30,000 G for 10 to 60 min. After a plug forms, the supernate
contains the majority of soluble impurities, is decanted and replaced with pure
solvent. The latex particles are then redispersed mechanically or with the aid of ultr
and the process is repeated. Centrifugation and washing was used by Harmia et
purify 98 nm polybutylcyanoacrylate nanoparticles prior to absorption of pilocarp
particles were centrifuged at 30,000 rpm and 10°C for 1 h (Du Pont Instruments,
OTD75). The sediment was separated and redispersed in a mixture of water and
(1:1), and the process was repeated three times.

This method is especially useful for dispersing into water a colloid originally syr
in an organic solvent. A solvent miscible with both the original continuous phase a
is usually used as an intermediate vehicle in the process. This method of solvent e
was used by Tarcha et al.[26] to prepare polyacrylamide and poly(*N*-vinyl pyrrolidinone
from dispersions originally prepared in toluene. First, the nonionic surfactants, u
monomer, and initiators were removed by centrifugation and washing with fresh
Then *N*-methyl pyrrolidinone was substituted for the toluene, and finally, water w
Dialysis with pure water was used to remove final traces of the intermediate solve

D. ULTRAFILTRATION

Ultrafiltration is a process in which a semipermeable membrane separates the
liquid sample (macromolecular solution or colloidal suspension) from the effluen
which may contain soluble impurities. In laboratory scale units, the sample is circu
one side of the membrane in either a turbulent flow or in a direction tangenti
membrane surface, so as to prevent build-up of a cake which can reduce the flov
the permeate. A membrane, which retains the latex particles and allows electrol
other soluble molecules to pass through, must be used. Purification is achieved by co
replacing the permeate's volume with fresh solvent. Such a system can also be
increase the concentration of a suspension. Since latexes are often destabilizec
application of shear, precautions should be taken to insure maximum colloidal stabil

circulating pumps are used in the system.[34] Ultrafiltration has seen substantial use in the large-scale disposal of colloidal waste,[35] and laboratory-scale units have recently become available. It is expected that this technique will find increased application in future colloidal drug delivery research.

E. SIMPLE FILTRATION

Purification of cyanoacrylate polymer colloids and nanocapsules is usually done by filtration through a sintered glass funnel.[27,36,37] The use of a 0.8 μm filter was also reported for nanocapsules.[38] However, it should be noted that simple filtration will not eliminate surfactants or unreacted monomers. Thus, it is surprising that so many studies, both *in vivo* and *in vitro*, have been reported using polycyanoacrylates without any apparent purification or analysis of residuals. This is likely due to the fact that removal of the stabilizing agents usually results in particle aggregation.[39]

F. DETERMINATION OF PARTICLE SIZE DISTRIBUTION

Characterization of the latex particle size and its distribution can be made by a variety of methods, including transmission and scanning electron microscopy, and light scattering. Quasielastic light scattering is rapidly replacing conventional light-scattering methods for particle size measurements, since commercially available instruments now eliminate the labor-intensive, angular-dependent measurements that were once the standard method. Quasielastic light scattering monitors the time-frequency fluctuations of light in a suspension, which is the result of the constant change in particle position due to Brownian motion. The velocity of motion is related to the diffusion constant of the particle, which is in turn related to the hydrodynamic particle size. This method works best for monodisperse systems; to date, systems are not available which can accurately determine more than a bimodal size distribution.

Absolute distributions can be accurately determined using transmission electron microscopy. However, the primary drawback of this technique is that the sample must first be dried, and the images observed may not accurately reflect the true morphology of the suspension. To reduce the likelihood that the particles will degrade under the electron beam, and hence give a false image of their diameter, the dried preparation should be shadowed with carbon at a defined angle, prior to examination. Size measurements are then made of the shadows, not of the actual particle images. Figure 4 shows latex particles shadowed using a platinum-carbon deposition method.[40,41] Alternatively, latex particles can be stained with phosphotungstic acid. Upon drying, the electron-dense stain concentrates around the circumference of the particle, and greatly increases the contrast and stability of the image. Figure 5 shows a transmission electron micrograph of a 126 nm chloramphenicol acrylate latex prepared using this staining technique.[41]

G. DETERMINATION OF SURFACE CHARGE DENSITY AND POLYMER DEGRADATION

The surface concentration of titratable groups, such as amines, carboxylic acids, thiols, phosphates, and sulfates, etc., can be determined using conductometric or potentiometric titration methods. The latex must first be purified so that the solution phase and weakly bound species will not contribute to the analysis. In addition, the particle size and solids content must be known. It is advisable to purge the suspension with nitrogen prior to titration. Examples of such analysis methods are found in numerous papers[4,42,43] and have proved useful for the study of polymer degradation[44] and polymer colloid pro-drug hydrolysis.[5]

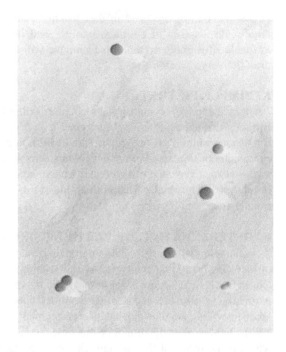

FIGURE 4.   Transmission electron micrograph of carbon-shadowed latex particles. Average particle size is 70 nm. (From Scholsky, K., unpublished results, 1982. With permission.)

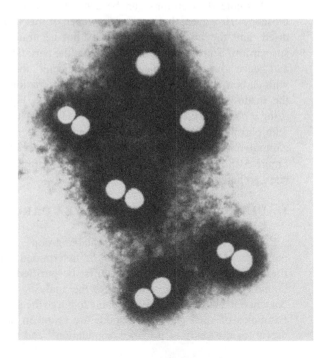

FIGURE 5.   Transmission electron micrograph of chloramphenicol acrylate latex illustrating the results of staining with phosphotungstic acid. Average particle size is 126 nm.

TABLE 2
Degradation Rates of Cyanoacrylate Polymers at 37°C

Poly-alkyl cyano acrylate side chain	Mn	Degradation rate 10^{-10}kg m^{-2} sec^{-1}	pH
Ethyl	1332	10.56	7.88
Ethyl	1332	7.96	7.40
Ethyl	1332	5.33	6.81
Ethyl	1332	3.27	5.97
n-Butyl	894	1.507	7.88
n-Butyl	894	0.686	6.99
n-Butyl	894	0.176	5.97
n-Hexyl	1017	1.105	7.88
n-Hexyl	1017	0.384	6.99
n-Hexyl	1017	0.071	5.97

From Vezin, W. R. and Florence, A. T., *In-vitro* degradation rates of biodegradable poly-n-alkyl cyanoacrylates, *Pharm. Pharmacol.*, 30, 5P, 1978. With permission.

IV. CHEMICAL AND BIOLOGICAL DEGRADATION OF CYANOACRYLATE

Vezin and Florence[45] showed that polycyanoacrylate degradation increases with pH and decreases with the alkyl side-chain length (Table 2). Relatively little information has been published on the degradation mechanism of polycyanoacrylate particles, however, a detailed study of both chemical and enzymatic degradation of polyisobutylcyanoacrylate nanoparticles was prepared by Lenearts et al.[44] They studied the reaction *in vitro* at pH 7, 10.5, and 12, and analyzed the degradation products by gas chromatography and automatic titration using a pH stat. After 24 h at pH 7, formaldehyde was detected corresponding to 5% of theory, if the chains were to quantitatively degrade to formaldehyde and butyl-1-cyanoacetate. During the same time period at pH 12, formaldehyde was detected at 7% of theory, and the chains became 94% hydrolyzed, as verified by the amount of base needed to maintain constant pH. Proposed degradation mechanisms are shown in Figure 6.

Enzymatic degradation was studied in a phosphate-buffered (0.05 N, pH 7) iso-osmolar sucrose solution containing various concentrations of rat liver microsomes as seen in Figure 7. Once again, it was found that, for the most part, the chains remain intact, and that pendant group hydrolysis is the predominant degradation pathway. By this mechanism, water-soluble polymer chains are produced which may be eliminated from the body if their molecular weights are sufficiently low. Couvreur et al.[19] synthesized polyisobutylcyanoacrylate nanoparticles comprised of polymer chains with molecular weights of 500 to 1000, within the size range for renal excretion.

V. DRUG LOADING

A. POLYCYANOACRYLATE LATEXES AND NANOCAPSULES

Loading of polycyanoacrylate particles has been performed using three different methods; *in situ* polymerization of the monomer in the presence of drug, sorption of drug into preformed particles, and encapsulation. A typical example of an *in situ* procedure, using doxorubicin as a model, employed an aqueous reaction medium with 1% and 0.075% of monomer and drug, respectively. After completion of the reaction, 89 ± 5% of the added drug was found to be associated with the particles.[46] Other examples of drug incorporation via *in situ* polymerization have been tabulated by Couvreur,[47] and are given in Table 3.

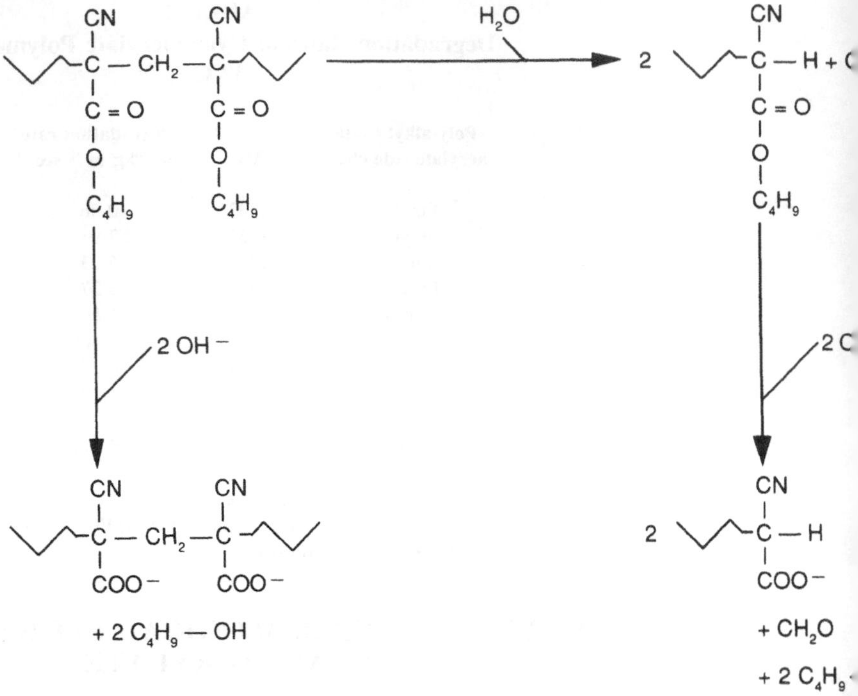

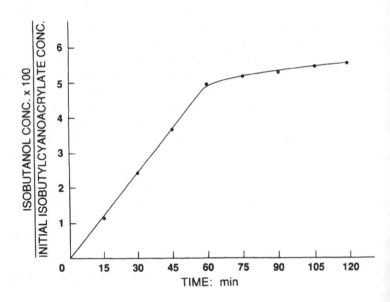

FIGURE 6.   Proposed degradation mechanism of cyanoacrylates. (From Lenearts, V. et al., Degr of poly(isobutyl cyanoacrylate) nanoparticles, *Biomaterials*, 5, 65, 1984. With permission.)

FIGURE 7.   Isobutanol produced by ester hydrolysis of poly(isobutyl cyanoacrylate) nanoparticles in the presence of rat liver microsomes (1.88 mg protein/ml) as a function of time. (From Lenearts, V. et al., Degradation of poly(isobutyl cyanoacrylate) nanoparticles, *Biomaterials*, 5, 65, 1984. With permission.)

TABLE 3
Drug Payload on (PACA) Nanoparticles

Drug	Conc in the polymerization medium (μg/ml)	Absorption (%)				
		PMCA	PECA	PIBCA or PBCA	PIHCA or PHCA	Ref.
Doxorubicin	1,000	—	—	94		7
Dactinomycin	55	92	86	70	—	53
Vinblastine	1,000	58	66	46	—	53
Vincristine	300	—	—	57	—	16
5-Fluorouracil	10,000	—	—	ND	—	56
Methotrexate	100	25	24	—·	—	8
Penicilline V	1,000	50	37	—	—	15
Ampicillin	1,000	—	—	72	78	29
Vidarabine	125	—	—	17	70	75
Insulin	12 IU	40	44	40	—	62
Dehydroemetine	1,000	—	—	—	81	68
Vincamine	2,000	—	—	—	42	55
Triamcinolone	400	79	—	—	—	31
Pilocarpine	5,000	—	—	20	—	72
Progestrone	12	—	—	99	—	74

Note: PACA = Polyalkylcyanoacrylate; PMCA = polymethylcyanoacrylate; PECA = polyethylcyanoacrylate; PIBCA = polyisobutylcyanoacrylate; PBCA = polybutylcyanoacrylate; PIHCA = polyisohexylcyanoacrylate; PHCA = polyhexylcyanoacrylate: ND = not determined.

Several studies have been performed to measure the effect of pH, temperature, ionic strength, stabilizer concentration, and other factors on the sorption of various model drug compounds. El Egakey and Speiser[18] demonstrated Langmuir sorption behavior for Verapamil hydrochloride with poly(butylcyanoacrylate). Illum et al.,[37] using rose bengal as a model with poly(butylcyanoacrylate) nanoparticles, showed that under certain conditions, 35% by weight loading is possible. They also made a distinction between drug loading by adsorption, and drug loading by incorporation, showing that much higher levels can be obtained by the latter method.

Insulin, dissolved in Miglyol, was encapsulated by isobutylcyanoacrylate by Damge et al.[38] using the method of Al Khouri Fallouh.[20] The amount of insulin per unit weight of nanocapsule was not given, but suspensions of nanocapsules containing 2 to 20 U (U = international unit) per ml were used in their studies.

El Samaligy et al.[27] showed that greater than 50% of the doxorubicin HCl, dissolved in water as a 0.50% solution, could be encapsulated. In addition, the level of drug entrapped could be increased by increasing the wall thickness of the nanocapsule.

B. POLYACRYLAMIDE LATEX LOADING

Latexes made from crosslinked, water-soluble polymers such as polyacrylamide and poly(N-vinylpyrrolidinone), exhibit unique properties, since they are sterically self-stabilized in water and certain organic solvents, presumably by the attached loops and tails of the base polymer. This gives them the ability to be reconstituted as a suspension of singlet particles, even after freeze-drying. The usual precautions associated with electrostatically-stabilized colloids, such as avoidance of organic solvents, high ionic strength continuous phases, and freezing do not generally apply to these latexes.

In view of these properties, the trapping of water-insoluble drugs inside the particle is possible. For example, Tarcha et al.[26] loaded a polyacrylamide latex with amphotericin B to a level of 67 μmg/mg with respect to latex solids. By this procedure Amphotericin B (10

mg) was first dissolved in 0.100 ml of morpholine. This solution was then added
of freeze-dried polyacrylamide latex (assumed to be 12% crosslinked, based on
linking monomer used) and stirred mechanically to form a fairly rigid paste, w
allowed to equilibrate overnight. Then 2.0 ml of diethyl ether was added to prec
drug and extract out the morpholine. The sample existed as a coarse suspension af
and was allowed to settle by gravity. The supernate was removed and the ethe
procedure was repeated. Finally, the ether was removed from the particles by ai

Using the method described, it is impossible to completely sequester all of the
drug inside the particles, since there will always be some solution present on
surfaces of the particles. In fact, observation of a dried sample under a pola
microscope revealed the presence of some free drug crystals. Indirect evidence
portion of the drug was entrapped inside the particle matrix was provided by th
gently centrifugation of the suspension in ether produced a uniformly-colored, ye

Water-soluble proteins can also be trapped inside these types of water-swella
and microparticles by *in situ* polymerization, as demonstrated by Ekman and .
Using this technique, they immobilized L-asparaginase inside polyacrylamide **r**
cles.[48] The enzyme was dissolved in phosphate buffer along with the monomers
in-oil emulsion was then formed in toluene/chloroform, and the reaction was c
using standard inverse emulsion polymerization techniques (Section IIB). The
biological properties of the immobilized enzyme were found to remain intact.

VI. *IN VITRO* RELEASE OF DRUGS FROM SYNTHET LATEXES

The kinetics of *in vitro* drug delivery can be studied by either static or dynami
Gurney et al.[30] have described a static method of monitoring drug release from bio
latexes. By this method, a dialysis bag containing the suspension of the radiola
was placed in a magnetically stirred Krebs buffer maintained at 37°C. Samples of
solution (0.5 ml) were then removed periodically and analyzed using a scintillatic

Scholsky and Fitch[5] have also described static methods for monitoring dru
from acrylic latex particles in phosphate buffered saline at pH 7.4 and 37°C. By th
samples of the suspension were removed periodically and flocculated by mixir
equivalent volume of a high ionic strength solution. The mixture was then fi
analyzed using ultraviolet or visible spectroscopy. A detailed description of **r**
kinetics was later published.[49]

Scholsky and Warner[50] have described an automated device for measuring d
kinetics from acrylic latex particles in dynamic environments. A simplified sche
gram of the device is shown in Figure 8. In this device, the latex, maintained at
temperature and pH, is circulated in a loop (1) through the outside section of a h
dialysis unit (B) by means of a peristaltic pump (D). Pure buffer at the same te
is circulated in a countercurrent fashion through the inside of the dialysis unit by
a second loop and pump. As the drug is released from the latex particles, it dif
loop (1) across the dialysis membranes into loop (2). Loop (2) then carries th
through a flow cell (F) inside a UV-visible spectrophotometer (A), which then m
concentration and plots it in real time by means of a Turbo Pascal software rout
9 shows a plot of the release kinetics of salicylic acid from polysalicylacrylate late
at 37°C and various pH values, as determined using this device.

For polycyanoacrylate latexes, a good correlation has been observed between
of drug and the degradation rate of the particles. Using ^{14}C-labeled nanopartic
with [3H] actinomycin, Lenearts et al.[44] observed this correlation for all pH val
namely, pH = 4.9, 7, and 9 (Figure 10). This observation suggests that the drug is

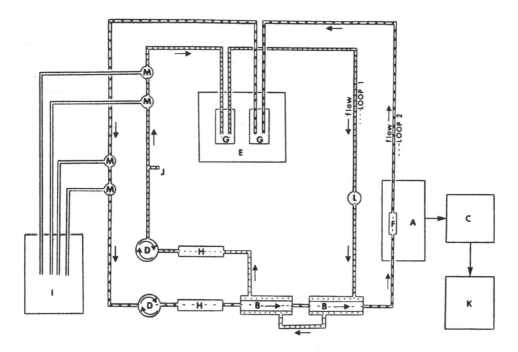

FIGURE 8. Schematic diagram of automated device for studying drug release kinetics. (A) UV-visible spectrophotometer; (B) hollow fiber dialysis cartridges; (C) IBM personal computer; (D) peristaltic pump; (E) thermostatically controlled temperature bath; (F) quartz flow cell; (G) debubbling chambers; (H) rotameter; (I) cleaning reservoir; (J) injection port; (K) Digital VAX mainframe computer; (L) thermocouple; (M) three-way valve.

distributed throughout the particle matrix. Consistent with the fact that longer chain length results in slower degradation, Couvreur et al.[51] showed that in calf serum at 37°C, using [³H] dactinomycin, polymethylcyanoacrylate was degraded almost entirely after 18 h, while polyethylcyanoacrylate retained 50% of the drug after 2 d. These same investigators also showed that for the release of dactinomycin from polymethyl- and polyethylcyanoacrylate particles, a longer side chain results in slower release. The same effect of alkyl chain length was reported by other research groups as well.[52,44] Treating diffusion in the absence of degradation, Vezin and Florence[53] found that for five model compounds (salicylic acid, *p*-nitroaniline, trinitrophenol, procaine, and fluphenazine), diffusivity increased with longer side-chain length, as seen in Table 4.

The release of rose bengal from dextran 70 stabilized polybutyl (2-cyanoacrylate) nanoparticles, loaded by adsorption or incorporation, exhibited biphasic rates.[37] Figure 11 shows an initial fast release, followed by a slower first-order release region. The profiles were described using a biexponential function:

$$P_1 = Ae^{-at} + Be^{-bt},$$

where P_1 is the concentration of compound remaining in the nanoparticle at time t. The constants A and B, and the two rate constants a and b, can be determined from the first-order plots of the data. A value for the constant [a] of 3.6 min^{-1} was reported for adsorbed rose bengal, while 1.2 min^{-1} was determined for incorporated dye. Both adsorbed and incorporated rose bengal exhibited a value of 1.1 h^{-1} for the constant [b].

El-Samaligy and Rohdewald[54] studied the *in vitro* release of drugs from polyacrylamide microbeads. Tetracycline HCl and theophylline were entrapped in the beads by a water-in-

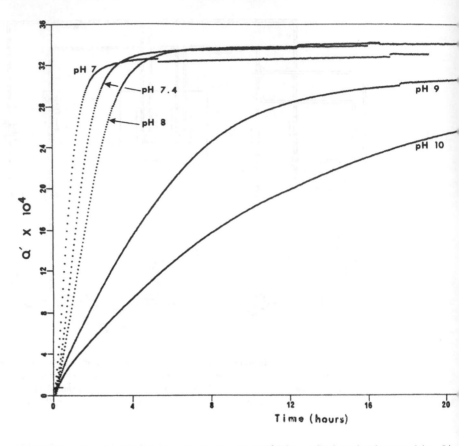

FIGURE 9.   Plot of release kinetics of salicylic acid at 37°C from salicyl acrylate latex particles. Q′
of drug released per gram of polymer.

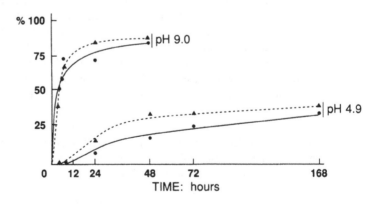

FIGURE 10.   Quantities (%) of ^{3}H (▲) and ^{14}C (●) released from ^{3}H-actinomycin-
D loaded ^{14}C-poly(isobutyl cyanoacrylate) nanoparticles as a function of time at
pH 9.0 and 4.9. (From Lenearts, V. et al., Degradation of poly(isobutyl cyanoacrylate) nano particles, *Biomaterials*, 5, 65, 1984. With permission.)

oil emulsion polymerization. Drug release in acid and alkaline media was studied
initial release was observed due to dissolution of drug particles dried on the m
surface, or initial diffusion through cracks and pores. Thereafter, two types of release
were observed, consistent with drug pH/solubility properties. In an acid medium, tetr
HCl (which is soluble in acidic media) showed a first-order release mechanism:

TABLE 4
Diffusion Coefficients at Zero
Concentration (D₀) in Two Poly-
***N*-Alkyl Cyanoacrylates**

| | $\log_{10} D_0$, m^2s^{-1} | |
| | poly-alkyl cyano-acrylate at 37°C | |
Compound	*n*-Hexyl-	*n*-Butyl-
Salicylic acid	-11.57	-13.47
p Nitroaniline	12.24	-13.72
Trinitrophenol	-13.43	-14.66
Procaine	-13.29	—
Fluphenazine	-14.40	-15.72

From Venzin, W. R. and Florence, A. T.,
Diffusion of small molecules in poly-*n*-alkyl-
cyanoacrylate, *J. Pharm. Pharmacol.*, 30, 20,
1978. With permission.

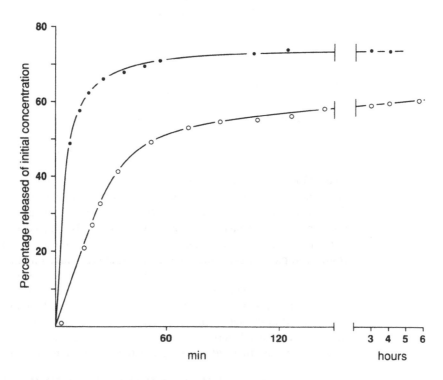

FIGURE 11. Release profile for rose bengal (RB) adsorbed onto (3.1 mg RB/100 mg nanoparticles) ●—●, and incorporated into (2.0 mg RB/100 mg nanoparticles) o—o poly(butyl 2-
cyanoacrylate) nanoparticles stabilized with dextran 70 (number of replicates = 2), from Illum,
L. et al., Evaluation of carrier capacity and release characteristics of poly(butyl-2-cyanoacrylate)
nanoparticles, *Int. J. Pharm.*, 30, 7, 1986. With permission.)

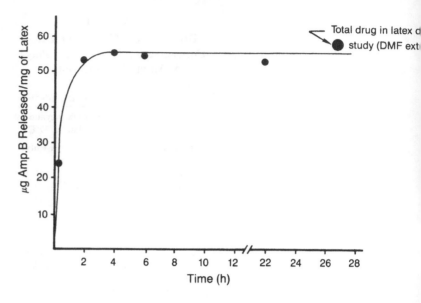

FIGURE 12.   *In vitro* dissolution in dog plasma of amphotericin B in 12% cross-linked polyacry
latex.

$$\log Q_t = \log Q_o - (kt)/2.303,$$

where Q_t is the amount of the drug remaining at time t; Q_o is the total drug amo
is the first-order dissolution rate constant. In alkaline media, tetracycline release
vs. the square root of time according to the Higuchi equation[55]:

$$Q = [D \; \epsilon/\tau(2A-C_s)C_s t]^{1/2},$$

where Q is the amount of drug released per unit area at time t; D is the diffusion
of the drug in the dissolution medium; C_s is the solubility of the drug in the me
the porosity of the matrix; τ is the tortuosity of the matrix; and A is the total amc
drug present in the matrix. Theophylline release also agreed with the Higuchi re
in both acid and alkaline media. This equation can be used to describe the releas
from hydrophobic, insoluble, and hydrophilic crosslinked matrices.[56]

The release of amphotericin B from polyacrylamide latex particles prepar
laboratory[26] was determined in dog plasma. At specified time points, with consta
at 37°C, plasma samples were withdrawn and centrifuged, and the released amph
was assayed in the supernantant by HPLC or spectrophotometically. The results
that release of amphotericin B from the polyacrylamide particle can be approx
monoexponential first-order release kinetics, with a rate constant of 0.52 h^{-1} (F

VII. *IN VIVO* DRUG DELIVERY

Latex systems have been widely investigated for delivery of parentera
tions,[26,46,48,57,58] oral protein drugs,[38] drug release from implants,[59,60] and ocula
tions.[29,33,61] The unfavorable distribution and elimination properties of the late
have precluded their use for *in vivo* drug products.

A. DISTRIBUTION

Latex and other nano/microparticle delivery systems introduced into the
system are rapidly cleared by the reticuloendothelial system (RES). Most of the late

TABLE 5
Lung and Liver Concentration of
Radioactivity 4 h after i.v.
Administration of
[^{14}C]Polyisobutylcyanoacrylate
Nanoparticles (2.5 μCi) to Healthy (A)
and Tumor-Bearing Mice (B)

	Lung	Liver	Lung/Liver
A	10.7 ± 1.9	26.4 ± 5.0	0.41 ± 0.13
B	67.9 ± 10.5	12.9 ± 1.0	5.26 ± 1.11

Note: The values represent the mean and the SD of
7 animals in each group.

From Girislain, L. et al., Pharmacokinetics and distribution of a biodegradable drug-carrier, *Int. J. Pharm.*,
15, 355, 1983. With permission.

are found deposited in the liver (Kupffer cells), spleen, bone marrow, and lung. Sjoholm and Edman[23] found that, after the intravenous (i.v.) or intraperitoneal (i.p.) injection of polyacrylamide latex particles (0.25 to 0.30 μm) in mouse and rat, the particles were cleared rapidly from circulation ($t_{0.5} \sim$ 40 min), and approximately 80% were deposited in the liver and spleen. Unless liver and spleen are the sites of therapy, this unfavorable distribution property is a main disadvantage of nano/microparticle drug delivery systems.[62]

Using polystyrene particles as the model system, Kanke et al.[63] demonstrated that particles smaller than 3 to 5 μm were freely cleared from the lung capillary bed and relocated in the phagocytic cells of the liver, bone marrow, spleen, and kidney. Their studies showed that 7 to 12 μm appears to be the critical size limit for nondeformable particles to pass through the pulmonary vascular bed.

The effects of administration routes on the distribution of micro/nanoparticles have also been studied.[63,64] Kanke et al.[63] showed that distribution and clearance patterns of polystyrene particles of various sizes (3 to 12 μm) after intra-arterial administration were not significantly different from that of intravenous administration. Radiolabeled cyanoacrylate nanoparticles (< 1 μm), administered intravenously,[64] were rapidly cleared from the circulation system ($t_{0.5}$ = 6.63 min) and concentrated in the RES. Nearly all of the radioactivity disappeared in less than 7 d. These same particles, administered subcutaneously or intramuscularly, concentrated in the gut wall and avoided the liver or spleen.

Grislain et al.[64] also showed that polyisobutyl cyanoacrylate particles were localized in the lung of Lewis Lung carcinoma-bearing mice, but not in the lung of healthy mice (Table 5). However, Gipps et al.[65] investigated the distribution of polyhexyl cyanoacrylate nano-particles in mice bearing human osteosarcoma, and found insignificant localization in the tumor site (generally <1% of the injected dose). They also noticed that the accumulation of radioactivity into tumor sites was variable, depending on size, viability, and vascularization of the tumor tissues. The mechanisms of transfer of nanoparticles into tumor tissues are still unknown.

Several attempts to modify the distribution pattern of microparticles have been reported. Blocking of the RES with inert macromolecules or blank particles prior to the administration of therapeutic microparticles was investigated.[66,67,68] This method is not desirable because repeated RES suppression may lead to impairment of normal RES functions. Coating of particles to increase surface hydrophilicity and decrease adhesion between macroparticles and phagocytic cells via steric repulsion[69,70,71] has been reported, but inconsistent results

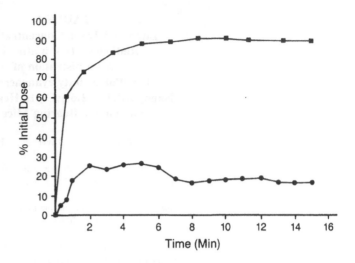

FIGURE 13.   Activity-time profiles for liver/spleen region after administration of [^{131}I]-labeled polystyrene microspheres; (■) uncoated, and (●)
poloxamer 407-coated. (From Illum, L and Davis, S. S., Targeting of colloidal particles to the bone marrow, *Life Sci.*, 40, 1553, 1987. With permission.)

have been observed. Illum and Davis[69] were able to reduce the distribution of pol
beads (60 nm) to the liver by coating the beads with a polyethylene oxide/polyp
oxide block copolymer (Poloxamer 407) (Figure 13). After modification, these
were rapidly taken up by the bone marrow, instead of the liver, as compared to un
particles. Further increases in the hydrophilicity of microparticles by coating the
with an even more hydrophilic polymer, Poloxamine 908 (Illum et al.[70]), resulted in
carrier circulation in the vascular compartment with little uptake by the RES (Fig
As shown in Figure 14, similar activities were obtained in the liver and in the liv
pool (which was determined to be 25% of circulating activity). In contrast, Dougla
showed that the distribution pattern of polybutyl 2-cyanoacrylate particles coated
block copolymer Poloxamer 338 or Poloxamine 908 was not significantly differe
uncoated particles when measured in rabbits (Figure 15).

The tissue distribution of cytotoxic drugs may be modified by adsorption or er
Attaching ligands to the surface of microparticles to induce receptor-media
cesses,[72,73] or coating particles with monoclonal antibodies[74,75] have also been inve
Cartlidge et al.[72] showed that by incorporating galactosamine-terminated side ch
soluble crosslinked HPMA copolymers, the distribution of the copolymer in hep
after i.v., i.p., and subcutaneous (s.c.) administration was increased. Hepatocytes ar
to recognize galactose residues in the circulatory system. *In vivo* studies of mo
antibody-coated polyhexylcyanoacrylate particles have indicated that the total live
of the particles was not reduced.[75]

The tissue distribution of cytotoxic drugs may be modified by adsorption or er
into latex particles. Couvreur et al.[63] found that the changes occurred mainly in
distribution phase. The distribution patterns in various tissues of dactinomycin and
tine, adsorbed to polyalkylcyanoacrylate particles, were modifed initially, but we
to be similar to the respective free drug 3 h after injection. Verdun et al.[46] determ
the distribution of doxorubicin into cardiac muscles was significantly reduced when
was adsorbed or incorporated to polyisobutylcyanoacrylate nanoparticles (Figure 1

B. ELIMINATION

The elimination half-life of latex particles is a function of their susceptibilit
degradation. The elimination $t_{0.5}$ of radiolabeled polyacrylamide particles (0.25 to 0

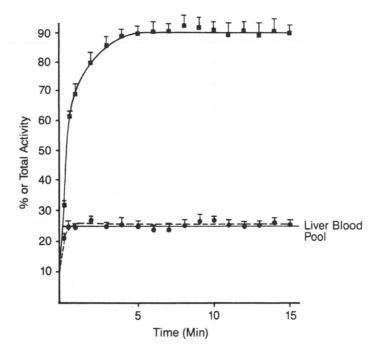

FIGURE 14. Activity-time profiles for the uptake of uncoated and poloxamine 908-coated particles (60 nm) in the liver (number of relicates — 3, mean ± standard error of mean); (■) uncoated, (●) poloxamine 908 coated. (From Illum, L. et al., The organ distribution and circulation time of intravenously injected colloidal carriers sterically stabilized with a block copolymer — Poloxamine 908, *Life Sci.*, 40, 367, 1987. With permission.)

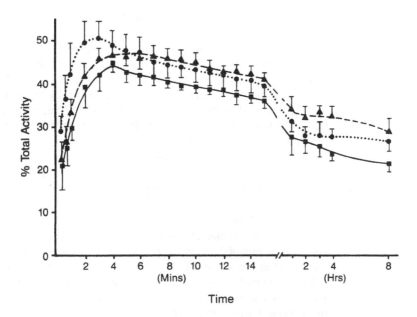

FIGURE 15. Activity-time profiles for the liver/spleen region of interest following injection of uncoated (●), poloxamer 338-coated (■), and poloxamine 908-coated (▲) polybutyl 2-cyanoacrylate nanoparticles labeled with ^{99m}Tc-dextran 10 (number of replicates = 3, bar = 1SD. (From Douglas, S. J. et al., Biodistribution of poly(butyl 2-cyanoacrylate) nanoparticles in rabbits, *Int. J. Pharm.*, 34, 145, 1986. With permission.)

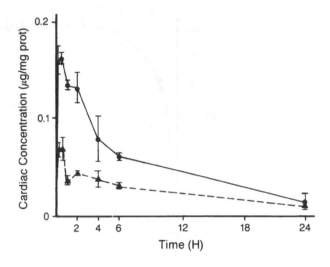

FIGURE 16.   Cardiac concentration of free (—) and nanoparticle-bound (---) doxorubicin after i.v. administration to mice (dose of drug administered: 7 mg/kg). (From Verdun, C. et al., Development of a nanoparticle controlled release formulation for human use, *J. Controlled Release*, 3, 205, 1986. With permission.)

in mouse and rat was 10 to 14 weeks in the liver and 15 to 24 weeks in the sp
i.v. and i.p. administration, respectively.[23] The extremely slow elimination of polya
particles is due to the resistance of the particles to degradation. Radioactivity
detected in the gut and gut walls 2 months after injection. It was believed that polya
particles were slowly metabolized by hydrolysis of the amide bonds yielding p
acid and ammonia. Other hypotheses, such as secretion through bile into gut,
discussed. It should be noted that in their study, the assay method could not di
parent particles from metabolites.

As discussed earlier in this chapter, the degradation rate of polycyanoacrylate
of the length of the alkyl chain. Polymethyl and polyethyl analogs degrade faste
higher alkyl analogs. Studies[36,58,62] have shown that polyalkylcyanoacrylate pa
culating in the system are also rapidly taken up by the liver and other macro
organs, degraded in the organs or in the circulation, and finally eliminated in
feces. Grislain et al.[64] showed that after i.v. administration, the plasma eliminatic
of polyisobutyl-2-cyanoacrylate nanoparticles (0.254 μm) was less than 20 min
of the radioactivity was recovered in 7 d (urine 67%, feces 27%). Kante et al.[36]
that the observed toxicity of polymethylcyanoacrylate was probably a result of
mulation of the toxic degradation products due to the fast degradation rate of the

C. *IN VIVO* USE

Edman and Sjoholm[48] used polyacrylamide particles to deliver L-asparag
enzyme was immobilized inside particles during the polymerization, and three diff
were used in the studies, i.e., 0.34, 18, and 36 μm. Compared to the untreate
solution, the biological activities of the immobilized enzyme were essentially ret
its stability was significantly improved. When administered by i.p. injection, the
the enzyme lasted significantly longer than the free enzyme solution; however
particles were taken up by the RES (2 weeks after administration), the enzyme th
unavailable to the circulating L-asparagine. Similarly, after i.v. administration
particle preparations), no improvement in bioavailability over free enzyme was
We have recently incorporated amphotericin B into polyacrylamide latex pa

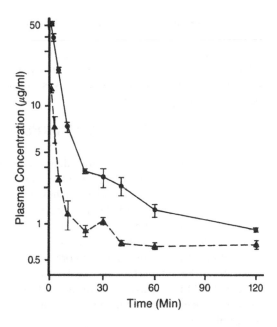

FIGURE 17. Plasma concentrations of free doxorubicin (▲) and nanoparticle-bound doxorubicin (●) after intravenous administration to mice (dose of doxorubicin administered: 7 mg/kg). (From Verdun, C. et al., Development of a nanoparticle controlled release formulation for human use, *J. Controlled Release*, 3, 205, 1986. With permission.)

to 1 μm).[26] The system was evaluated against a commercial drug product in mice infected with *Candida albicans*. The results showed that the LD_{50} of amphotericin B was improved about threefold when the drug was administered intravenously. When this system was administered subcutaneously, the ED_{50} was practically unchanged, but the LD_{50} was improved more than sixfold. The improved therapeutic index is probably due to the absence of transient high plasma concentration immediately after i.v. administration of unmodified drug.

Davis[60] showed that a polyacrylamide implant, having incorporated insulin, was able to sustain a positive effect on diabetic rats for a few weeks, when administered subcutaneously; however, modification of this delivery system to provide for biodegradability is necessary before this system can be favorably considered for parenteral use.

Due to their presumed biodegradability, considerable interest has developed in the production of polyalkylcyanoacrylates for colloidal delivery systems. Couvreur[47] recently reviewed current investigations in detail. Promising results have been obtained in several studies. For example, the therapeutic index of doxorubicin was significanly improved by encapsulating the drug in polyisobutylcyanoacrylate nanoparticles.[46] The area under the plasma concentration curve was significantly greater than that of unmodified drugs (Figure 17), and the cardiac concentration of the drug was also significantly lowered (Figure 16). Using polymethylcyanoacrylate nanoparticles as carrier for actinomycin-D, Brasseur et al.[76] also found that the drug activity toward subcutanous sarcoma in rats was improved. In addition, [75Se]Norcholestenol, bound to polybutylcyanoacrylate nanoparticles, showed prolonged $t_{0.5}$ in the rabbit compared to a commercial micellar solution.[58] Damge et al.[38] showed that insulin encapsuled in polyisobutylcyanoacrylates was orally bioavailable to a certain extent, suggesting that peptides (or proteins) may be protected from proteolytic enzymes when administered orally. Additionally, prolonged activity of the same insulin preparation

was also observed when administered subcutaneously, which is consistent with th
of Davis.[60]

Harmia et al.[33] showed that the myotic activity of pilocarpine was slightly prol
rabbits when the drug was adsorbed onto polybutylcyanoacrylate nanoparticles; ▶
no improvement in myotic acitivity was observed when the drug was incorpor∢
particles during polymerization.

VIII. ADVANTAGES AND LIMITATIONS

The development of latex drug delivery systems offers exciting benefits for t
with selected drugs. These opportunities, however, are not without significant ch
When the particle delivery system reaches circulation, a majority of the particles ar∢
taken up by the reticuloendothelial system, which leaves very little opportunity for
exert activity. Targeting to the sites of action and retaining the system in these site
as major challenges of *in vivo* use of acrylic latex systems. Another major cha∢
elimination of the carrier. Furthermore, studies have shown that a build-up of de∢
products in the cytoplasm can be potentially toxic.[36] A well-designed biodegrada∢
system should be capable of controlled release, degradation, and elimination. Tox
to the presence of residual monomers should not be a concern if careful purification
are employed.

If the above problems are overcome, a latex-based drug product can be repr
manufactured on a large scale and sterilized by autoclaving. In the case of unstab∢
the system could be filtered, lyophilized, and sterilized by radiation. The lyophili
systems can be so designed to retain their integrities, and be easily redispersed at
of administration. Due to their chemical structure, this category of delivery system ∢
is low in immunogenicity and toxicity.[77,78] The long-term potential of developin∢
latex particles into commercial drug products is quite significant.

IX. FUTURE DIRECTIONS

As mentioned earlier, one of the biggest problems facing most synthetic la∢
delivery systems is their inherent lack of biodegradability. This is especially true for
based systems. Incorporation of biodegradable units such as ester linkages into the
backbone offers a possible solution to this problem. Bailey et al.[79] have used cycl
acetal monomers to form polymers containing biodegradable ester linkages. Ba∢
suggested that under appropriate conditions such monomers could be utilized in ∢
copolymerization reactions.[80]

Another possible means of incorporating biodegradable linkages involves cop
zation of carbon dioxide into the polymer backbone. Generally CO_2 is regareded as a ▶
inert, unreactive substance. However, in 1969, Inoue et al.[81,82] demonstrated that
capable of reacting with alkelene oxides to form alternating copolymers of polyc∢
Since that time numerous other monomers have been copolymerized with CO_2, ▶
butadiene, isoprene, and ethyl vinyl ether.[83,84]

Copolymerization reactions involving CO_2 are generally done in bulk or in s∢
super-atmospheric pressure. Soga et al.[84] found that up to 23 wt% CO_2 could be
merized with ethyl vinyl ether, and the resulting polymers exhibited strong infrar∢
at 1730 and 1100 to 1300 cm^{-1}, indicative of linear ester linkages. On this basis,
reasonable that CO_2 could be copolymerized with vinylic monomers in a pressur
using emulsion polymerization techniques. High pressure emulsion polymerizat∢
niques have been used extensively for the preparation of ethylene vinyl acetat∢
copolymers. Use of similar processes offer the potential for producing acrylic la
delivery devices containing biodegradable polymer backbones.

REFERENCES

1. **Roseman, T. and Mansdorf, S., Eds.,** *Controlled Release Delivery Systems,* Marcel Dekker, New York, 1983.
2. **Julano, R.,** Controlled delivery of drugs: an overview and prospectus, in *Drug Delivery Systems,* R. Juliano, Ed., Oxford University Press, 1980.
3. **Kreuter, J.,** nanoparticles and nanocapsules — new dosage forms in the nanometer size range, *Pharm. Acta Helv.,* 53, 33, 1978.
4. **Gregoriadis, G.,** *Liposome Technolgoy,* Vol. 3, CRC Press, Boca Raton, FL, 1984.
5. **Scholsky, K. and Fitch, R. M.,** Controlled release of pendant bioactive materials from acrylic polymer colloids, *J. Controlled Release,* 3, 87, 1986.
6. **Marty, J. and Oppenheim, R.,** Colloidal systems for drug delivery, *Aust. J. Pharm. Sci.,* 6, 65, 1977.
7. **Guiot, P. and Couvreur, P.,** *Polymeric Nanoparticles and Microspheres,* CRC Press, 1986.
8. **Gurny, R.,** Controlled drug delivery with colloidal polymeric systems, *NATO ASI Ser. E.,* 106, 195, 1986.
9. **Blackley, D.,** Emulsion Polymerization, John Wiley & Sons, New York, 1975.
10. **Vanderhoff, J., Bradford, E., Tarkowski, H., Shaffer, J., and Wiley, R.,** *Adv. Chem. Ser.,* 32, 32, 1962.
11. **Singer, J. and Plotz, C.,** The latex fixation test. 1. Application to the serological diagnosis of rheumatoid arthritis, *Am. J. Med.,* 21, 888, 1956.
12. **Harkins, W.,** A general theory of emulsion polymerization, *J. Am. Chem. Soc.,* 69, 1428, 1947.
13. **Smith, W. and Ewart, R.,** Kinetics of emulsion polymerization, *J. Chem. Phys.,* 16, 592, 1049.
14. **Fitch, R., Prenosil, M., and Sprick, K.,** Mechanism of particle formation in polymer hydrosols. I. Kinetics of aqueous polymerization of methyl methacrylate, *J. Polym. Sci. Polym. Symp.,* 27, 95, 1969.
15. **Fitch, R., and Tsai, C.,** Particle formation in polymer colloids, III: Prediction of the number of particles by a homogeneous nucleation theory, in *Polymer Colloids,* R. M. Fitch, Ed., Plenum Press, New York, 1971, 73.
16. **Napper, D.,** Steric stabilization, *J. Colloid Interface Sci.,* 58, 390, 1977.
17. **Donnelly, E., Johnston, D., Pepper, D., and Dunn, D.,** Ionic and zwitterionic polymerization of *n*-alkyl 2-cyanoacrylates, *J. Polym. Sci. Polym. Lett. Ed.,* 15, 399, 1977.
18. **El Egakey, M. and Speiser, P.,** Drug loading studies on ultrafine solid carriers by sorption procedures, *Pharm. Acta Helv.,* 57, 236, 1982.
19. **Couvreur, P., Lenaerts, V., Leyh, D., Guiot, P., and Roland, M.,** Design of biodegradable poly(alkylcyanoacrylate) nanoparticles as a drug carrier, in *Microspheres and Drug Therapy, Pharmaceutical, Immunological, and Medical Aspects,* Davis, S. S., Illum, L., Mc Vie, J. G., and Tomlinson, E., Eds., Elsevier, Amsterdam, 1984.
20. **Al Khouri Fallouh, N., Robolt-Treupel, L., Fessi, H., Ph Devissaguet, J., and Puisieux, F.,** Development of a new process for the manufacture of poly(isobutylcyanoacrylate) nanocapsules, *Int. J. Pharm.,* 28, 125, 1986.
21. **Barrett, K.,** Dispersion polymerization in organic media, *Br. Polym. J.,* 5, 259, 1973.
22. **Birrenbach, G. and Speiser, P.,** Polymerized micelles and their use as adjuvants in immunotherapy, *J. Pharm. Sci.,* 65, 1763, 1976.
23. **Sjoholm, I. and Edman, P.,** Acrylic microspheres *in vivo.* I. Distribution and elimination of polyacrylamide microparticles after intravenous and intraperitoneal injection in mouse and rat, *J. Pharmacol. Exp. Ther.,* 211, 656, 1979.
24. **Ekman, B. and Sjoholm, I.,** Improved stability of proteins immobilized in microparticles prepared by a modified emulsion polymerization technique, *J. Pharm. Sci.,* 67, 693, 1978.
25. **Visioli,, D.,** Formation and Stabilization of Inverse Emulsion Polymers, Ph.D. thesis, Lehigh University, Bethlehem, PA, 1984.
26. **Tarcha, P., Misun, D., and Hsu, A.,** Unpublished results.
27. **El-Samaligy,M., Rohdewald, P., and Mahmoud, H.,** Polyalkylcyanoacrylate nanoparticles, *J. Pharm. Pharmacol.,* 38, 216, 1986.
28. **Vanderhoff, J., El-Asser, M., and Ugelstad, J.,** Polymer emulsification process, U.S. Patent 4,177,177, 1979.
29. **Gurny, R.,** Preliminaary study of prolonged acting drug delivery system for the treatment of glaucoma, *Pharm. Acta Helv.,* 56, 130, 1981.
30. **Gurny, R., Peppas, N., Harrington, D., and Banker, G.,** Development of biodegradable and injectable latices for controlled release of potent drugs, *Drug Dev. Ind. Pharm.,* 7, 1, 1981.
31. **McCarvill, W., and Fitch, R.,** The surface chemistry of polystyrene latices initiated by the persulfate/bisulfite/iron system, *J. Colloid Interface Sci.,* 67, 204, 1978.
32. **Vanderhoff, J., van den Hul, J., Tausk, R., and Overbeek, J.,** *Clean Surfaces: Their Preparation and Characterization for Interfacial Studies,* G. Goldfinger, Ed., Marcel Dekker, New York, 1970.

33. **Harmia, T., Kreuter, J., Speiser, P., Boye, T., Gurny, R., and Kubis, A.,** Enhancement o response of rabbits with pilocarpine-loaded polybutylcyanoacrylate nanoparticles, *Int. J. Pharr* 1986.

34. **Zahka, J. and Mir, L.,** Ultrafiltration of latex emulsions, *Chem. Eng. Prog.,* 73, 53, 1977.

35. **Kirjassoff, D., Pinto, S., and Hoffman, C.,** Ultrafiltration of waste latex solutions, *Chem.* 76, 58, 1980.

36. **Kante, B., Couvreur, P., Dubois-Krack, G., DeMeesler, C., Guiot, P., Roland, M., M and Speiser, P.,** Toxicity of polycyanoacrylate nanoparticles, *J. Pharm. Sci.,* 71, 786, 1982

37. **Illum, L., Khan, M., Mak, E., and Davis, S.,** Evaluation of carrier capacity and release cl for poly(butyl-2-cyanoacrylate) nanoparticles, *Int. J. Pharm.,* 30, 7, 1986.

38. **Damge, C., Michel, C., Aprahanian, M., and Couvreur, P.,** New approach of oral admii insulin with polycyanoacrylate nanoparticles as drug carriers, *Diabetes,* 37, 246, 1988.

39. **Kreuter, J.,** Physicochemical characterization of polyacrylic nanoparticles, *Int. J. Pharm.,* 1-

40. **Fitch, R.,** Polymer Colloids, NATO Advanced Study Institute, University of Trondheim, N 1978.

41. **Scholsky, K.,** Unpublished results, 1982.

42. **Fitch, R., Gajria, C., and Tarcha, P.,** Acrylic polymer colloids: kinetics of autocatalyzed h *Colloid Interface Sci.,* 71, 107, 1979.

43. **Stone-Masui, J. and Watillon, A.,** Characterization of surface charge on polystyrene latice: *Interface Sci.,* 52, 479, 1975.

44. **Lenearts, V., Couvreur, P., Christiaens-Leyh, D., Joiris, E., Roland, M., Rollman, B., ₴ P.,** Degradation of poly(isobutyl cyanoacrylate) nanoparticles, *Biomaterials,* 5, 65, 1984.

45. **Vezin, W. R. and Florence, A. T.,** *In vitro* degradation rates of biodegradable poly-*n*-alkyl cy₴ *Pharm. Pharmacol.,* 30, 5P, 1978.

46. **Verdun, C., Couvreur, P., Vranckx, H., Lenaerts, V., and Roland, M.,** Development of a controlled release formulation for human use, *J. Controlled Release,* 3, 205, 1986.

47. **Couvreur, P.,** Polyalkylcyanoacrylates as colloidal drug carriers, in *CRC Critical Reviews in Drug Carrier Systems,* 5(1), 1, 1988.

48. **Edman, P. and Sjoholm, I.,** Acrylic micropsheres *in vivo.* II. The effect in rat of l-asparagin microparticles of polyacrylamide, *J. Pharm. Exp. Ther.,* 211, 663, 1979.

49. **Fitch, R. and Scholsky, K.,** Polymer colloids as controlled release devices, in *Microspheres: Biological Applications,* Rembaum, A. and Tokes, Z., Eds., CRC Press, Boca Raton, FL, 1

50. **Scholsky, K. and Warner, R.,** Automated device for analyzing drug release kinetics fr particles, *Rev. Sci. Instrum.,* 58, 1545, 1987.

51. **Couvreur, P., Kante, B., Roland, M., and Speiser, P.,** Adsorption of antineoplastic drugs cyanoacrylate nanoparticles and their release in calf serum, *J. Pharm. Sci.,* 68, 1521, 1979.

52. **Leonard, F., Kulkarni, R., Brandes, G., Nelson, J., and Cameron, J.,** Synthesis and d₤ poly(alkylcyanoacrylates), *J. Appl. Polym. Sci.,* 10, 259, 1966.

53. **Vezin, W. R. and Florence, A. T.,** Diffusion of small molecules in poly-*n*-alkylcyano acryla₤ *Pharmacol.,* 30, 20, 1978.

54. **El-Samaligy, M. and Rohdewald, P.,** Polyacrylamide microbeads, a sustained release drug del *Int. J. Pharm.,* 13, 23, 1983.

55. **Higuchi, T.,** Mechanism of sustained-action medication, theoretical analysis of rate of rel drugs dispersed in solid matrices, *J. Pharm. Sci.,* 52, 1145, 1963.

56. **Lapidus, H. and Lordi, M.,** Drug release from compressed hydrophilic matrices, *J. Phar* 1292, 1968.

57. **Couvreur, P., Kante, B., Lenaerts, V., Scailteur, V., Roland, M., and Speiser, P.,** Tissu of antitumor drugs associated with polyalkylcyanoacrylate nanoparticles, *J. Pharm. Sci.,* 69,

58. **Kreuter, J., Mills, S. N., Davis, D. D., and Wilson, C. G.,** Polyalkylcyanoacrylate nan₤ the delivery of [^{75}Se] norcholestenol, *Int. J. Pharm.,* 16, 105, 1983.

59. **Firsov, A. A., Nazarov, A. D., and Fomina, I. P.,** Biodegradable implants containing gen release and pharmacokinetics, *Drug Dev. Ind. Pharm.,* 13, 1651, 1987.

60. **Davis, B. K.,** Control of diabetes with polyacrylamide implants containing insulin, *Experien* 1972.

61. **Ticho, U., Blumenthal, M., Zonis, S., Gal, A., Blank, I., and Mazor, Z. W.,** *Annal.* 11, 555, 1979.

62. **Oppenheim, R.,** Solid colloidal drug delivery systems: nanoparticles. *Int. J. Pharm.,* 8, 21

63. **Kanke, M., Simmons, G. H., Weiss, D. L., Bivins, B. A., and de Luca, P. P.,** Clearan labelled microspheres from blood and distribution in specific organs following intravenous an administration in beagle dogs, *J. Pharm. Sci.,* 69, 755, 1980.

64. **Grislain, L., Couveur, P., Lenaerts, V., Roland, M., Deprez-Decampeneere, D., and** Pharmacokinetics and distribution of a biodegradable drug-carrier, *Int. J. Pharm.,* 15, 335,

65. **Gipps, E. M., Arshady, R., Kreuter, J., Groscurth, P., and Speiser, P. P.,** Distribution of polyhexyl cyanoacrylate nanoparticles in nude mice bearing human osteosarcoma, *J. Pharm. Sci.,* 75, 256, 1986.
66. **Bradfield, J. W. B. and Wagner, H. N., Jr.,** The relative importance of blood flow and liver phagocytic function in the distribution of Technetium^{99m} sulfur colloid, *J. Nucl. Med.,* 18, 620, 1977.
67. **Gregoriadis, G., Neerunjun, E. D., and Hunt, R.,** Fate of a liposome-associated agent injected into normal and tumour-bearing rodents. Attempts to improve localization in tumour tissues, *Life Sci.,* 21, 357, 1977.
68. **Illum, L., Thomas, N. W., and Davis, S. S.,** Effect of a selected suppression of the reticuloendothelial system on the distribution of model carrier, *J. Pharm. Sci.,* 75, 16, 1986.
69. **Illum, L. and Davis, S. S.,** Targeting of colloidal particles to the bone marrow, *Life Sci.,* 40, 1553, 1987.
70. **Illum, L., Davis, S. S., Muller, R. H., Mak, E., and West, P.,** The organ distribution and circulation time of intravenously injected colloidal carriers sterically stabilized with a block copolymer — Poloxamine 908, *Life Sci.,* 40, 367, 1987.
71. **Douglas, S. J., Davis, S. S., and Illum, L.,** Biodistribution of poly (butyl 2-cyanoacrylate) nanoparticles in rabbits, *Int. J. Pharm.,* 34, 145, 1986.
72. **Cartlidge, S. A., Duncan, R., and Lloyd, J. B.,** Soluble, crosslinked *N*-(2-hydroxypropyl)methacrylamide co-polymers as potential drug carriers. 3. Targeting by incorporation of galactosamine residues. Effect of route of administration, *J. Controlled Release,* 4, 265, 1987.
73. **Gregoriadus, G., Poste, G., Senior, J., and Trouet, A., Eds.,** *Receptor-Mediated Targeting of Drugs,* Plenum Press, New York.
74. **Illum, L., Jones, P. D. E., Kreuter, J., Baldwin, R. W., and Davis, S. S.,** Adsorption of monoclonal antibodies to polyhexylcyanoacrylate nanoparticles and subsequent immunospecific binding to tumor cells *in vitro, Int. J. Pharm.,* 17, 65, 1983.
75. **Illum, L., Jones, P. D. E., Baldwin, R. W., and Davis, S. S.,** Tissue distribution of poly(hexyl 2-cyanoacrylate) nanoparticles coated with monoclonal antibodies in mice bearing human tumor xenografts, *J. Pharmcol. Exp. Ther.,* 230, 733, 1984.
76. **Brasseur, F., Couvreur, P., Kante, B., Deckers-Passau, L., Roland, M., Deckers, C., and Speiser, P.,** Actinomycin-D adsorbed on polymethylcyanoacrylate nanoparticles: increased efficiency against an experimental tumor, *Eur. J. Cancer,* 16, 1441, 1980.
77. **Drewes, P. A., Kamp, A. O., and Winkelman, J. W.,** Radio immunoassay of polyacrylamide, *Experientia (Basel),* 34, 316, 1978.
78. **Sjoholm and Edman, Kopecek, J., Sprincl, L., Bazilova, H., and Vacik, J.,** Biological tolerance of poly(*N*-substituted acrylamides), *J. Biomed. Mater. Res.,* 6, 111, 1973.
79. **Bailey, W., Ni, Z., and Wu, S.,** Free radical ring opening polymerization of 4, 7-dimethyl-1,3-dioxepane, *J. Polym. Sci.,* 20, 3021, 1982.
80. **Bailey, W.,** personal communication, 1984.
81. **Inoue, S., Koinuma, H., and Tsurata, T.,** Copolymerization of carbon dioxide and epoxide, *J. Polym. Sci. Polym. Lett. Ed.,* 7, 287, 1969.
82. **Inoue, S., Koinuma, H., and Tsurata, T.,** Copolymerization of carbon dioxide and epoxide with organometalic compounds, *makromol. Chem.,* 130, 210, 1969.
83. **Soga, K., Hosoda, S., and Ikeda, S.,** Copolymerization of carbon dioxide and some diene compounds, *Makromol. Chem.,* 176, 1907, 1975.
84. **Soga, K., Sato, M., Tazaki, Y., and Ikeda, S.,** Copolymerization of carbon dioxide and ethyl vinyl ether, *J. Polym. Sci. Polym. Lett. Ed.,* 13, 265, 1975.

Chapter 10

POLOXAMERS IN THE PHARMACEUTICAL INDUSTRY

Irving R. Schmolka

TABLE OF CONTENTS

I. INTRODUCTION

Over the past several years much interest has developed in designing new dr
forms in order to enhance the effectiveness of existing medications.[1] These have enc
a variety of delivery vehicles such as microemulsions, nanoparticles, gels, ps
coatings, and other controlled or sustained release delivery systems. They have
veloped in order to provide enhanced bioavailability, to increase the solubility of
drugs, to enhance drug effectiveness, to lengthen the duration of contact and/or
specific delivery to selected sites in the body while maintaining the physical and
stability of the drug. The use of any one of these could lead to a reduction in the
of applied drugs, thereby minimizing systemic effects.

These new processes have often entailed the preparation and use of newer (
including surface active agents. While the use of surface active agents in pharm
dosage forms has been recognized, it is only in the past few years that the safety and
of properties possessed by one particular family of surface active agents, the po
have become better known.[2] They are one of the few surfactant types that have
directly for medicinal purposes. This chapter will summarize many of the diffe
cations of the poloxamers that have been disclosed in over 1000 articles in m
pharmaceutical publications. The poloxamers have been, and continue to be,
internally and externally in products that are designed for animal and human use

II. TECHNICAL PRINCIPLES

A. SYNTHESIS

The poloxamer series are but one of several hundred commercially availab
active agents, more frequently referred to as surfactants.[3] They are more accurately
as block copolymer surfactants because they comprise three segments or block
derived from the sequential polymerization of propylene and ethylene oxides. The p
are only one of a few series of all block copolymer surfactants in which the h
consists of a propylene oxide block and the hydrophile consists of ethylene oxi
A segment may also be formed by the simultaneous polymerization of a mixture
more alkylene oxides, in which case it is referred to as a heteric. Other surfactar
entirely from alkylene oxides are formed by combining two or more heteric segm
a combination of heteric and block segments.[4]

First offered commercially in the U.S. in 1950 under the Pluronic® polye
Corporation) trade name, they are now made in several countries and under man
trade names.[5] The poloxamers are made by the addition of propylene oxide, at a
temperature and pressure in an anhydrous and inert atmosphere in the presence of a
catalyst, to a propylene glycol initiator to form a polyoxypropylene glycol hydrophe
a minumum molecular weight of 900, as measured by its hydroxyl number.[6-9] A
propylene oxide has been reacted, it is followed by the controlled addition of ethy
to form two polyoxyethylene blocks which function as the hydrophile. The latter can
from 10% to 90% of the total molecular weight of the finished surfactant. The
then neutralized with acid to a pH of about 7.0. Although phosphoric acid is gene
other inorganic or organic acids may be employed for use in an application
presence of a phosphate salt is undesirable. The neutralized catalyst is generally
the finished polymer, although it may be removed. The structure of the resulting
surfactant is shown by Equation 1:

$$HO(C_2H_4O)_a(C_3H_6O)_b(C_2H_4O)_cH$$

in which a and c are statistically equal, b is a minimum of 15, and the sum of a ar

TABLE 1
Molecular Weights of Poloxamers

Poloxamer No.	Av mol wt	Av values		
		a	b	c
401	4,400	6	67	6
402	5,000	13	67	13
403	5,750	21	67	21
407	12,000	98	67	98
331	3,800	7	54	7
333	4,950	20	54	20
334	5,850	31	54	31
335	6,000	38	54	38
338	15,000	128	54	128
282	3,650	10	47	10
284	4,600	21	47	21
288	13,500	122	47	122
231	2,750	6	39	6
234	4,200	22	39	22
235	4,600	27	39	27
237	7,700	62	39	62
238	10,800	97	39	97
212	2,750	8	35	8
215	4,150	24	35	24
217	6,600	52	35	52
181	2,000	3	30	3
182	2,500	8	30	8
183	2,650	10	30	10
184	2,900	13	30	13
185	3,400	19	30	19
188	8,350	75	30	75
122	1,630	5	21	5
123	1,850	7	21	7
124	2,200	11	21	11
101	1,100	2	16	2
105	1,900	11	16	11
108	5,000	46	16	46

from 10 to 90% of the total weight of the polymer. This arrangement of the hydrophile water soluble blocks and water insoluble blocks allows for many variations of the total molecular weight of the surfactants, as well as in the ratio of the weight of the hydrophile to the hydrophobe. This structure allows for the preparation of a family of similar products with a systematic variation in their physical properties. This then permits the development of polymers with an optimization of properties, which can be established by the use of screening methods.[10] However, their chemical properties, as ether alcohols, are essentially identical. The surfactants thus obtained are produced as liquids, pastes, or solids.[11] The solid products are not hygroscopic, and are hard and brittle, allowing them to be powdered, flaked, prilled, or supplied as cast solids. Table 1 lists the poloxamers, with their approximate molecular weight and their ethylene oxide and propylene oxide content in moles.

It is theoretically possible to make many different series of block copolymer surfactants from two or more alkylene oxides. By using an initiator with three active hydrogens (glycerol) or four active hydrogens (ethylene diamine), surfactant series with three or four hydrophile blocks can be produced. An example of the latter are the commercially available poloxamines, the structure of which is shown by Equation 2:

$$(H(C_2H_4O)_a(C_3H_6O)_b)_2NC_2H_4N((C_3H_6O)_b(C_2H_4O)_aH)_2 \qquad (2)$$

By reversing the order of the alkylene oxide addition, surfactant series are prepared
the hydrophobe blocks are at the end of the products, rather than in the middle. T
commercially available surfactant series are the meroxapols and the minoxapols, t
tures of which are seen in Equation 3 and 4, respectively:

$$HO(C_3H_6O)_a(C_2H_4O)_b(C_3H_6O)_cH$$

$$(H(C_3H_6O)_b(C_2H_4O)_a(C_3H_6O))_2NC_2H_4N((C_3H_6O)(C_2H_4O)_a(C_3H_6O)_bH)_2$$

Many variations are possible by using a mixture of alkylene oxides to form e
hydrophile or the hydrophobe, or both. An example of a commercially available
surfactants representative of the latter are the hetomers, which are derived from a trifu
initiator.[12] Still other surfactant polymers have been prepared in which the hydro
derived from the polymerization of tetrahydrofuran and from 1,2 butylene oxide
the polymeric surfactants previously mentioned are made in the same way as that d
for the poloxamers. However, only the applications of the poloxamers will be disc
this chapter.

B. MOLECULAR STRUCTURE

As an aid in understanding why the poloxamers often exhibit properties unlike
the more widely known surfactants, such as the fatty alcohol ethoxylates or the alky
ethoxylates, it is informative to examine their structure. Four essential differences
noted.

1. The poloxamers exhibit a molecular weight range of from about 1,000 to
    Most other surfactant series have much lower weights.
2. The poloxamers have two hydrophiles, whereas most nonionic surfactants h
    one hydrophile.
3. The poloxamers have ether oxygen atoms in their hydrophobe, as well as
    hydrophile. This enables the polymers to form hydrogen bonds in their hyd
    which is not possible in ethoxylated fatty alcohols or alkyl phenols.
4. The micellar arrangement of aqueous poloxamer solutions appears to be uni
    celles are colloid-sized clusters of surface active compounds in a solvent.[15] The
    formed by the poloxamers appear to be unlike the hydrated spherical fo
    exhibited by other nonionic surfactants. This will be covered in a later secti

Since there are more than 30 different poloxamers, a nomenclature system w
lished by the original manufacturer, the Wyandotte Chemicals Corporation, to aid
tifying each polyol and to distinguish each from the other members of the series.
system, shown in Figure 1, explains the relationship between the nomenclature
composition of each member of the series. It is patterned after the original Pluronic
grid developed by the original manufacturer. The approximate hydrophobe molecul
is obtained by multiplying the first two digits of a poloxamer number, by 100.
proximate wt% of the hydrophile is obtained by multiplying the last digit by ten. Th
subtracted from 100, gives the wt% of the hydrophobe. Thus, poloxamer 188, se
right side of the grid in Figure 1, is derived from a 1750 mol wt hydrophobe, and
polyoxyethylene hydrophile comprises the remainder of the mol wt.

C. TOXICITY

Before considering the use of a chemical for any pharmaceutical application, e
toxicity data must first be available. Considerable toxicity data have been reported
of the poloxamers.[17] This includes acute and chronic oral toxicity studies, skin

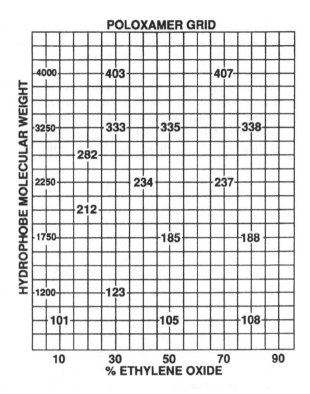

FIGURE 1. The poloxamer grid displays the relationship between the nomenclature and the composition of the members of a family of ethylene oxide, propylene oxide block copolymer surfactants. The hydrophobe (polyoxypropylene) mol wt are shown as the approximate midpoints of their ranges. The first two digits of a poloxamer number on the grid, multiplied by 100, give the approximate mol wt of the hydrophobe. The last digit, times 10, gives the approximate wt% of the hydrophile (polyoxyethylene) content of the surfactant. For e.g., poloxamer 407, shown in the upper right corner of the grid, is derived from a 4000 mol wt hydrophobe with the hydrophile comprising 70% of the final mol wt.

sensitivity studies, acute i.v. studies, a three-generation reproduction study, and other toxicological data.[1] Additionally, the results of some independent investigators have confirmed the safety of these polyols.[18,19] In summarizing the toxicity data that are available, it can be concluded that the higher the hydrophobe molecular weight, and the greater percent of ethylene oxide content and the lower the use level, the safer the poloxamer is for use in a drug product. One of the manufacturers of the poloxamers, the BASF Corporation, maintains toxicity studies in master files at the Bureau of Foods and the Bureau of Drugs. The Bureau of Foods has issued a number of regulations providing for the use of many of the poloxamers in indirect food applications, as well as in some direct food uses. In addition, the Bureau of Drugs has granted approval to selected poloxamers for use in specific drug formulations. Further verification of the safe use of the poloxamers will be seen in the following pages, in which experiments on animals and humans, as well as commercial usages, are described.

III. APPLICATIONS

A. INTRODUCTION

The poloxamers vary widely in their physical properties, so that it is usually not feasible to interchange one polymer for another. Their physical properties, which are utilized in the evaluation of pharmaceuticals, in drug delivery systems, and in other drug and medical

studies, may include one or more of the following: emulsifying, wetting, thickening
solubilizing, dispersing, and foaming. In many applications, two or more function
utilized. Some of these properties, such as wetting, do vary in a logical manner a
upon the hydrophobe molecular weight and the percent of ethylene oxide in the total
Other properties, such as solubilizing water-insoluble chemicals, appear not to vary
Although focusing primarily on the use of the poloxamers in drug delivery systems
thickening), application areas are described in which the polymers themselves
function as drugs (in blood). The applications of the poloxamers, as disclosed in
publications, will be divided according to the apparent primary function of the p
is used.

B. EMULSIFYING

An emulsion is a two-phase system consisting of two incompletely miscible li
one being dispersed as finite droplets in the other and having a minimum diame
μm, but a maximum, preferably, of 1 to 2 μm.[20] Emulsions used in pharmacy and
can include oil-in-water (o/w), or water-in-oil (w/o), or multiple emulsions such
in-oil-in-water (w/o/w), which are formed by the re-emulsification of an o/w or a w
The use of microemulsions, which are transparent, thermodynamically stable syst
prising swollen micelles, is also feasible. The dispersed phase in microemulsior
of droplets with a diameter in the range of 0.01 to 0.1 μm. Many stable emuls
been prepared with various members of the poloxamer series.

The first poloxamer-containing commercial product in clinical use was Lipo
(Upjohn).[21] It was a stable o/w emulsion of refined cottonseed oil in isotonic dex
used a combination of 0.3% poloxamer 188 and a purified soya lecithin as the
system. The product was designed to be given to malnourished patients and to
were unable to ingest food orally. A similar fat emulsion for i.v. feeding, Infonutro
Hewlett), also contained poloxamer 188 at 0.3% (w/v).[22] However, both proc
eventually withdrawn, after having been successfully administered to several hr
tients.

The emulsifying properties of a series of poloxamers, each containing 80%
oxide, but varying in total molecular weight from 5,000 to over 14,000, were co
a fat emulsion (o/w) in rats and rabbits.[23] All the polymers were found to be nor
the higher molecular weight emulsifiers, the 238, 288, and 338 grades, decrease
of removal of the emulsion from the blood compared to the lower molecular weight
the 108 and the 188 grades, which gave normal removal rate curves. A mor
summary of the many publications which describe the numerous trials with ex
i.v. fat emulsions in animals and humans, in which the poloxamers were utilized
previously reported.[24]

Studies were designed to develop the potential of w/o/w multiple emulsions
for the controlled release of drugs. The physical interaction occurring between the
and a macromolecule at the interface was used to form a stable system. The
comprised bovine serum albumin in the internal aqueous phase, poloxamer 331
phase, and poloxamer 403 in the external aqueous phase. A membrane, which
in a few days, formed at the interface between the albumin and the poloxamers,
a more effective barrier, as shown by optical microscopy measurements of the re
of some model compounds.[25] A group of poloxamers was evaluated in subseque
into the effect of varying both the internal (primary) hydrophobic surfactant and th
(secondary) hydrophilic surfactant used. The lipophilic polymers, the 331 or 4
were preferable to the 181 or 231 grades in forming a stable w/o and subsequ
emulsion. The more hydrophilic poloxamers, the 188 and 403 grades, were bett
101 and 105 members for re-emulsifying the initial w/o emulsions into the w/o/

Other multiple w/o/w emulsions have been prepared in which (1) poloxamer 188 was the emulsifier in the secondary phase and sesame oil was the oil phase, or (2) in which a 50:50 blend of poloxamers 237 and 238 emulsified the secondary phase in which isopropyl myristate was the oil phase.[27] The prolonged release behavior of an oily lymphography agent, Lipiodol, was studied in a w/o/w emulsion in which polyol 188 was in the internal phase and polymer 184 was used in the inner oil phase.[28]

The influence of varying the emulsifier was studied on the phagocytosis of soybean oil lipid emulsions by macrophages. Systems containing anionic lipids and poloxamer 338 were taken up more slowly than those emulsions stabilized by simple phosphatide mixtures. It was suggested that this was due to the hydrophilic coating on the emulsified particles from the poloxamer.[29] Because the duration of action of physostigmine is short, attempts have been made to prolong its ability to reverse the toxic effects associated with overdoses of other drugs. Stable emulsions containing physostigmine salicylate were prepared from a mixture of poloxamer 188 and anionic phospholipid surfactants. When studied in rabbits, the emulsion greatly increased the bioavailability of the drug compared with the i.m. conventional means of injection. It was suggested that this was due to the presence of poloxamer micelles in the aqueous phase.[30,31]

A laboratory study was undertaken to prepare emulsions of anesthetic agents, which were then evaluated on several species of animals. A stable emulsion of methoxyflurane (1,1-difluoro- 2,2-dichloroethyl methyl ether) was finally prepared in water, using 0.25% poloxamer 188 as the coemulsifier. After completion of the animal studies, a limited number of clinical trials were successfully completed. It was the first time that a volatile anesthetic agent was injected i.v. in man.[32]

C. FLUOROCARBON EMULSIONS

The emulsifying properties of the poloxamers, together with their history of use in blood, led to studies on their use with fluorocarbons for the preparation of intravenously injectable oxygen delivery systems. These microemulsions have been referred to as artificial or synthetic blood or as a red blood cell substitute. Several fluorocarbons had been found to have a good gas-carrying capacity, especially for oxygen and carbon dioxide, but it was necessary to select only those that could be shown to exhibit biological tolerance for further study. After initial studies had eliminated all but the most hydrophilic polyols as potential emulsifiers, an investigation centered on the use of poloxamers 188 and 338. Fluorocarbon microemulsions were compared in a rat study. The 338 polyol gave a more stable emulsion than that prepared with poloxamer 188. However, the higher molecular weight polymer was removed more slowly from the blood stream than the 188 grade.[33]

Poloxamer 188 proved to be superior to dog albumin and more hydrophobic polymers as an emulsifier, in experiments on dogs. It provided the colloid osmotic characteristics needed to maintain adequate plasma volume, and enabled the animals to recover more quickly.[34] Stable emulsions of perfluorotributylamine and perfluorotripropylamine were prepared with the polymer 188. Although not toxic, these fluorocarbons had excessively long retention time in the liver and spleen, and their clinical use had to be limited or abandoned.

The first commercial product developed, Fluosol® DA-20% (Green Cross), contained 2.7% poloxamer 188 and 0.4% egg yolk phospholipids as emulsifiers, and 20% of a blend of perfluorotripropylamine and perfluorodecalin. It has been used on several hundred patients over the past 10 years.[35] However, the product has some serious limitations, since it must be stored frozen to remain stable. Some adverse reactions have been reported, believed due to complement activation by the polyol, although premedication with corticosteroid will prevent them.[36] Perfluorodecalin had satisfactory retention times, but it could not be prepared as a stable emulsion without the addition of another perfluorocarbon. This led to synthesis programs to prepare other nontoxic fluorocarbons with good gas-carrying capacity which could form emulsions with small particles (less then 0.1 μm), were stable at temperature, and had a short retention time in the body.

The alternate approach was to modify or replace the surfactant system. In on poloxamer 188 was converted to its perfluroroalkyl diester. Aqueous emulsions of a of perfluorodecalin and perfluorotripropylamine were prepared with the poloxamer d and compared with the same emulsion using poloxamer 188 in the control. The rooctanoyl diester of poloxamer 188 was found to substantially improve the emul bility.[37]

Recent studies to improve the stability of a perfluorocarbon emulsion led to th a combination of poloxamer 188 with a perfluoroalkylated polyhydroxylated surf; the emulsifying system. This combination of surfactants, which exhibited a sy stabilization, produced perfluorodecalin emulsions which exhibited good stability peratures ranging from 4°C to 50°C.[38]

Emulsions of perfluoroctyl bromide have been tested in animals as radiographic agents in conjunction with radiography and in computed tomography scanning. A administration, the emulsions localize in malignant neoplasms. A 5% solution of po 188 in Ringer's lactate is used as the emulsifier. Radiopaque perfluoroctyl bromic sions appear useful in clinical applications for detecting abnormal tissue such as m tumors, and for total body angiography. The emulsions are also suggested to be t diagnostic radiography of the lungs and gastrointestinal tract, the central nervous lymph nodes, the liver and spleen, and the vascular system.[39]

D. DISPERSING AND STABILIZING

The dispersing or stabilizing properties of the poloxamers have been utilized different ways. It is suggested that the polymers function in either of two ways. T "coat" the dispersed particles, and are held in place by Van der Waals forces or by l bonding. In so doing, they prevent or delay the coalescence of these particles whic occur in their absence. Or, they may preferentially coat the surface of a container preventing the adsorption of a dispersed material from agglomerating on its surface. of the multiplicity of surfaces and materials used in many applications in the pharm industry, both the hydrophilic and the hydrophobic polymers are finding utility as di: or stabilizers, as will be seen in the following paragraphs.

An improved calamine lotion was developed using poloxamer 188 as the surf; stabilized the product while also acting as the wetting agent.[40] The poloxamers h found useful in preparing physically stable suspensions of parenterally useful dru as sulfadiazine, which can be injected with hypodermic syringes without cloggin; ringes.[41] The addition of poloxamer 188 in lysine has been reported to increase the of a streptokinase-activated plasminogen solution.[42] The same polymer was fou especially effective in preventing the precipitation of proteins in tissue cell cultures horse or human serum. The polyol appears to function as a dispersing and so agent.[43]

The addition of 1.0 g of poloxamer 188 per l to a submerged culture of baby kidney cells proved valuable in increasing yields. It protects mammalian cells agains due to excessive agitation, reportedly by stabilizing the cell-liquid interface.[44] The four hydrophilic polymers — the 188, 217, 238, and 338 grades — was studie growth of two human lymphocyte cell lines. Poloxamers 188 and 238 were fou slightly superior to the 217 and 338 grades at concentrations of 0.05 to 0.1%. In to their protective effect against mechanical damage, the polymers were reported to transport of metabolites into cells, and thus increase the growth rate.[45] A dilute po 188 solution was used to stabilize a suspension culture in which lymphoma L51 were grown.[46] In a study on mice to determine whether or not cross tolerance between ethanol and delta-9-tetrahydrocannabinol, the drug was administered as a suspension in 1% poloxamer 188. The use of the poloxamer was found to have had no effect on tetrahydrocannabinol-induced impairment of rotarod performance.[47]

Poloxamer 188, at a dosage range of 0.1 to 3.0 mg, was used clinically as a stabilizing agent for suspensions of $^{99}Tc^m$-labeled colloids, given i.v. for liver scintigraphy. The study showed that the 0.5 mg level gave the most satisfactory results in terms of background level, renal excretion, liver:spleen ratio, stability, and consistent performance.[48] The same polyol has been used as a stabilizer in a stannous microaggregated albumin colloid test, Microlite® (NEN) for reticuloendothelial imaging.[49] It has also been used for stabilizing normal serum albumin (human) tin microspheres (3 *M*) for gamma scintillation imaging of the lungs, following i.v. administration.[50]

The aggregation of insulin and of insulin protected with surfactants was studied by shaking in containers of different materials. Whereas polymer 188 was effective in preventing aggregation, meroxapols 17R8 and 25R5 (reverse poloxamers, PO/EO/PO) hastened the aggregation which developed in all the containers of unprotected insulin. The activity of the insulin containing the poloxamer 188 was unchanged even after 8 d of shaking.[51]

A hydrophobic poloxamer, the 181 grade, Genapol® PF 10 (Hoechst), has been used clinically with a programmable delivery device for the continuous infusion of insulin for treating diabetics.[52] At a continuous concentration of only 0.10%, the polymer prevents both the adsorption of dissolved proteins to the various hydrophobic surfaces in the device as well as the resultant aggregation. Examination of one device after 1 year of insulin infusion revealed surfaces clean of precipitated insulin along the entire delivery pathway.[53] This is due to the preferential adsorption of polymer on hydrophobic surfaces, thus forming a hydrophilic surface coating.

The surface of a commonly used hydrophobic medical material, low density polyethylene, was converted to produce a hydrophilic surface onto which proteins would not adsorb. The studies were designed to modify surfaces onto which blood comes in contact, since proteins adsorb to most surfaces during the first few minutes of blood exposure.[54] In studying poloxamers with varying molecular weight hydrophobes, a 1750 mol wt hydrophobe (30 mol PO) was found to be the maximum that can exist in linear form in aqueous solution that will bind strongly onto a hydrophobic surface. It was suggested that lower mol wt hydrophobes (shorter PO chains) bind less strongly due to fewer binding sites, while hydrophobe molecular weights greater than 1750 (longer PO chains) readily form intra-aggregates in solution, resulting in weaker suface binding.[55] Other factors which were found to effect adsorption and desorption were found to include the length of the polyoxyethylene chain and the surfactant structure. Thus, a polymer with a 5-link polyoxytheylene chain at each end of a 30-mol PO chain, was found to be less effective at adsorption than a poloxamer with a 3-link polyoxyethylene chain at each end of a 30-mol PO link chain.

E. WETTING

All the poloxamers function as wetting agents, but those members with a lower oxyethylene content and a higher hydrophobe molecular weight are better than those polymers with a higher oxyethylene content and a lower hydrophobe molecular weight. However, other factors, such as physical form, taste, or solubility, have to be considered in selecting a polyol for use as a wetting agent. Poloxamer 188, a tasteless solid, has been extensively used in commercially available fecal stool softeners because of its wetting action. This allows the fecal masses to be penetrated by water, thereby reducing their desiccation and maintaining them in a pliable, easily moved condition while passing through the large bowel. A very early product, Polykol Drops (Upjohn) contained a 20% solution of poloxalkol, a name previously assigned to Pluronic® F-68 by Upjohn.[56] The drops were recommended for children under 3 years of age, as well as older children and adults. In a controlled trial of

laxatives containing poloxamer 188 on several hundred elderly patients, no to׳
reported and no interference was found with the absorption of beneficial nutrie
poloxamer 188 has been a component of several other laxatives, both liquids and
such as Magcyl® (Elder), Dorbanex® (Riker), Alaxin® (Delta), Casakol® (Up)
Geriplex® FS (Parke Davis). A poloxamer of unknown composition was used as t
agent in a clinical trial of Haemosol® (Eisai) for the treatment of idiopathic hem׳
The poloxamer 188 also found use as a wetting agent in eye drops, including
(Ayerst) and Neosporin® (Burroughs Wellcome).

A cerumolytic pharmaceutical preparation for removing cerumen from the
Cerumenex® (Purdue Frederick), utilized pharmacologically active substances in a
glycerol or polyoxyethylene glycol solution and contained 1% of poloxamer 1
wetting agent.[59]

Poloxamer 188 has been used clinically as a wetting agent in formulations d׳
dissolve bile duct and kidney stones. Used either in solutions with mineral-disso׳
stances or in o/w emulsions of glyceryl-1-monooctanoate, in which it also funct׳
coemulsifier, high success rates were reported.[60-63] The wetting property of the po
combined with their record of biological compatibility, resulted in an unusual c׳
plication. The cleansing action of poloxamer 188 is utilized in a skin wound clea׳
Clens® (Biosyntec), which contains the surfactant at a 20% level. It was appro׳
FDA for use in humans, and has been recommended as a safe cleanser for
lacerations.[64]

Of all the commercial nonionic surfactants, the block copolymers were reporte
the lowest binding activity of chlorhexidine. The highest foaming member of the po
the 237 grade, is used at a 25% level as a component of a surgical scrub, Hibi
Hibiscrub® (ICI), which contains chlorhexidine gluconate for the disinfection of
and has been recommended for treating neonates against staphylococcal infectio׳

F. SOLUBILIZING

Surface active agents exhibit the property of solubilizing water-insoluble drug׳
materials when their concentration is equal to or exceeds their critical micelle cor
(cmc), which is the lowest concentration at which a surfactant forms micelles. M
properties of a surfactant are first manifested at its cmc value. The question as t
or not poloxamers form micelles and what their cmc values are, has been revie׳
earlier publication.[66] Different cmc values for the polymers, measured in sev׳
continue to be reported, and will not be reviewed here. Variation in sample sourc
used, concentration range studied, and temperature used may all play a role in ׳
for these differences. Despite the anomalies that appear to exist, there is no qu׳
the poloxamers have the property to solubilize many drugs and other macromole

The nature and shape of the poloxamer micelles have been the subject of ׳
vestigations. A recent study on the association behavior of aqueous poloxamer
using light-scattering, concluded that, depending upon temperature, polymer 188
as unimers (single molecules), transition, and polymolecular micelles. Above ׳
polymolecular micelles exist, which are composed of a relatively compact core o׳
blocks and a highly swollen shell of soluble blocks.[67] Other investigators have al׳
that the poloxamers form monomolecular micelles at very low concentration׳
conventional polymolecular aggregates develop at higher concentrations.[68] Ultr
locity and light-scattering studies on very dilute poloxamer 407 solutions revea
gregation number of six molecules per micelle at 10°C, increasing to 44 at ׳
confirms, in principle, that aggregation increases as the temperature rises, but
disagree with the unimolecular micelle theory as proposed by others.[69]

Nine different poloxamers were evaluated as solubilizers for tropicamide, a po׳

soluble drug. Solubility was found to increase as the oxyethylene content increased. When drug solubilization was expressed as the amount solubilized per ethylene oxide group, the solubilizing capacity of the polyol decreased with an increasing oxyethylene chain length. After the successful completion of rabbit studies showed that the polymers tested were capable of increasing the drug bioavailability, a limited clinical trial was initiated, using poloxamers 235 and 237 at a 20% concentration. The experimental formulations were better tolerated and sometimes more effective than the standard 1% tropicamide collyria in inducing mydriatic and cycloplegic effects.[70]

The solubilization of *para*-substituted acetanilides was studied in aqueous solutions of a group of five different polymers with the same hydrophobe, but with the ethylene oxide content increasing from 20 to 80%. Solubilization increased linearly with polyol concentration. When the increased solubility of the drugs was expressed as moles solubilized per ethylene oxide equivalent, solubilizing capacity of the polymers decreased as the oxyethylene increased. When calculated as moles of drug solubilized per mole of poloxamer, solubility of the polar drugs increased with polyol hydrophilicity, but for the hydrophobic drugs, solubility decreased with increasing oxyethylene content.[71]

Poloxamer 188 has been reported to increase the aqueous solubility of sulfadiazine, sodium cetaben, aspirin, and Vitamins K_1 and K_2.[72-75] Studies on the solubility of diazepam in polymer aqueous solutions showed the 188, 238, and 338 grades were effective in increasing its solubility, with the 338 being the most effective. However, the 188 grade was the most effective in preventing the loss of potency of the diazepam solution stored in PVC.[76,77] The same three polyols were used to study the aqueous solubility of indomethacin, an anti-flammatory drug. The 338 gave the greatest increase in solubility, while the 188 gave the least increase. Drug solubility increased with an increase in poloxamer concentration and with temperature.[78]

A study was used to develop a stable nontoxic parenteral vehicle for three poorly water-soluble anti-cancer drugs, taxol, 3,5-dichloro-2,4-dimethoxy-6-(trichloromethyl)-pyridine, and 2-(*s*-chloromethyl)-mercapto quiniline. A 60% solution of polyol 184 was used to simulate drug administration by i.v. bolus or by slow infusion. The vehicle was found to be nonhemolytic compared to normal saline, and the drugs remained stable in it for 3 months.[79] Several intravenous test solutions were prepared and evaluated by an *in vitro/in vivo* screening procedure for their hemolytic potential. The solutions, which contained a drug with very low intrinsic aqueous solubility, were given i.v. to rats and evaluated for their bioavailability. Poloxamer 184 was used in one of the formulations utilized to solubilize the dihydropyridine.[80]

The aqueous solubility of a potential antidepressant drug, 7-chloro-5,11-dihydrodibenz(*b*,*e*)(1,4)-oxazepine-5-carboxamide, was greatly increased by incorporating polymer 407 in a coating of the capsule containing the drug. As a result, the drug's bioavailability was found to increase in dogs and humans.[81] Many mouth rinses utilize polymers to solubilize the flavors, thus preventing them from coming out of solution and causing turbidity to develop when the products are cooled.

In a study of the water-soluble poloxamers in the upper left quadrant of the grid, the 284 grade was found to be the best to use in a diluent composition for measuring factor VIIIRAg by laser nephelometry because of its ability to potentiate the reaction without precipitating sparingly soluble proteins. The level of Factor VIIIRAg is an important diagnostic parameter for differentiating between classical haemophilia and von Willebrand's disease, and helps improve the detection of female carriers in hemophilic A carriers.[82]

Three poloxamers, the 181, 184, and 188 grades, were among 61 surfactants used to solubilize 124 water-insoluble drugs that were included in a study for their action on amine oxidase. Although all three polymers exhibited no inhibitory effects on canine intestinal diamine oxidase, a combination of the 181 polyol with an anionic surfactant was only one

of five systems found suitable for solubilizing drugs in studies on diamine oxidase a₍
The use of the poloxamers as surfactants for time release control medications ₍
suggested from a study on the dissolution kinetics of benzoic acid. The addition of
188 to the dissolving fluid increased the apparent solubility of the acid. As the
concentration increased, the dissolution rate of the benzoic acid decreased.[84]

G. THICKENING

A unique property of concentrated aqueous solutions of many of the poloxamer₍
ability to form gels that are thermally reversible. The gels liquify upon cooling, bu
upon rewarming.[85] These two properties of the gels, namely, their aqueous natur₍
allows them to be readily removed, and the reversible gel-liquid transition behavi
distinctive application advantages over other gel systems. The gels will also liqui₍
heated to high (over 80°C) temperatures. The gel-liquid transition temperature w
depending upon the poloxamer concentration, the pH, and the composition of t
ingredients in the formulation.[86] The phase change phenomenon is reversible innu
times. Only those polyols with a hydrophobe molecular weight of 1750 or greater fo
As the hydrophobe molecular weight increases, the concentration needed to for
decreases. Poloxamer 407 forms a gel at only 20% in water, at 25°C, while ₍
concentration is needed for the other members of the series. Several water-insoluble
chemicals, mostly aromatic, were found to increase the yield strength of the gel₍
means that they made the gel stronger or allowed for the preparation of a gel with
polymer content. The addition of glycerol, but not propylene glycol, also had ₍
effect. Gels have been made with as little as 10% (w/w) poloxamer 407. On the oth
other additives are effective in lowering the yield strength. This includes other sur
which form mixed micelles with the polyol, as well as several solvents, such as
and ketones. The addition of 1% polyoxyethylene glycol 10,000 to a poloxamer
caused a weakening of the microviscosity of the system, but had no significant ₍
the *in vitro* release of a range of model drugs.[88] The minimum poloxamer 407 conc₍
needed to form a gel depends upon the other components present in the formulat
minimum temperature at which a liquid poloxamer composition gels upon warmin₍
adjusted by using proper formulating techniques.

The explanations for the formation of gels by an aqueous poloxamer solution h₍
reviewed in a recent publication.[89] The first potential clinical application disclose₍
poloxamer gel was as a carrier for silver salts, for the treatment of topical burn₍
were presented from several experiments on the use of gels on 18 to 22% surface
thickness burns on rats.[91] Additional data, obtained from treating third degree burn
on pigs, corroborated the usefulness of these gels for treating burns. It was sugge
the polymer 407 significantly enhanced the rate of wound healing by stimulatio
epithelial growth factor.[92] A dispersion of silver sulfadiazine in a poloxamer 4₍
reported to be microbiologically as effective as two commercial products, also base
silver salt, for treating burns.[93]

A further development in topical wound therapy has been the development of a₍
system for delivering a liquid polymer 407 formulation which gels upon body con
offers a facile method to deliver any skin treating agent or drug to an infected are₍
an artificial skin with a high moisture content. The use of a poloxamer 407 gel as an ₍
drug delivery system provides many advantages. Since it contains a surfactant, the
seek every body contour and provide a medium in which water, protein, and ele
will be able to come into equilibrium with the underlying tissue, while allowing
exchange of oxygen and carbon dioxide. Desireable additives such as medication₍
readily incorporated in the gels to further enhance their effectiveness in treating skin d
The gels have a low degree of toxicity and have high loading characteristics.[95] The p₍

gel system is especially useful in dispensing drugs that are water insoluble, since they may be dispersed or solubilized in the surfactant micelles.

Stable hydrogen peroxide gels, which are useful for treating poison ivy and other dermatological conditions, have been prepared with polyol 407.[96] A stable hydrogen peroxide dental gel has been prepared for the treatment of gingivitis and periodontitis, and the prevention of caries and other diseases of the oral cavity.[97] A dental gel, based on poloxamer 407, Protect® (Butler Brush), designed for patients with sensitive teeth and gums, has been availabe for over 10 years.[98] The fluoride uptake of a polymer 407 gel containing 1% fluoride was compared with that of two commercial gels in a study on children. The experimental gel produced a significantly higher fluoride uptake than did the conventional gels.[99]

Topically, the gels have been used as drug carriers for treating athlete's foot, Blis-to-sol® (Chattem), as well as acne.[100,101] In the latter, the antimicrobial effects of a blend of three antimicrobial agents in an 18% poloxamer 407 gel were compared *in vitro* to clinical studies *in vivo*. The product was stable after storage for one month at 55°C. Poloxamer 407 gels containing various drugs have been used successfully to treat patients with a variety of ocular conditions, including red eye, corneal edema, and dry eye syndrome.[102] Formulations with dexamethasone USP, used for treating inflammatory ocular conditions caused by chemical burns, and containing only half the drug, were as effective as Decadron® (Merck). The reduction in intraocular pressure by a polymer 407 gel containing 0.5% pilocarpine hydrochloride, for treating glaucoma, was equal to or better than liquid products containing four times as much of the drug. A 25% poloxamer 407 gel containing pilocarpine nitrate was evaluated for use as a vehicle for ophthalmic drug delivery. Based on the miotic response in rabbits, the gel appeared to enhance the pilocarpine activity compared to a control in water.[103] The same gel containing 4% pilocarpine hydrochloride was reported to show an increase in bioavailability when inserted into the cul de sac of the eye, in comparison with an isotonic solution of the drug.[10] A 25% poloxamer 407 gel containing 1% adrenaline bitartrate was reported to increase the intraocular pressure compared to an aqueous solution of the drug.[105]

A poloxamer 338 gel has been evaluated as a potential vehicle for alloplastic kerato-refractive surgery in rabbits. Refractive flattening of approximately 3 diopters was observed compared to no change in a control group.[106] The poloxamer 407 gels have been used for the topical application of prostaglandins, radiological contrast agents, and antibiotics, as well as the anti-cancer agents 5-fluorouracil and adriamycin, and have been reported to enhance the therapeutic effects of interleukin-2.[107-109] Topical gels of two anti-inflammatory drugs, diclofenac and hydrocortisone, have been made with poloxamer 407.[110] The *in vitro* efficacy of lidocaine release from a poloxamer 407 gel has been reported. It showed the largest percent of drug release and apparent diffusion coefficient for release of the drug, in comparison with commercial and other experimental products.[111] Measuring the diffusion of lidocaine hydrochloride and its base in a 25% poloxamer 407 gel indicated that it took place in the water channels between the polyol segments. A comparison with traditional methods indicated a possible influence of the partition coefficient and the interfacial barrier in the diffusion process.[112,113]

In a study measuring drug release from 20, 25, and 30% poloxamer 407 gels, the release rate of butobarbitol was found to decrease as the poloxamer concentration increased. The diffusion rate of similar drugs was found to increase with a decrease in drug molecular weight.[114] An increase in the lipophilicity of a series of *p*-hydroxybenzoate esters resulted in a decrease in the rate of drug release from the poloxamer 407 gels. This was attributed to a greater partitioning into the polymer micellar region within the gel structure.[115] Similar results were obtained in a study of *in vitro* release of nicotinic acid alkyl esters.[116] Clear gels, designed for use as analgesics, have been prepared with poloxamer 407 and an analgesic agent such as treithanolamine salicylate.[117]

Poloxamer 407 gels, containing the anthelmintic, levamisole, when fed to ca
reported to provide advantages over other forms of oral administration of the dru
adheres to the animal's tongue so that it dissolves slowly as it is gradually swa
Gamma scintigraphy has been used to study release rates from 30% poloxamer 4
rats by the use of technetium labelling. The loss of activity was measured at the
site, and the gain in activity in the kidneys. Release rates from implants in the ge
significantly affected by the molecular characteristics of the polymer.[119] An inv
into the muscle toxicity of concentrated solutions of several poloxamers in rabbits
conclusion that gels of the 238 and 407 grades appeared suitable as vehicles for intr
use, whereas the 335 and 403 grades appeared unsuited.[120]

A new spermicidal compound was evaluated in a poloxamer 407 gel in st
macaques. *In vivo* results showed it was bioequivalent at a 0.1% concentratic
superior at a 1.0% use level to a commercial product based on nonoxynol-9.[121]
407 gel containing 5% silver nitrate was found to be effective as a fibrosing ag
applied to the fallopian tubes, thereby blocking them.[122] A novel method for
intravaginal contraception uses an aerosol system to delivery a liquid poloxame
mulation containing a spermicidal agent such as nonoxynol-9. Upon contact v
tissue, a gel forms.[123]

Several types of dosage forms, such as suppositories, enemas, and gelatin cap
useful for the rectal administration of drugs. Of these, the poloxamers have be
for use in enemas and in suppositories. Three hydrophilic polymers, the 288, 33
grades, were evaluated in a rabbit study. Indomethacin gels were administered re
plasma levels were determined. The use of a 25% poloxamer 407 gel appeared
most suitable because of its prolonged action and minimal side effects.[124] Polox
was one of three components in a suppository base in a study on the release
absorption of aminopyrine in rabbits. Increasing the polymer concentration from
to 20% (w/w) decreased the bioavailability from 100 to 47.2%. This agrees with
the greater the polymer concentration, the slower is the rate of drug release.[125] A
polyols 124 and 188 was used to prepare aspirin suppositories which had a disi
time of about 25 min in water at 37°C. They could be stored for several month
temperature in closed glass containers, without showing signs of deterioration.[126] To
suppositories, designed for rectal or vaginal use, were prepared from poloxam
molecular weight greater than 7500. The products were stable and remained s
stored below 50°C.[127]

Dilute aqueous solutions of polymers with an ethylene oxide content of 70%
such as 188 or 238, have been gelled by exposure to X-rays. Solutions of poly
lesser ethylene oxide content do not gel. Their use as sustained drug release delive
was studied using acetanilide. The release rate of 0.01% acetanilide from a
poloxamer 188 solution was much lower than from a 2% aqueous poloxamer 188 s
The poloxamer 407 gel has been used as a solid culture media for the enrichment
and growth of micro organisms. The gel is more transparent than the agar norm
and was suggested for isolating heat-sensitive organisms.[129] Solidified melt prep
1 to 20% of griseofulvin and poloxamer 188 were chemically and physically s
solid melt, containing 20% of the drug, gave after administration to volunteer
urinary excretion rate of total 6-dimethylgriseofulvin than the corresponding physic
or the micronized drug without surfactant.[130]

Reaction products of the poloxamers (with diisocyanates to produce polyure
with acryloyl chloride, for example), have been evaluated for the preparation of
release microparticles. These hydrophilic water-swelling polymers, known as
have been covered in a previous chapter. These systems are especially desira
controlled release of lower molecular weight drugs, for use in delivering medi
oral, pediatric, and geriatric applications because of their high biocompatability

H. COATINGS

Although the subjects of latex systems and enteric coatings are covered elsewhere in this book, a few examples on the use of the poloxamers can be cited. A number of factors have contributed to the development of new techniques for coatings used in controlled release drug tablets. Latex or pseudolatex coatings offer one of the better methods to eliminate the use of solvents. In a study to show the effect of surfactants on the dissolution of theophylline from pellets coated with the latex coating Surelease® (Colorcon), the addition of a poloxamer (of unknown composition) considerably enhanced the release of the theophylline in simulated intestinal fluid and caused no damage in simulated gastric fluid.[132] The development of aqueous colloidal dispersions of enteric polymers was studied for use in tablet film coatings. The phase inversion technique was utilized for preparing a pseudolatex in which poloxamer 188 was used to produce physically stable o/w emulsions.[133] In a study designed to develop biodegradable and injectable latices for the controlled release of drugs, a formulation was prepared which contained poly-d,l-lactic acid as the drug carrier and testosterone as the drug marker. The use of poloxamer 188 was found to be a suitable surfactant for preparing the latex into which the drug carrier and marker were molecularly dispersed.[134] A study was conducted to evaluate drug-containing matrix films prepared from aqueous colloidal polymer dispersions. The addition of salts of two basic drugs, propranolol hydrochloride or chlorpheniramine maleate, to ethylcellulose pseudolatices resulted in flocculation or coagulation. By replacing the anionic surfactant-containing cellulosic latex system used with an o/w emulsion of a methylene chloride solution of ethylcellulose pseudolatex and dibutyl sebacate in water, and using poloxamer 333 as the emulsifier, no flocculation or coagulation occurred, and films were successfully prepared.[135]

I. ADJUVANTS

An interesting property reported for a few of the poloxamers is that of functioning as an adjuvant. An immunological adjuvant is any material, usually of a high molecular weight, that increases the specific immune reponse to an antigen when combined with the antigen. Poloxamer 401 has been found to be a powerful antigen for increasing antibody formation to bovine serum albumin in mice when injected as an o/w emulsion. Poloxamer 331 was less effective, more so than several more hydrophilic polyols, such as the 101, 333, and 338 grades.[136] When tested in mice while studying the adjuvant activity of dimethyl dioctadecyl ammonium bromide (DDA), both polymer 401 and the DDA were found to enhance the primary antibody response to sheep red blood cells, while poloxamers 101, 188, and 331 were found to suppress this response. The secondary humoral response to sheep red blood cells was also enhanced by the poloxamer 401. The mechanism responsible for the difference in abilities of poloxamer 331 and 401 was unknown.[137]

The structures of a series of seven ethylene oxide propylene oxide block copolymers were studied in relation to their ability to enhance antibody formation and inflammation. Hydrophobic poloxamers — the 231, 282, 331, 401, and 402 grades — were compared with each other and with two meroxapols (PO-EO-PO), the 25R1 and 31R1 grades, in the form of an o/w emulsion injected into the hind foot pad of mice. Each polymer produced a distinct immune response and inflammation pattern. The most hydrophobic polyols, the 331 and 401 grades, were the most effective for increasing antibody formation. They also activated complement and induced the release of chemotactic factors from serum. Increasing the oxyethylene content decreased the adjuvant activity and inflammation. The meroxapols induced glaucoma instead of antibodies. The antigen activity of the polymers was believed to be due to their ability to form adsorptive surfaces on various plasma proteins.[138]

A nontoxic tumor antigen formulation has been developed which elicits cell mediated and humoral responses against a variety of antigens. It contains poloxamer 401 and N-acetylmuramyl-L-threonyl-D-isoglutamine. Adjuvant activity is claimed to be comparable to Freund's

complete adjuvant but lacking in its undesirable effects. Using killed feline leuken
antigens produced in cell cultures, it protected the great majority of cats again
challenge.[139] Since previous investigators had used mineral oil emulsions, which
acceptable for human injections, a stable o/w emulsion was prepared with poloxar
which incorporated only those ingredients authorized for pharmaceutical usage. A hy
suggested for the cause of the antigen activity of the polyol in stimulating immune re
was similar to that described previously, namely, the surfactants concentrate at the
interface and retain the antigens at this interface through their surface activity and t
bonding ability.[140] Additional experiments were conducted on monkeys, since
studies had been on mice and guinea pigs.[141] Induction of simian-acquired immune de
syndrome by inoculation of a type D retrovirus was prevented by immunizatioi
retrovirus containing an adjuvant of threonyl muranyl-dipeptide emulsified with pc
401 in saline. After additional testing on guinea pigs, it was concluded that the
formulation was effective, and thought to be useful for both humans and animals.

The ability of several poloxamers to stimulate a humoral immune response
haptenated liposomes was tested in mice. Humoral immune response was measure
spleen as the number of antibody-secreting cells detected by the plaque-forming cell
and, in the serum, as the amount of circulating antibodies detected by a hemagglu
All the polymers tested significantly increased both the PFC and the hemagglutinat
titer. Poloxamers 331, 401, and 402 were found to display low adjuvant activit
polymers 212, 231, and 282 exhibited high adjuvant activity. It was concluded tha
of the poloxamers are strong adjuvants for stimulation of the antibody response
haptenated liposomes.[143]

Immunodulation with adjuvants has proven to be valuable in increasing the i
genecity of modern semi(synthetic) vaccines. The current pneumococcal polysa
vaccine is poorly immunogenic in young children because of the behavior of polysac
as thymus-independent type-2 antigens. Poloxamer 331, incorporated in an o/w e
changed the kinetics of generated antibody responses against pneumococcal hexasae
protein conjugates, resulting in prolonged immunoglobulin M and immunoglobu
sponses. Incorporating a poloxamer in an o/w emulsion vaccine may be the first step
the future development of a single injection vaccine which would give long-lasting p
to infants.[144]

J. HYPOLEMIC AGENTS

Several investigators have studied the effect of incorporating various poloxame
diet of animals. The following paragraphs summarize their findings. The acute i
of intestinal lipid transport in rats was measured using poloxamer 231. Lymph tri
and cholesterol outputs were found to be greatly impaired, compared to controls
not impair digestion and absorption. The rats regained their ability to transport li
after ending the polyol feeding.[145] The poloxamer 231 was found to produce a
inhibition in the intracellular transport of chylomicron-sized particles, thereby
secretion of chylomicrons by the erythrocytes. Poloxamer 234 was less effective.

The effect of feeding hydrophobic detergents on fat absorption in animals
reported. Initial experiments on rats with poloxamers that had an oxyethylene c
from 10 to 70%, showed that only those with a 90% hydrophobic content were
inhibit fat absorption.[147] Sterol and fat balance studies were then conducted on sv
poloxamer 231. It was concluded that a hydrophobic surfactant could have an i
effect on intraluminal and intracellular events of fat absorption.[148] A comparative
study of poloxamer 188 and 331 on rats revealed that the 331 was a potent *in vitro*
of human pancreatic lipase, while the 188 was a poor inhibitor. Excretion of dieta
the feces was significantly enhanced during the 331 feeding, but not during the 188 fe

The dibenzoyl ester of poloxamer 231 was reported to be a more effective hypolemic agent than the 231 itself. Plasma cholesterol levels were lower in rabbits, without affecting plasma triglycerides. Hepatic total lipid and cholesterol were significantly decreased with the dibenzoyl ester, but not in the controls. The same applied to aortic and heart muscle cholesterol content. It also prevented the development of experimental atherosclerosis.[150] A lipid emulsion containing the 231 ester was administered intraduodenally to rats. The changes in lipid and protein content of apolipoproteins produced by the ester resulted in increased ratio of lipids to intestinal triglyceride-rich lipoproteins. The inhibition of lipid transport by the poloxamer ester was not a result of apolipoprotein deficiency.[151]

The poloxamer 213, poloxalene (SmithKline), also successfully prevented experimentally produced atherosclerosis in rabbits. This same surfactant has been used in veterinary medicine for over a decade, as a feed additive to prevent gastric bloating in cattle, Bloatguard® (SmithKline).[152] The effect of poloxamer 213 on lipid absorption was then studied in rats. It was concluded that it affects lipid absorption, food intake, and serum cholesterol concentration, but results of the feeding are affected by dietary factors.[153] Feeding poloxamer 213 to rabbits showed it had a systemic effect on lipoproteins which may contribute to its antiatherogenic effect.[154] The results obtained from all these animal studies have shown promise for potential human use, but have not yet reached the clinical stage.

K. MICROSPHERES

Microspheres, or nanoparticles, are but one of a multiplicity of colloid systems that are being evaluated as drug carriers. A review of this subject has listed the various types and their requirements, as well as the properties of the colloids that influence drug targeting and the methods that can be used to evaluate drug targeting.[155] The poloxamers are used in nanoparticles in different capacities; they function as dispersants, or as emulsifiers, or as coating agents. The following paragraphs will exemplify each of these application areas.

Poloxamer 188 has been used as the emulsifier in an emulsion (w/o) polymerization process for polymerizing acrylamide to form spherical microparticles of an acrylamide gel. Various additives such as enzymes, proteins, or other macromolecules can be entrapped in the gel or immobilized on the surface without loss of biological activity of the additive.[156-158] The same poloxamer has been utilized as an emulsifier (o/w) in an emulsion for the preparation of polyacryl starch microspheres.[159] In a comparison of albumin and casein microspheres as a carrier for doxorubicin, poloxamer 231 was used together with other surfactants to form a (w/o) emulsion.[160]

Poloxamer 183 has been used as the dispersant in the suspension polymerization preparation of polybutylcyanoacrylate microspheres containing radioactive actinomycin D.[161] Poloxamer 188 has been utilized as the suspending or dispersing agent in several studies in which nanoparticles of different compositions were successfully suspended in aqueous media and injected i.v. in mice or rats or placed in the cul de sac of rabbits.[162-164] In some of the studies, the microspheres encapsulated a drug or radiological tracer which was used to study the path the nanoparticles took after i.v. injection.[165] Poloxamer 144 has been used in a meltable dispersion procedure to prepare 5-fluorouracil wax microspheres, while poloxamer 338 was utilized to prepare nanoparticle suspensions of poly(butyl-2- cyanoacrylates).[166,167] Although utilized as an emulsifying or as a suspending agent, the poloxamer could often end up as part of the outer layer of the microsphere.

A big disadvantage in using colloids as intravenous drug carriers has been their rapid uptake and clearance by the liver and spleen within cells of the RES. This is thought to be due to interfacial adsorption of plasma proteins onto the colloid, or opsonization, followed by adherence of the opsonized particles to the phagocyte surface, and internalization or phagocytosis. The technique of preferentially coating the microspheres with a poloxamer has led to some interesting results, as will be seen in the following paragraphs.

A study of the effects of surface characteristics when poloxamer 338 was us
small polystyrene microspheres showed that the measured zeta potential differ
reduced. It was postulated that the hydrophobic polyoxypropylene portion of the
anchors to the colloidal particle surface, while the hydrophilic polyoxyethylene chai
in the aqueous phase to provide stability by repulsion and steric hindrance of simila
particles. In a comparison of the 188 and 338 grades, the higher molecular wei
338 results in a thicker adsorbed layer than that of the 188 grade, which con
greater colloid stability with minimal adhesive properties. Similar results wer
earlier in a study on the clearance of fat emulsions.[23] The 338 emulsion (o/w)
stable than the one in which polyol 188 was the emulsifier. By coating the colloid
with an agent that adsorbs strongly to the surface, it has been found possible to
nanoparticles to target organs without their being completely taken up by the liver
(RES), which is the fate of uncoated particles. It was suggested that this may be
complement activation property exhibited by the poloxamers, which causes them to
rapidly by the liver and spleen, leading to the possibility of drug-carrying nat
reaching their target sites.[168-170]

A limited study compared the coating effect of varying the hydrophile size o
molecular weight poloxamer hydrophobes on the nanoparticle size. Average di
70 to 250 nm were obtained. It was found that size increased with a decre
polyoxyethylene chain length due to smaller steric stabilization. It was not feasible
the effect of a varying hydrophobe chain length on nanoparticle size due to the
effect of unequal oxyethylene chain lengths. However, it was concluded that it
possible to obtain microspheres with a controlled average particle size and a lo
perisity index by using the proper poloxamer.[171]

Further investigations with poloxamers 188 and 388 as a coating for polyst
oparticles led to the finding that it was possible to divert the microspheres awa
liver after i.v. injection into rabbits. The use of polymer 338 resulted in a 48%
in the liver uptake of coated nanoparticles and a concurrent uptake by the bon
The effect on drug phagocytosis was studied *in vitro*. In the presence of serum,
338, but not 188, maintained the ability to suppress phagocytosis. The powerful an
properties of the 338 polymer were attributed to its two large hydrophilic grc
prevented cell adhesion and minimized opsonization.[172] The effect of coating sm
colloidal particles with poloxamers 188, 338, or 407 was studied on the uptake
when given i.v. to rabbits. This resulted in a combined liver and spleen uptake,
of the particles injected to 70%, 45%, and 15%, respectively. A significant uptake
in the bone marrow occurred with poloxamers 338 and 407, which suggests
systems might be useful for drug targeting to the bone marrow. Evaluation of
11 polyols with varying hydrophile and hydrophobe chain lengths clearly estab
the thickness of the adsorbed layer depends directly on the oxyethylene con
independent of the propylene oxide content. The zeta potential was reduced fro
for uncoated particles to about $-18mV$ for the poloxamer 407-coated particles
also indicated that the particle-macrophage interaction can be significantly redu
high molecular weight poloxamer with large oxyethylene chains is used to coa
particles.[173]

The design of novel drug delivery systems should take into account the
delivery system at, or on its way to, its destination in the body for the better t
a disease.[174] As a better understanding of all the factors involved is develope
appear that the coating of microspheres with a poloxamer, or a chemical modif
poloxamer, could lead the way for the creation of drug carrier systems that w
practical, efficient, and cost effective.

L. NATURAL BLOOD

Another interesting and unusual application area of the poloxamers has been due to the antihemolytic effect observed with at least one member of the series, the 188 grade. The effects produced by the poloxamers when used with natural blood have been extensively studied and reported in the literature. An earlier publication has summarized many of the investigations reported through the early 1970s.[175] To summarize, based on animal studies, the polyol 188 showed promise for clinical use, since it was concluded that it

1. Decreased hemolysis and aided the urinary excretion of hemoglobin in extracorporeal circulation.
2. Lowered whole blood viscosity.
3. Raised blood flow in the microcirculation and in the venous return to the pump.
4. Markedly decreased platelet adhesiveness.
5. Lowered vascular resistance in isolated splenic perfusion and increased successful perfusion from 1 to 6 h.
6. Showed no toxic effects.[176]

The same poloxamer was reported to have been used clinically for treating frostbite, and was routinely added to blood used in the pump oxygenator for all clinical cases at the Department of Surgery, Vanderbilt University School of Medicine.

Isolated rabbit kidneys were perfused with an ionic composition similar to that of rabbit plasma and containing various colloids, including poloxamer 338 or bovine serum albumin. Good glomerular filtration rates and low protein leakage were observed with the polymer, but a high degree of protein leakage was observed in the albumin-perfused kidney.[177] The same poloxamer was evaluated as a plasma expander in a study on the permeability of the glomerular capillary wall to neutral macromolecules in isolated perfused rat kidneys. No significant differences were found between the fractional clearance of the poloxamer obtained with concentrations ranging from 15 to 35 g/l, and therefore with largely different osmotic pressures.[178]

The effect of poloxamer 188 as a prophylactic for hemolysis in extracorporeal circulation was studied by the double blind method in 83 patients. At a level of 1 mg/cc, the hemolytic effect was more noticeable when circulation time exceeded 60 min. No adverse effects on serum lipids, kidney, liver, pancreas, blood coagulation, and serum enzymes were observed.[179] The same polymer has been reported to inhibit the *in vitro* adherence and migration of polymorphonuclear leukocytes obtained from some species of animals.[180] The influence of polyol 188 was studied on the rheology and adhesion of sickle cells saturated with oxygen and carbon monoxide.

A 5% (v/v) concentration of the polymer was effective in improving the filtration of washed sickle cells by 25% (filtered through 5 μm diameter pores at wall shear stresses of up to 1000 dyn/cm²). Adherence of gravity-sedimented sickle cells to endothelial monolayers in the presence of saline or plasma was eliminated. The poloxamer was reported to have no effect on normal adult red cells. Instead, the lubricating effect of the polyol on cell surfaces was believed responsible for all the rheological observations.[181]

The infusion of poloxamer 188 on the injury induced by intratracheal bleomycin instillation was studied in rats. The data obtained showed that the poloxamer can affect polymorphonuclear leukocyte traffic both *in vitro* and *in vivo*.[182] An improved fibrinolytic composition for treating thrombi and emboli is claimed to consist of a hydrophilic poloxamer, such as the 188, together with a proteolytic enzyme such as tissue plasminogen activator, urokinase, prourokinase, or streptokinase.[183] The poloxamer 188 appears to inhibit coronary thrombosis after stent placement in swine and appears beneficial for use in coronary angioplasty.[184]

Poloxamer 108 has been reported to be potentially useful for application in the large

scale fractionation of human plasma proteins at ambient temperatures. The same po
has been used to precipitate immunoglobulin for a range of antisera as an initial st
preparation of diagnostic reagents. The ability of the poloxamer to form insoluble co
with macromolecules is believed to be the cause of this phenomenon.[185]

M. LUBRICATING

An unusual application of poloxamer 188 is its use as a lubricant coating for a s
polyglycolic acid suture, Dexon® (Davis & Geck). This poloxamer is gradually a
in the body and results in an uncoated suture with increased knot security.[185] The
188 was specifically selected because it does not damage the tissue defenses of the
invite infection, and because it had a history of safety in experimental animals and hu
The Dexon Plus, when compared to another coated suture, displayed a lower coeff
friction, encountered less tissue drag forces, and exhibited less flexural rigidity.[187]

IV. CONCLUSION

The selected, but necessarily limited, examples of the published uses of the po
block copolymer surface active agents that have been described for the medical a
maceutical industries can be augmented by a perusal of the items listed in the re
that follow. The uniqueness of these high molecular weight polymers, together w
long and varied history of safety in so many different clinical applications, will e
lead to further study of poloxamers and their derivatives in related disciplines.

REFERENCES

1. **Swarbrick, J.,** Drug delivery systems of the future, *Aust. J. Pharm. Sci.,* 55, 73, 1976.
2. **Rieger, M. M.,** Surfactants, in *Pharmaceutical Dosage Forms: Disperse Systems,* Vol. 1, H. A., Rieger, M. M., and Banker, G. S., Eds., Marcel Dekker, New York, 1988, 349.
3. *McCutcheon's Emulsifiers and Detergents,* North American Ed., M C Publishing, Glen Rock,
4. **Schmolka, I. R.,** Polyalkylene oxide block copolymers, in *Nonionic Surfactants,* Schick, I Marcel Dekker, New York, 1967, chap. 10.
5. **Vaughn, T. H., Suter, H. R., Lundsted, L. G., and Kramer, M. G.,** Properties of some newly nonionic detergents, Am. Oil Chemists' Soc. Meet., San Francisco, September 26, 1950.
6. **Lundsted, L. G.,** U.S. Patent 2,674,619, 1954.
7. **Vaughn, T. H., Suter, H. R., Lundsted, L. G., and Kramer, M. G.,** Properties of some newl nonionic detergents, *J. Am. Oil Chemists' Soc.,* 28, 294, 1951.
8. **Am. Soc. for Testing Materials,** Method D 1638-67T, E222, E 326-69.
9. **Ogg, C. L., Porter, W. L., and Wittlets, C. O.,** Determining the hydroxyl content of cer compounds, macro and semi-micro methods, *Ind. Eng. Chem. Anal. Ed.,* 17, 395, 1945.
10. **Wyandotte Chemicals Corp.,** The Pluronic® Grid, 6th ed., Wyandotte, MI, 1968.
11. **Pacifico, C. R., Lundsted, L. G., and Vaughn, T. H.,** Flake form nonionic detergents, *So Chem.,* 26, 40, 1950.
12. **Schmolka, I. R.,** Block polymer surfactants in cosmetic creams and lotions, *Cosmet. Toiletr* 1980.
13. **Kuwamura, T., Takahashi, H., and Hatori, T.,** Surface active copolymers. I. Preparatio surface active properties of block copolymers of tetrahydrofuran and ethylene oxide, *J. Am. O Soc.,* 48, 29, 1971.
14. **Schmolka, I. R.,** New surfactants for shampoo formulations, *Cosmet. Toiletries,* 97, 61, 198
15. **Rosen, M. J.,** Surfactants and Interfacial Phenomena, John Wiley & Sons, New York, 1978,
16. **Wyandotte Chemicals Corporation,** Tech. Bull., Presenting the Pluronic® Grid, Wyandotte, 1956.
17. **BASF Wyandotte Corporation,** Industrial Chemicals Group, Pluronic® Polyols, Toxicity a Data, Wyandotte, MI. May 1976.

18. **Fukumoto, M.,** Acute oral and acute dermal toxicity study of poloxamer 407 in rats and rabbits, *Nippon Kontakuto Renzu Gakkai Kaishi,* 22, 161, 1980.
19. **Case, M. T., Smith, J. K., and Nelson, R. A.,** Acute mouse and chronic dog toxicity studies of danthron, dioctyl sodium sulfosuccinate, poloxalkol and combinations, *Drug Chem. Toxicol.,* 1, 89, 1977.
20. **Schmolka, I. R.,** Theory of emulsions, *Fed. Proc.,* 29, 1717, 1970.
21. **Artz, C. P.,** Newer concepts of nutrition by the intravenous route, *Ann. Surg.,* 149, 841, 1959.
22. **DeLuca, P. P. and Boylan, J. C.,** Formulation of small volume parenterals, in *Pharmaceutical Dosage Forms: Parenteral Medications,* Vol. 1, Avis, K. E., Lachman, L., and Lieberman, H. A., Eds., Marcel Dekker, New York, 1984, 175.
23. **Geyer, R.,** Parenteral emulsions — formulations, preparation, and use in animals, in *Parenteral Nutrition,* Meng, H. C. and Law, D. H., Eds., Thomas, Springfield, MA, 1970.
24. **Lundsted, L. G. and Schmolka, I. R.,** The applications of block copolymer polyol surfactants, in *Block and Graft Copolymerization,* Vol 2, Ceresa, E. J., Ed., John Wiley & Sons, New York, 1976, 185.
25. **Law, T. K., Florence, A. T., and Whateley, T. L.,** Release from multiple w/o/w emulsions stabilized by interfacial complexation, *J. Pharm. Pharmacol.,* 36, 50P, 1984.
26. **Law, T. K., Whateley, T. L., and Florence, A. T.,** Stabilisation of w/o/w multiple emulsions by interfacial complexation of macromolecules and nonionic surfactants, *J. Controlled Release,* 3, 279, 1986.
27. **Davis, S. S. and Walker, I. M.,** Multiple emulsions as targetable delivery systems, *Methods Enzymol.,* 149, 51, 1987.
28. **Lin, T. H. and Lin, S. Y.,** Encapsulation and prolonged release behavior of w/o/w type multiple emulsions, *J. Chin. Chem. Soc. (Taipei),* 35, 463, 1988.
29. **Davis, S. S. and Hansrani, P.,** The influence of emulsifying agents on the phagocytosis of lipid emulsions by macrophages, *Int. J. Pharm.,* 23, 69, 1985.
30. **Benita, S., Friedman, D., and Weinstock, M.,** Physostigmine emulsion: a new injectable controlled release delivery system, *Int. J. Pharm.,* 30, 47, 1986.
31. **Benita, S., Friedman, D., and Weinstock, M.,** Pharmacological evaulation of an injectable prolonged release emulsion of physostigmine in rabbits, *J. Pharm. Pharmacol.,* 38, 653, 1986.
32. **Krantz, Jr., J. C., Cascarbi, H. F., Hebrich, M., Burgison, R. B., Gold, M. I., and Rudo, F.,** A note on the intravenous use of anesthetic emulsions in animals and man with special reference to methoxyflurane, *Anesthesiology,* 22, 491, 1961.
33. **Geyer, R. P.,** Whole animal perfusion with fluorocarbon dispersions, *Fed. Proc.,* 29, 1758, 1970.
34. **Nose, Y., Kon, T., Weber, D., Mrava, G., Malchesky, P., MacDermott, H., Williams, Jr., C., Lewis, L., Hoffman, G., Willis, C., Deodhar, S., Harris, G., and Anderson, R.,** Physiological effects of intravascular fluorocarbon liquids, *Fed. Proc.,* 29, 1789, 1970.
35. **Mitsuno, T., Ohyanagi, H., and Yokoyama, K.,** Development of perfluorochemical emulsion as a blood gas carrier, *Artif. Organs,* 8, 25, 1984.
36. **Vercellotti, G. M., Hammerschmidt, D. E., Craddock, P. R., and Jacob, H. S.,** Activation of plasma complement by perfluorocarbon artificial blood: probable mechanism of adverse pulmonary reactions in treated patients and rationale for corticosteroid prophylaxis, *Blood,* 59, 1299, 1982.
37. **Gangoda, M., Fung, B. M., and O'Rear, E. A.,** Modifications of nonionic surfactants with perfluorinated terminal groups, *J. Colloid Interface Sci.,* 116, 230, 1987.
38. **Zarif, L., Manfredi, A., Varescon, C., LeBlanc, M., and Riess, J. G.,** Synergistic stabilization of perfluorocarbon-Pluronic F-68 emulsion by perfluoroalkylated polyhydroxylated surfactants, *J. Am. Oil Chemists' Soc.,* 66, 1515, 1989.
39. **Young, S. W., Enzmann, D. R., Long, D. M., and Muller, H. H.,** Perfluoroctylbromide contrast enhancement of malignant neoplasms: preliminary observations, *Am. J. Roentgenol.,* 137, 141, 1981.
40. **Willits, L. W. and Holstius, E. A.,** Calamine lotion-suggested improvements, *J. Am. Pharm. Assoc.,* 17, 87, 1956.
41. **Nash, R. A. and Haeger, B. E.,** U.S. Patent 3,457,348, 1969.
42. **Richard, M. N. and Sanders, B. E.,** Effect of lysine and wetting agents on activated plasminogen solutions, *Can. J. Biochem. Physiol.,* 41, 211, 1963.
43. **Swim, H. E. and Parker, R. F.,** Effect of Pluronic F-68 on growth of fibroblasts in suspension on rotary shaker, *Proc. Soc. Exp. Biol. Med.,* 103, 252, 1960.
44. **Radlett, P. J., Telling, R. C., Stone, C. J., and Whiteside, J. P.,** Improvements in the growth of baby hamster kidney-21 cells in submerged culture, *Appl. Microbiol.,* 22, 534, 1971.
45. **Mizrahi, A.,** Pluronic polyols in human lymphocyte cell line cultures, *J. Clin. Microbiol.,* 2, 11, 1975.
46. **Evans, H. H., Ricanati, M., Horng, M., and Mencl, J.,** Relationship between topoisomerase II and radiosensitivity in mouse L5178Y lymphoma strains, *Mutation Res.,* 217, 53, 1989.
47. **Sprague, G. L. and Craigmill, A. L.,** Ethanol and delta-9-tetrahydrocannabinol: mechanism for cross-tolerance in mice, *Pharmacol. Biochem. Behavior,* 5, 409, 1976.
48. **Clarke, M. B., Tyrrell, D. A., and Barrett, J. J.,** Normal volunteer studies with modified $^{99}Tc^m$ tin colloid, *Nucl. Med. Commun.,* 6, 641, 1985.

49. **New England Nuclear Corp.**, Microlite® ⁹⁹Tcᵐ albumin colloid kit, Medical diagnostics divi

50. Albumin Microspheres (Human), 3M Company Tech. Bull., Minneapolis, 1975.

51. **Chawla, A. S., Hinberg, I., Blais, P., and Johnson, D.**, Aggregation of insulin, containin in contact with different materials, *Diabetes*, 34, 420, 1985.

52. **Irsigler, K., Kritz, H., Hagmüller, G., Franetzki, M., Prestele, K., Thurow, H., and** Long-term continuous intraperitoneal insulin infusion with an implanted remote-controlled in device, *Diabetes*, 30, 1072, 1981.

53. **Grau, U. and Saudek, C. D.**, Stable insulin preparation for implanted insulin pumps, la animal trials, *Diabetes*, 36, 1453, 1987.

54. **Lee, J. H., Kopecek, J., and Andrade, J. D.**, Protein-resistant surfaces prepared by PE block copolymer surfactants, *J. Biomed. Mater. Res.*, 23, 351, 1989.

55. **Thurow, H. and Geisen, K.**, Stabilisation of dissolved proteins against denaturation at interfaces, *Diabetologia*, 27, 212, 1984.

56. *USAN and the USP Dictionary of Drug Names*, U.S. Pharmacopeial Convention, Inc., Ro 1980, 303.

57. **Christopher, L. J.**, A controlled trial of laxatives in geriatric patients, *Practitioner*, 202, 8

58. **Akande, B.**, Treatment of hemorrhoids: controlled clinical trial of haemosol and placebo, *Res.*, 40, 369, 1986.

59. **Sasmor, E. J.**, U.S. Patent 3,422,186, 1969.

60. **Fenner, O., Von Der Beek, T. H., Kallistratos, G., and Timmerman, A.**, Dissolutic components in chemolysis of kidney stones, *Arzneim. Forsch.*, 18, 1348, 1968.

61. **Leuschner, U., Baumgärtel, H., and Wurbs, D.**, Resolution of cholesterine-bilestone wi Capmul 8210-emulsion and with an EDTA solution, *Leber Magen Darm*, 10, 284, 1980.

62. **Leuschner, U., Wurbs, D., Baumgärtel, H., Helm, E. B., and Classen, M.**, Alternating common bile duct stones with a modified glyceryl-1-monooctanoate preparation and a bil solution by nasobiliary tube, *Scand. J. Gastroenterol.*, 16, 497, 1981.

63. **Leuschner, U. and Baumgärtel, H.**, Gallstone dissolution in the biliary tract: *in vitro* inv inhibiting factors and special dissolution agents, *Am. J. Gastroenterol.*, 77, 222, 1982.

64. **Bryant, C. A., Rodeheaver, G. T., Reem, E. M., Nichter, L. S., Kenney, J. G., and F** Search for a nontoxic surgical scrub solution for periorbital lacerations, *Ann. Emerg. Med.*, 1

65. **Lowbury, E. J. L. and Billy, H. A.**, Use of 4% chlorhexidine detergent solution (Hibiscr methods of skin disinfection, *Br. Med. J.*, 1, 510, 1973.

66. **Schmolka, I. R.**, A review of block polymer surfactants, *J. Am. Oil Chemists' Soc.*, 54, 1

67. **Zhou, Z. and Chu, B.**, Light-scattering study on the association behavior of triblock polyme oxide and propylene oxide in aqueous solution, *J. Colloid Interface Sci.*, 126, 171, 1988.

68. **Prasad, K. N., Luong, T. T., Florence, A. T., Paris, J., Vaution, C., Seiller, M., and** Surface activity and association of ABA polyoxyethylene-polyoxypropylene block copolyme solution, *J. Colloid Interface Sci.*, 69, 225, 1979.

69. **Rassing, J. and Attwood, D.**, Ultrasonic velocity and light scattering studies on the pol polyoxypropylene copolymer Pluronic F-127 in aqueous solution, *Int. J. Pharm.*, 13, 47, 1

70. **Saettone, M. F., Giannaccini, B., Delmonte, G., Campigli, V., Tota, G., and LaMar** bilization of tropicamide by poloxamers: physicochemical data and activity data in rabbits anc *J. Pharm.*, 43, 67, 1988.

71. **Collett, J. H. and Tobin, E. A.**, The solubilization of some *para*-substituted acetanilid solutions of polyoxyethylene-polyoxypropylene block copolymers, *J. Pharm. Pharmacol.*, 2

72. **Reddy, R. K., Khalil, S. A., and Gouda, M. W.**, Effect of dioctyl sodium sulfosuccinate a 188 on dissolution and intestinal absorption of sulfadiazine and sulfisoxazole in rats, *J. Pho* 115, 1976.

73. **Chow, S. and Sims, B. E.**, Micellar solubilization of cetaben sodium in surfactant and lipi *Pharm. Sci.*, 70, 924, 1981.

74. **Collett, J. H., Rees, J. A., and Buckley, D. L.**, The influence of some structurally relate the hydrolysis of aspirin, *J. Pharm. Pharmacol.*, 31, 80P, 1979.

75. **Hollander, D., Rim, E., and Muralidhara, K. S.**, Vitamin K₁ intestinal absorption *in vivc* luminal contents on transport, *Am. J. Physiol.*, 232, E69, 1977.

76. **Prancan, A. V., Ecanow, B., Bernardoni, R. J., and Sadove, M. S.**, Poloxamer 188 as injectable diazepam, *J. Pharm. Sci.*, 69, 970, 1980.

77. **Lin, S. and Kawashima, Y.**, Pluronic surfactants affecting diazepam solubility, compatib sorption from i.v. admixture solutions, *J. Parenter. Sci. Technol.*, 41, 83, 1987.

78. **Lin, S. and Kawashima, Y.**, The influence of three poly(oxyethylene)poly(oxypropylene) block copolymers on the solubility behavior of indomethacin, *Pharm. Acta Helv.*, 60, 339,

79. **Tarr, B. D. and Yalkowsky, S. H.**, A new parenteral vehicle for the administration of som soluble anticancer drugs, *J. Parenter. Sci. Technol.*, 41, 31, 1987.

80. **Fu, R. C., Lidgate, D. M., Whatley, J. L., and McCullough, T.,** The biocompatibility of parenteral vehicles — *in vitro/in vivo* screening comparison and the effect of excipients on hemolysis, *J. Parenter. Sci. Technol.*, 41, 164, 1987.

81. **Gibbs, I. S., Heald, A., Jacobson, H., Wadke, D., and Weliky, I.,** Physical characterization and activity *in vivo* of polymorphic forms of 7-chloro-5,11-dihydrodibenz(b,e)(1,4)oxazepine-5-carboxamide, a potential tricyclic antidepressant, *J. Pharm. Sci.*, 65, 1380, 1976.

82. **Fergusson, M. J. C., Munro, A. C., and Gabra, G. S.,** Measurement of factor, VIIIRAg-1. A method for use in the hyland laser nephelometer, *Thromb. Res.*, 34, 175, 1984.

83. **Sattler, J., Hesterberg, R., Schmidt, U., Crombach, M., and Lorenz, W.,** Inhibition of intestinal diamine oxidase by detergents: a problem for drug formulations with water insoluble agents applied by the intravenous route, *Agents Actions*, 20, 270, 1987.

84. **Parrott, E. L. and Sharma, V. K.,** Dissolution kinetics of benzoic acid in high concentrations of surface-active agents, *J. Pharm. Sci.*, 56, 1341, 1967.

85. **Schmolka, I. R. and Bacon, L.,** Viscosity characteristics of aqueous solutions of block copolymers of propylene and ethylene oxides, *J. Am. Oil Chemists' Soc.*, 44, 559, 1967.

86. **Schmolka, I. R.,** Artificial skin I. Preparation and properties of Pluronic F-127 gels for treatment of burns, *J. Biomed. Mater. Res.*, 6, 571, 1972.

87. **Schmolka, I. R.,** Gel cosmetics, *Cosmet. Toiletries*, 99, 69, 1984.

88. **Gilbert, J. C., Richardson, J. L., Davies, M. C., Palin, K. J., and Hadgraft, J.,** The effect of solutes and polymers on the gelation properties of Pluronic F-127 solutions for controlled drug delivery., *J. Controlled Release*, 5, 113, 1987.

89. **Henry, R. L. and Schmolka, I. R.,** Burn wound coverings and the use of poloxamer preparations, *Crit. Rev. Biocompatibility*, 5, 207, 1989.

90. **Schmolka, I. R.,** U.S. Patent 3,639,575, 1972.

91. **Nalbandian, R. M., Henry, R. L., and Wilks, H. S.,** Artificial skin. II. Pluronic F-127 silver nitrate or silver lactate gel in the treatment of thermal burns, *J. Biomed. Mater. Res.*, 6, 571, 1972.

92. **Nalbandian, R. M., Henry, R. L., Balko, K. W., Adams, D. V., and Neuman, N. R.,** Pluronic F-127 gel preparation as an artificial skin in the treatment of third-degree burns in pigs, *J. Biomed. Mater. Res.*, 21, 1135, 1987.

93. **Kolling, W. M.,** Studies on silver sulfadiazine poloxamer 407 gels, M.S. thesis, University of Illinois, Chicago, 1984.

94. **Adams, D. V., Cremers, N. J., and Henry, R. L.,** U.S. Patent 4,534,958, 1985.

95. **Miyazaki, S., Yokouchi, C., Nakamura, T., Hashiguchi, N., Hou, W., and Takada, M.,** Pluronic F-127 gels as a novel vehicle for rectal administration of indomethacin, *Chem. Pharm. Bull.*, 34, 1801, 1986.

96. **Schmolka, I. R.,** U.S. Patent 3,639,574, 1972.

97. **Ng, S., Mei, K., and Wieckowski, S.,** Eur. Pat. Appl. EP 288,420, 1988.

98. **Zinner, D. D., Duany, L. F., and Lutz, H. J.,** A new desensitizing dentifrice: preliminary report, *J. Am. Dent. Assoc.*, 95, 982, 1977.

99. **Wei, S. H. Y., and Connor, Jr., C. W.,** Fluoride uptake and retention *in vitro* following topical fluoride applications, *J. Dent. Res.*, 62, 830, 1983.

100. **Shevlin, E. J.,** private communication, 1978.

101. **Silverman, H. I. and Himathongkham, T.,** Evaluation of an anti-microbial gel using microbiological studies *in vitro* and clinical studies *in vivo*, Abstr. SCC Annu. Sci. Meet., New York, 1972.

102. **Krezanoski, J. Z.,** U.S. Patent 4,188,373, 1980.

103. **Miller, S. C. and Donovan, M. D.,** Effect of poloxamer 407 gel on the miotic activity of pilocarpine nitrate in rabbits, *Int. J. Pharm.*, 12, 147, 1982.

104. **Gurny, R., Ibrahim, H., Boye, T., and Buri, P.,** Latices and thermosensitive gels as sustained delivery systems to the eye, *Fidia Res. Ser.*, 11, 27, 1987.

105. **Habib, F. S. and Attia, M. A.,** Comparative study of the ocular activity in rabbit eyes of adrenaline bitartrate formulated in carbopol and poloxamer gels, *Arch. Pharm. Chem., Sci. Ed.*, 12, 91, 1984.

106. **Kim, J. P., Peiffer, R. L., and Holman, R. E.,** Pluronic polyol: a potential alloplastic keratorefractive material, *J. Cataract Refract. Surg.*, 14, 312, 1988.

107. **Better, B., Grosse, E., Zimmerman, I., and Tack, J. W.,** PCT Int. Appl. WO 86 00,813, 1986.

108. **Miyazaki, S., Takeuchi, C., Yokouchi, C., and Takada, M.,** Pluronic F-127 gels as a vehicle for topical administration of anticancer agents, *Chem. Pharm. Bull.*, 32, 4205, 1984.

109. **Morikawa, K., Okada, F., Hosokawa, M., and Kobayashi, H.,** Enhancement of therapeutic effects of recombinant interleukin 2 on a transplantable rat fibrosarcoma by the use of a sustained release vehicle, Pluronic gel, *Cancer Res.*, 47, 37, 1987.

110. **Tomida, H., Shinohara, M., Kuwada, N., and Kiryu, S.,** *In vitro* release characteristics of diclofenac and hydrocortisone from Pluronic F-127 gels, *Acta Pharm. Suec.*, 24, 263, 1987.

111. **Chen-Chow, P. and Frank, S. G.,** *In vitro* release of lidocaine from Pluronic F-127 gels, *Int. J. Pharm.*, 8, 89, 1981.

112. **Chen-Chow, P. and Frank, S. G.,** Comparison of lidocaine release from Pluronic F-127 gels formulations, *Acta Pharm. Suec.,* 18, 239, 1981.

113. **Rassing, J.,** A new ultrasonic differential method for measuring diffusion coefficients of drugs in gel samples. Application to the diffusion of lidocaine hydrochloride and lidocaine base inside a 25% F-127 gel, *J. Controlled Release,* 1, 169, 1985.

114. **Hadgraft, J. and Howard, J. R.,** Drug release from Pluronic gels, *J. Pharm. Pharmacol.,* 34,

115. **Gilbert, J. C., Hadgraft, J., Bye, A., and Brookes, L. G.,** Drug release from Pluronic F-127 *J. Pharm.,* 32, 223, 1986.

116. **Wu, H. S.,** Poloxamer Drug Delivery Systems for Topical Applications. I. *In Vitro* Release of Acid Alkyl Esters, Ph.D. thesis, University of Minnesota, Minneapolis, 1986.

117. **Schmolka, I. R.,** U.S. Patent 4,511,563, 1985.

118. **Demchak, R. J. and Corso, Jr., V.,** U.S. Patent 4,287,176, 1981.

119. **Attwood, D., Collett, J. H., Davies, M. C., and Tait, C. J.,** The effect of batch variability properties and *in vivo* release characteristics of Pluronic F-127 gels, *J. Pharm. Pharmacol.,* 37,

120. **Johnston, T. P. and Miller, S. C.,** Toxicological evaluation of poloxamer vehicles for intramu *J. Parenter. Sci. Tech.,* 39, 83, 1985.

121. **Zanevold, L. J. D., Burns, J. W., Goodpasture, J. C., and Vickery, B. H.,** Evaluation of efficacy of a new vaginal contraceptive agent in stumptailed macaques, *Fertil. Steril.,* 41, 455

122. **Corey, H.,** U.S. Patent 4,185,618, 1980.

123. **Schmolka, I. R.,** U.S. Patent 4,585,647, 1986.

124. **Miyazaki, S., Nakamura, T., Yokouchi, C., and Takada, M.,** Effect of Pluronic gels on absorption of indomethacin in rabbits, *Chem. Pharm. Bull.,* 35, 1243, 1987.

125. **Itoh, S., Morishita, N., Yamazaki, M., Suginaka, A., Tanabe, K., and Sawanoi, M.,** Biophar characteristics of a suppository base containing poly(oxyethylene)-poly(oxypropylene) copolyme I. Effects of a suppository base containing unilube .70DP-950B on release and rectal absorpti nopyrine in rabbit, *J. Pharmacobio-Dyn.,* 10, 173, 1987.

126. **Neville, J. and Swafford, W. B.,** Pluronics as a suppository base, *Am. J. Pharm.,* 132, 301,

127. **Buckwalter, F. H.,** U.S. Patent 2,854,378, 1958.

128. **Al-Saden, A. A., Florence, A. T., and Whateley, T. L.,** Cross-linked hydrophilic gels from copolymeric surfactants, *Int. J. Pharm.,* 5, 317, 1980.

129. **Gardener, S. and Jones, J. G.,** A new solidifying agent for culture media which liquifies on *Gen. Microbiol.,* 130, 731, 1984.

130. **Heyer, K. and Frömming, K. H.,** Solidified melts of griseofulvin in Pluronic F-68, *Dtsch. A* 123, 859, 1983.

131. **Gander, B., Gurny, R., Doelker, E., and Peppas, N. A.,** Cross-linked poly(alkylene oxide preparation of controlled release micromatrices, *J. Controlled Release,* 5, 271, 1988.

132. **Chang, R., Hsiao, C. H., and Robinson, J. R.,** A review of aqueous coating techniques and data on release from a theophylline product, *Pharm. Technol.,* 11, 56, 1987.

133. **Davis, M. B., Peck, G. E., and Banker, G. S.,** Preparation and stability of aqueous-based enter dispersions, *Drug Dev. Ind. Pharm.,* 12, 1419, 1986.

134. **Gurny, R., Peppas, N. A., Harrington, D. D., and Banker, G. S.,** Development of biodeg injectable latices for controlled release of potent drugs, *Drug Dev. Ind. Pharm.,* 7, 1, 1981.

135. **Bodmeier, R. and Paeratakul, O.,** Evaluation of drug-containing polymer films prepared fro latexes, *Pharm. Res.,* 6, 725, 1989.

136. **Hunter, R., Strickland, F., and Kezdy, F.,** The adjuvant activity of nonionic block polymer I. The role of hydrophile-lipophile balance, *J. Immunol.,* 127, 1244, 1981.

137. **Snippe, H., DeReuver, M. J., Strickland, F., Willers, J. M. N., and Hunter, R. L.,** Adju of nonionic block polymer surfactants in humoral and cellular immunity, *Int. Arch. Allergy Appl.* 65, 390, 1981.

138. **Hunter, R. L. and Bennett, B.,** The adjuvant activity of nonionic block polymer surfactants II formation and inflammation related to the structure of triblock and octablock copolymers, *J.* 133, 3167, 1984.

139. **Allison, A. C. and Schreiber, A. B.,** Applications of monoclonal antibodies to investigation factors, their receptors and tumor antigens, and an adjuvant formulation potentially useful for im against malignant diseases, *Symp. Mol. Cell. Biol. New Ser.,* 27, 397, 1985.

140. **Allison, A. C. and Byars, N. E.,** An adjuvant formulation that selectively elicits the formation o of protective isotypes and of cell-mediated immunity, *J. Immunol. Methods,* 95, 157, 1986.

141. **Marx, P. A., Pedersen, N. C., Lerche, N. W., Osborn, K. G., Lowenstine, L. J., Lackr Maul, D. H., Kwang, H., Kluge, J. D., Zaiss, C. P., Sharpe, V., Spinner, A. P., Allis and Gardner, M. B.,** Prevention of simian acquired immune deficiency syndrome with a for tivated type D retrovirus vaccine, *J. Virology,* 60, 431, 1986.

142. **Byars, N. E. and Allison, A. C.**, Adjuvant formulation for use in vaccines to elicit both cell-mediated and humoral immunity, *Vaccine*, 5, 223, 1987.

143. **Zigterman, G. J. W. J., Snippe, H., Jansze, M., and Willers, J. M. N.**, Adjuvant effects of nonionic block polymer surfactants on liposome-induced humoral immune response, *J. Immunol.*, 138, 220, 1987.

144. **Zigterman, G. J. W. J., Snippe, H., Jansze, M., Ernste, E. B. H., DeReuver, M. J., and Willers, J. M. N.**, Nonionic block polymer surfactants enhance immunogenicity of pneumococcal hexasaccharide-protein vaccines, *Infect. Immun.*, 56, 1391, 1988.

145. **Tso, P., Balint, J. A., and Rodgers, J. B.**, Effect of surfactant (Pluronic L-81) on lymphatic lipid transport in the rat, *Am. J. Physiol.*, 239, G348, 1980.

146. **Tso, P. and Gollamudi, S. R.**, Pluronic L-81: a potent inhibitor of the transport of intestinal chylomicrons, *Am. J. Physiol.*, 247, G32, 1984.

147. **Bochenek, W. J. and Rodgers, J. B.**, Effect of Pluronic detergents on lipid absorption, *Gastroenterology*, 72, 7, 1977.

148. **Brunelle, C. W., Bochenek, W. J., Abraham, R., Kim, D. N., and Rodgers, J. B.**, Effect of hydrophobic detergent on lipid absorption in the rat and on lipid and sterol balance in the swine, *Dig. Dis. Sci.*, 24, 718, 1979.

149. **Comai, K. and Sullivan, A. C.**, Antiobesity activity of Pluronic L-101, *Int. J. Obes.*, 4, 33, 1980.

150. **Kapuscinska, B., Bochenek, W. J., and Pikiewicz, K.**, Hypolipemic activity of benzoyl ester of polyoxypropylene-polyoxyethylene block copolymer (BEP) in rabbits, *Atherosclerosis*, 45, 235, 1982.

151. **Bochenek, W. J., Kapuscinska, B., Slowinska, R., and Rodgers, J. B.**, Alterations of secretory pattern of intestinal lipoproteins by the benzoyl ester derivatives of poloxalene surfactant (BEP), *Atherosclerosis*, 64, 167, 1987.

152. **Rodgers, J. B., Kyriakides, E. C., Kapuscinska, B., Peng, S. K., and Bochenek, W. J.**, Hydrophobic surfactant treatment prevents atherosclerosis in the rabbit, *J. Clin. Invest.*, 71, 1490, 1983.

153. **Rodgers, J. B., Kyriakides, E. C., and Bochenek, W. J.**, Effect of surfactant poloxalene 2930 on food intake, lipid absorption, and serum cholesterol in rats, *Exp. Mol. Pathol.*, 40, 214, 1984.

154. **Kapuscinska, B., Bochenek, W. J., Peng, S. K., and Rodgers, J. B.**, Poloxalene 2930, a hydrophobic surfactant that prevents atherosclerosis, alters composition of rabbit lipoproteins, *Atherosclerosis*, 57, 149, 1985.

155. **Illum, L. and Davis, S. S.**, The targeting of drugs parenterally by use of microspheres, *J. Parenter. Sci. Techno.*, 36, 242, 1982.

156. **Ekman, B., Lofter, C., and Sjöholm, I.**, Incorporation of macromolecules in microparticles: preparation and characteristics, *Biochemistry*, 15, 5115, 1976.

157. **Ekman, B. and Sjöholm, I.**, Improved stability of proteins immobilized in microparticles prepared by a modified emulsion polymerization technique, *J. Pharm. Sci.*, 67, 693, 1978.

158. **Ljungstedt, I., Ekman, B., and Sjöholm, I.**, Detection and separation of lymphocytes with specific surface receptors, by using microparticles, *Biochem. J.*, 170, 161, 1978.

159. **Laakso, T., Artursson, P., and Sjöholm, I.**, Biodegradable microspheres IV. Factors affecting the distribution and degradation of polyacryl starch microparticles, *J. Pharm. Sci.*, 75, 962, 1986.

160. **Chen, Y., Willmott, N., Anderson, J., and Florence, A. T.**, Comparison of albumin and casein microspheres as a carrier for doxorubicin, *J. Pharm. Pharmacol.*, 39, 978, 1987.

161. **Kante, B., Couvreur, P., Lenaerts, V., Guiot, P., Roland, M., Baudhuin, P., and Speiser, P.**, Tissue distribution of (^{3}H) actinomycin D adsorbed on polybutylcyanoacrylate nanoparticles, *Int. J. Pharm.*, 7, 45, 1980.

162. **Leu, D., Manthey, B., Kreuter, J., Speiser, P., and DeLuca, P. P.**, Distribution and elimination of coated polymethyl (2-^{14}C) methacrylate nanoparticles after intravenous injection in rats, *J. Pharm. Sci.*, 73, 1433, 1984.

163. **Harmia, T., Speiser, P., and Kreuter, J.**, Optimization of pilocarpine loading onto nanoparticles by sorption procedures, *Int. J. Pharm.*, 33, 45, 1986.

164. **Harmia, T., Kreuter, J., Speiser, P., Boye, T., Gurny, R., and Kubis, A.**, Enhancement of the myotic response of rabbits with pilocarpine-loaded polybutylcyanoacrylate nanoparticles, *Int. J. Pharm.*, 33, 187, 1986.

165. **Illum, L., Jones, P. D. E., Baldwin, R. W., and Davis, S. S.**, Tissue distribution of poly(hexyl2-cyanoacrylate) nanoparticles coated with monoclonal antibodies in mice bearing human tumor xenografts, *J. Pharmacol. Exp. Ther.*, 230, 733, 1984.

166. **Benita, S., Zouai, O., and Benoit, J. P.**, 5-Fluorouracil:carnauba wax microspheres for chemoembolization: an *in vitro* evaluation, *J. Pharm. Sci.*, 75, 847, 1986.

167. **Illum, L., Khan, M. A., Mak, E., and Davis, S. S.**, Evaluation of carrier capacity and release characteristics for poly(butyl 2-cyanoacrylate) nanoparticles, *Int. J. Pharm.*, 30, 17, 1986.

168. **Illum, L. and Davis, S. S.**, Effect of the nonionic surfactant poloxamer 338 on the fate and deposition of polystyrene microspheres following intravenous administration, *J. Pharm. Sci.*, 72, 1086, 1983.

169. **Illum, L. and Davis, S. S.,** The organ uptake of intravenously administered colloidal par altered using a non-ionic surfactant (poloxamer 338), *FEBS Lett.*, 167, 79, 1984.
170. **Illum, L. and Davis, S. S.,** Physiological aspects of small particle delivery systems, Excer Congr. Ser., 750 (Pharmacol.), 619, 1987.
171. **Douglas, S. J., Illum, I., and Davis, S. S.,** Particle size and size distribution of poly(butyl 2-c nanoparticles, *J. Colloid Interface Sci.*, 103, 154, 1986.
172. **Illum, L., Hunneyball, I. M., and Davis, S. S.,** The effect of hydrophilic coatings on ï colloidal particles by the liver and by peritoneal macrophages, *Int. J. Pharm.*, 29, 53, 1986.
173. **Illum, L., Jacobsen, L. O., Müller, R. H., Mak, E., and Davis, S. S.,** Surface character interaction of colloidal particles with mouse peritoneal macrophages, *Biomaterials*, 8, 113, ï
174. **Davis, S. S.,** Biopharmaceutical aspects of drug formulation, *Acta Pharm. Suec.*, 23, 305,
175. **Lundsted, L. G. and Schmolka, I. R.,** The applications of block copolymer polyol surfacta *and Graft Copolymerization*, Vol 2, Ceresa, E. J., Ed., John Wiley & Sons, London, 1976,
176. **Paton, B. C., Grover, F. L., Heron, M. W., Bess, H., and Moore, A. R.,** The use ï detergent added to organ perfusates, in *Organ Perfusion and Preservation*, Norman, J. C., Eï Century-Crofts, New York, 1964, chap. 11.
177. **Fuller, B. J., Pegg, D. E., Walter, C. A., and Green, C. J.,** An isolated rabbit kidney pï use in organ preservation research, *J. Surg. Res.*, 22, 128, 1977.
178. **Brink, H. M., Moons, W. M., and Slegers, J. F. G.,** Glomerular filtration in the isolated pe I. Sieving of macromolecules, *Pfluegers Arch.*, 397, 42, 1983.
179. **Ohishi, K., Hoshino, Y., Isamoto, Y., Nishimura, H., Yuda, T., Miyazaki, T., Yamashit K., Kaneko, H., Tachibana, N.,** Clinical evaluation of poloxamer 188 (Exocorpol) as a prï hemolysis in excorporeal circulation by double-blind method, *J. Jpn. Assoc. Thorac. Surg.*, 3ï
180. **Lane, T. A. and Lampkin, G. E.,** Paralysis of phagocytic migration due to an artificial blo *Blood*, 64, 400, 1984.
181. **Smith, C. M., II, Hebbel, R. P., Tukey, D. P., Clawson, C. C., White, J. G., and G. M.,** Pluronic F-68 reduces the endothelial adherence and improves the rheology of liï erythrocytes, *Blood*, 69, 1631, 1987.
182. **Williams, J. H., Jr., Chen, M., Drew, J., Panigan, E., and Hosseini, S.,** Modulation of rï traffic by a surface activie agent *in vitro* and bleomycin injury (42761), *Proc. Soc. Exp. Bio* 461, 1988.
183. **Hunter, R. L. and Duncan, A.,** U.S. Patent 4,801,452, 1989.
184. **Robinson, K. A., Roubin, G. S., King, S. B., III, Black, A. J., Stack, J. E., and Hï** Inhibition of coronary thrombosis after stent placement in swine by copolymer poloxamer 18ï *Suppl. II*, 78, 408, 1988.
185. **Spence, L. R., Chung, A., and Moore, B. P. L.,** Use of watersoluble polymers in the ï blood group diagnostic reagents, *Med. Lab. Sci.*, 42, 115, 1985.
186. **Rodeheaver, G. T., Foresman, P. A., Brazda, M. T., and Edlich, R. F.,** A temporary nont for a synthetic absorbable suture, *Surg. Gynecol. Obstet.*, 164, 17, 1987.
187. **Rodeheaver, G. T., Thacker, J. G., Owen, J., Strauss, R. A., Masterson, L. P., and Ï** Knotting and handling characteristics of coated synthetic absorbable sutures, *J. Surg. Res.*, 33

Chapter 11

ION-EXCHANGE RESIN DELIVERY SYSTEMS

Saul Borodkin

TABLE OF CONTENTS

I. INTRODUCTION

In the continuing search for novel drug delivery systems to optimize presenta
bioavailability of established therapeutic agents, ion exchange resins should be cc
as polymers with unique advantageous properties. Ion exchange resins may be de
high molecular weight water-insoluble polymers containing fixed positively or ne
charged fucntional groups in their matrix, which have an affinity for oppositely
counterions. Since the majority of drugs possess an ionic site in their molecule, th
of the resin provides a means to loosely attach such drugs to insoluble polymers.

Synthetic ion exchange resins have long been used in pharmacy and medicin
diverse uses include isolation of chemicals in processing operations, absorption of un
toxins in the body, aiding in tablet disintegration, controlled release of drugs, taste
of bitter drugs, and various applications in diagnostic procedures. Their long-term
strated safety, even when ingested in large dosages as in the the use of cholestyr
reduce cholesterol,[2] provides additional incentive to consider the use of such agent
carriers in formulation.

II. ION EXCHANGE RESIN PROPERTIES

A. TYPES OF RESINS

The ion exchange resins can contain either positively or negatively charged s
thus can be either cation or anionic exchangers.[3] Within each category they are
classified as strong or weak depending on their affinity for soluble counter-ions. Tl
cation exchangers contain sulfonic acid sites (e.g., Dowex®50, Amberlite®IR 12(
the weak cation exchange resins (e.g., Amberlite®IRC 50) are based on carbox
moieties. The strong anion exchange resins (e.g., Dowex®1, Amberlite®IR 4(
quaternary amine ionic sites attached to the matrix, while weak anion exchange
Amberlite®IR 4B, Dowex®2) have predominantly tertiary amine substituents.

B. POLYMER MATRIX

The most commonly used polymer backbone for the anion exchange and stro
exchange resins is based on polystyrene. Divinylbenzene(DVB) is included in the
merization for crosslinking the polymer chains. The amount of divinylbenzene
expressed as percentage by weight (wt%), has a major effect on the physical pr
The weak cation exchange resins are generally polyacrylic or polymethacrylic ac
with divinylbenzene as the crosslinking agent. Figure 1 illustrates representative st

C. EQUILIBRIA PHENOMENA

The principal property of these resins is their capacity to exchange bound or
ions with those in solution. Soluble ions may be removed from solution through
with the counterions absorbed on the resin as illustrated in Equations 1 and 2:

$$\text{Re-SO}_3^- \text{ Na}^+ + \text{DRUG}^+ \rightleftharpoons \text{Re-SO}_3^- \text{ DRUG}^+ + \text{Na}^+$$

$$\text{Re-}N(\text{CH}_3)_3^+ \text{ Cl}^- + \text{DRUG}^- \rightleftharpoons \text{Re-}N(\text{CH}_3)_3^+ \text{ DRUG}^- + \text{Cl}^-$$

These exchanges are equilibrium reactions in which the extent of exchange
governed by the relative affinity of the resin for particular ions. Relative affinity
ions may be expressed as a selectivity coefficient, derived from a mass action exp

$$K_{DM} = \frac{[D]_r[M]_s}{[D]_s[M]_r}$$

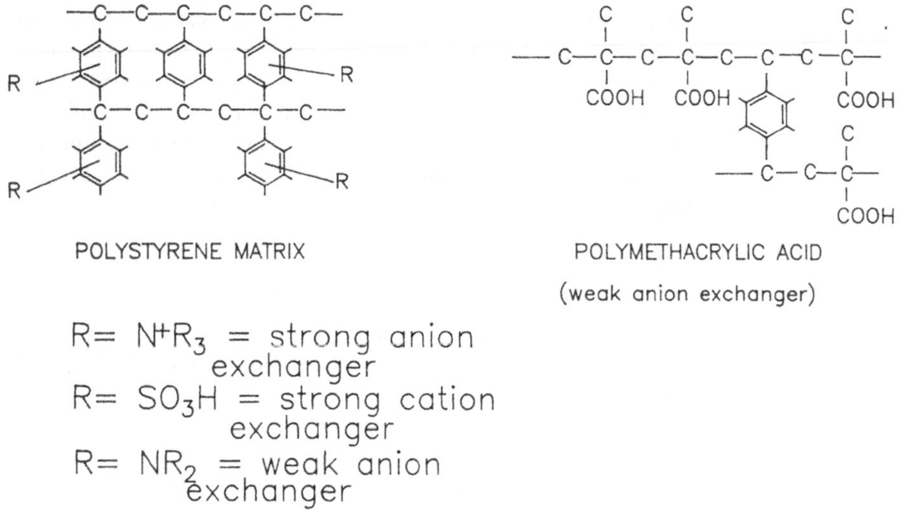

POLYSTYRENE MATRIX

POLYMETHACRYLIC ACID

(weak anion exchanger)

R= N^+R_3 = strong anion exchanger

R= SO_3H = strong cation exchanger

R= NR_2 = weak anion exchanger

FIGURE 1. Structures of ion exchange resins.

TABLE 1
Selectivity Coefficients for Amine Drugs with
Ambelite® IRP-88 at Various pH Levels
Using 0.154 N Na Concentrations

Drug	pH			
	4.5	5.0	5.5	6.0
Phenylpropanolamine	2.5	2.7	2.1	1.5
Desoxyephedrine	7.4	5.8	3.8	2.4
Ephedrine	5.4	4.5	2.8	1.7
Pseudoephedrine	5.6	3.9	2.6	1.6
Carbinoxamine	267	236	131	49
Chromonar	151	77	17	15
Quinidine	353	308	208	116
Methapyriline	179	122	61	24
Dextromethorphan	276	196	112	68
Thiamine	52	44	23	9
Neostigmine	6.4	4.2	2.2	1.1

From Borodkin, S. and Yunker, M. H., Interaction of Amine drugs with a polycarboxylic acid ion-exchange resin, *J. Pharm. Sci.*, 59, 486, 1970. With permission.

where K_{DM} is the selectivity coefficient for drug D and counterion M, $[D]_r$ is drug concentration absorbed on the resin, $[D]_s$ is drug concentration in solution, and $[M]_s$ and $[M]_r$ are counterion concentrations in the solution and resin phases, respectively.

Factors that influence selectivity include valence, hydrated size, pKa, and the pH of the solution. Table 1 lists selectivity coefficients for a series of drugs determined with a carboxylic acid ion exchange resin.[4] When loading the resin with the ion with less affinity, the exchange may be driven toward the direction of unfavorable equilibrium by flooding the influent with high concentrations or, alternatively, by using chromatographic column procedures.

D. EXCHANGE CAPACITY
The exchange capacity refers to the number of ionic sites per unit weight or volume

(meq per g or meq per ml). The weight basis value (meq per g) is generally mu
than the volume-based exchange capacity since the wet resin is highly hydrated. The
capacity may limit the amount of drug that may be absorbed on a resin and hence th
of a complex. Carboxylic acid resins derived from acrylic acid polymers have highe
capacities (about 10 meq/g) than the sulfonic acid (about 4 meq/g) or amine resins
to bulkier ionic substituents and the polystyrene matrix. Therefore, higher drug p
may often be achieved with the carboxylic acid resins.

E. CROSSLINKAGE

The degree of crosslinkage is controlled by the percent divinylbenzene u
copolymerization. This is generally designated with commercial resins by X, fo
the percentage DVB. The fraction DVB determines to what extent the ion exch
is free to swell and shrink. The swelling will in turn affect the rate of hydration, t
expansion of resin in a column, the rate of exchange of ions, and the capacity o
to absorb large molecules. Even after absorption, some large molecules may be
elute unless the DVB percentage is quite low. The swelling capacity of the ior
resins when wetted has been put to practical use with the potassium form of th
thacrylic acid resin, Amberlite® IRP-88, commercially available as a tablet dis
agent.[5]

F. PARTICLE SIZE

Ion exchange resins are available commercially in different size ranges, ge
pressed as mesh ranges. The most common, which are best for column oper
spherical beads of 20 to 50 mesh (297 to 840 μm). Smaller size ranges (50 to
100 to 200 mesh, 200 to 400 mesh) provide better chromatographic separations
be more appropriate for pharmaceutical applications. A series of pharmaceutical g
(e.g., Amberlite®IRP from Rohm & Haas) have ranges of 100 to 400 mesh
μm). Although useful when used directly in formulations, this size range does n
well in column absorption or filtration operations.

III. DRUG RESIN ABSORBATES

A. APPLICATIONS

Drugs absorbed onto ion exchange resins have been referred to as absorbates,
resinates, or sometimes as salts. The first three terms are used interchangeably
they do possess some properties similar to insoluble salts, the resinates differ fro
tional salts in a number of important respects. They are noncrystalline, usually
hydrate readily, have a totally insoluble, nonabsorbable cation or anion, can ha
percentages of drug, and can be prepared in controllable particle size ranges. Such
can strongly influence the release or dissolution behavior of the drug and, thus, th
applications. The ion exchange resin absorbates have been used for the followir

1. *Taste protection* — The slow elution process reduces the exposure of bitt
    the mouth before swallowing.
2. *Sustained release* — The equilibria-driven drug release process results
    dissolution of drug from the resin carrier during its transit in the gastrointes
3. *Controlled release* — Drug release may be effected at target sites by speci
    concentrations of counterions.
4. *Accelerated dissolution* — The noncrystalline, rapidly hydrating adsorbate
    provide faster dissolution of a poorly soluble drug than a crystalline salt.
5. *Carrier for microencapsulation* — The spherical nature and polymer matri

an advantageous substrate for microencapsulation or polymer coating. This process may be used to optimize any of the previous applications or simply as the best method for generating protected particles.

B. SELECTION OF ION EXCHANGE RESIN

Selecting the resin for a specific application requires consideration of a number of factors. Generally, the type charge (cation or anion exhcanger) is obvious, although some amphoteric compounds may allow use of either type. If we wish rapid dissolution in the gastrointestinal tract, we may select weak cation or anionic resins, low crosslinkage, small particle size, and/or high drug potency. Slow or gradual release or maximum taste protection may be obtained with strong cation or anion resins, high crosslinkage, large size range, and lower drug percentages.

If maximum potency is a priority with a low molecular weight drug, we may select a resin with a high exchange capacity (i.e., the carboxylic acid resins). High molecular weight often limits the ability to absorb the drug, and very low crosslinkage may be necessary to achieve meaningful loadings. Drug stability must often be a concern, where a sulfonic acid or quaternary amine may act as a catalyst for degradation even in the dry state. The hydrodynamics of the absorption process as well as the economics must also be factored into the selection process. It is often beneficial to begin with the larger commercial particle size range and mill the complex after loading.

Obviously, the considerations are many, but the options are likewise plentiful. In practice, the best approach is to select several alternatives, prepare the absorbates, and rely on *in vitro* and *in vivo* testing to aid in the decision.

C. PREPARATION OF ABSORBATES

The drug may be absorbed on the ion exchange resin by a batch or column process. Since the reaction is an equilibrium phenomenon, maximum potency and efficiency is best obtained using the column technique. However, the batch process is much simpler and quicker to carry out, and is the only alternative when starting with very fine particles. A typical batch procedure involves slurrying the resin in water, filtering or decanting the liquid on top, slurrying the resin with the desired acid, base, or salt solution to change cycle (if necessary), decanting and washing with water several times, and treating with the appropriate drug solution. After absorption, the complex formed should be washed with water and dried.

A typical column technique for preparing an absorbate of an amine drug with a strong cation exchange resin would be to slurry the resin in water, add the slurry to a column, backwash with water to eliminate air pockets and distribute the beads, add acid (e.g., 1 N HCl) to convert to H^+ cycle, wash with water, add salt solution of drug, wash with water, remove cake from column, filter with vacuum, and oven dry. An analogous procedure might be used to absorb a carboxylated drug to an anion exchange resin, using NaOH to convert the resin to the OH^- cycle.

Several recycling steps might be included before drug absorption to assure cleaning of the resin. Drug absorption onto the sodium form of the cation exchanger or chloride from the anion exchanger is often preferred. Excess drug may be used to saturate all the cationic sites on the resin and achieve maximum potency. Best hydrodynamic conditions will occur with larger size ranges and be almost impossible with too many fine particles. Smaller size ranges give better chromatographic exchange. The progress of absorption may be monitored by on-line pH measurements or chemical assays of the effluent.

D. *IN VITRO* TESTING

1. Potency

Determination of the percentage drug on the complex requires complete elution from the resin. This is often quite difficult when the affinity is strong. The high selectivity

TABLE 2
Iron Release from Iron
Polystyrenesulfonate Resinate in
Different Solvents and Resinate:
Solvent Ratios

Solvent	Volume/ 105 mg iron (ml)	% Iron dissolved at equilibrium
0.08N HCl	500	69.3%
0.08N HCl	100	39.3%
0.08N HCl	50	25.5%
0.08N HCl[a]	50	27.0%
0.9% NaCl	100	43.1%
0.9% NaCl	50	34.6%
0.45% NaCl	50	23.4%

[a]   Used liquifer suspension. Others used dry resinate.

coefficients associated with many drugs often require large excesses of competing cc
to approach complete displacement. Probably, the best method of assuring essential
titative recovery of the drug is through sequential slurries with high concentrations
terions. Alternatively, a continuous elution method may be set up using fresh dis
media. In questionable situations it may be advantageous to use different media in s
to achieve complete recovery.

2. Dissolution Rate Testing

Since the use of ion exchange resins is invariably associated with controlling dis
rate, *in vitro* testing is usually important to assess performance. Conventional dis
rate tests for dosage forms employ a fixed volume of solvent with sufficient solu
approximate sink-type conditions. Drug dissolution from an ion exchange resin on
hand is driven by exchange of ions toward an equilibirum, and sink-conditions (e
solubilization) are generally not possible. Equilibrium will likely occur with a su
percentage of drug still bound to the resin. This percentage will be dependent on co
in the dissolution solution, their concentrations, and the complex to solution ratio.
dissolution methods may be used for quality control purposes in assessing reproc
of batches or comparing release rates through rate-controlling membranes or coati

Predictions of *in vivo* release behavior may often be best estimated by a
dissolution studies employing varying ratios, solutions, and concentrations. Both
release and equilibrium distributions should be assessed. With uncoated resin partic
equilibrium is usually achieved in minutes. The results can give a clearer understa
the performance of the system than dissolution rate studies alone. Sample data from
polystyrenesulfonic acid adsorbate[6] is shown in Table 2.

A continuous dissolution process may alterntively be used to approach complete
The resin absorbate may be stirred in a fixed volume of buffer, and fresh fluie
pumped in continuously. Effluent from the chamber containing eluted drug may be
periodically or continuously using a spectrophotometer. This system may use a
influent solvent and rate, or may be modelled to use varying eluting solutions, ra
volumes to simulate gastrointestinal fluids the adsorbate would encounter when s
Figure 2 shows two continuous release curves from the iron-polystyrenesulfonate
described in Table 2.

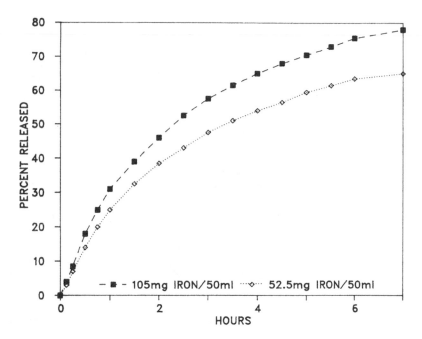

FIGURE 2. Dissolution of iron from resinate. Continuous flow — 75 ml/min of 0.08 *N* HCl.

E. GASTROINTESTINAL RELEASE MECHANISM

Bioavailability of drugs absorbed to ion exchange resins depends on both transit of the particles through the gastrointestinal tract and drug release kinetics. Drug release or dissolution from the resin can in turn occur only through replacement of the drug by another ion with the same charge. Since the exchange is an equilibrium process, it will depend on the ionic constitution and fluid volume of the body fluid. Additionally, release is not instantaneous, and the drug must diffuse through the resin from the internal exchange sites. Thus, agitation and time of exposure play a key role in drug release.

If the drug-resin complex is exposed to the mouth, a small amount of drug may be released. This would then be followed by significant release in the stomach when exposed to the high acid and chloride concentrations. Anionic exchange resins and the strong cation exchangers will release a limited amount of drug in the stomach through the competitive equilibrium route as shown in Equations 4 and 5.

$$Re\text{-}SO_3^- \ DRUG^+ \ + \ H^+ \ \rightleftharpoons \ Re\text{-}SO_3^- \ H^+ \ + \ DRUG^+ \tag{4}$$

$$Re\text{-}N(CH_3)_3^+ \ DRUG^- \ + \ Cl^- \ \rightleftharpoons \ Re\text{-}N(CH_3)_3^+ \ Cl^- \ + \ DRUG^- \tag{5}$$

In contrast, drug bound to weakly acidic carboxylic acids are released much more readily in the stomach as illustrated in Equation 6.

$$Re\text{-}COO^- \ DRUG^+ \ + \ H^+ \ \rightleftharpoons \ Re\text{-}COOH \ + \ DRUG^+ \tag{6}$$

The high effective pKa of the resin drives the equilibrium toward formation of undissociated acid in a low pH environment. This may be quite beneficial when rapid drug release is desired.

Stomach emptying with fine particles likely follows a first order or distributional process. In the intestine the neutral pH should keep all ionic sites on the resins ionized, and the

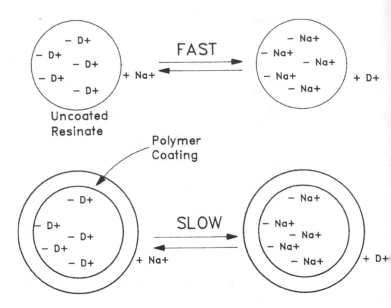

FIGURE 3.   Effect of microencapsulation or coating.

exchange process should occur continuously. The absorption into the body of
drug should drive the equilibrium further toward drug release. In the large int
sorption from the resin and absorption into the body may be slowed considera
low fluid content, entrapment in fecal matter, and poorer membrane absorption.

The highly insoluble resin never dissolves, and should not be absorbed. It v
be eliminated from the body with whatever counterions have replaced the drug.
complete dissolution of drug from the ion exchange resin during its gastrointest
is impossible due to the equilibrium mechanism of release. However, in practice,
complete bioavailability frequently occurs.

F. MICROENCAPSULATION/PARTICLE COATING

Without coating, the ion exchange process begins within seconds, and the dr
equilibrium is very rapid. Applying a polymer coating to the ion exchange resi
can delay and slow the elution process[7] (Figure 3). Taste coverage may be imp
a coating that delays drug dissolution in the mouth for the several minutes neede
clearance by swallowing.[8] Controlled release systems can be fine tuned using
semi-permeable membranes.[9] Acid labile drugs may be protected from stomach
radation by microencapsulation with an acid-insoluble enteric coating.[10]

Polymer coatings may be introduced by coacervation[11] or physical proce
suspension coating systems appear to be the most useful and versatile. The ior
resin particles offer a receptive substrate for this method, being compact, highl
polymers with fairly narrow particle-size ranges. Coatings may be further stabilize
against the tendency of ion exchange resins to swell when wet by using an im
agent such as polyethylene glycol.[12]

IV. PRODUCT APPLICATIONS

A. CONTROLLED RELEASE CAPSULES

Absorbing an ionic drug to an ion exchange resin and administering it in a
tablet dosage has long been considered as one alternative for controlled releas

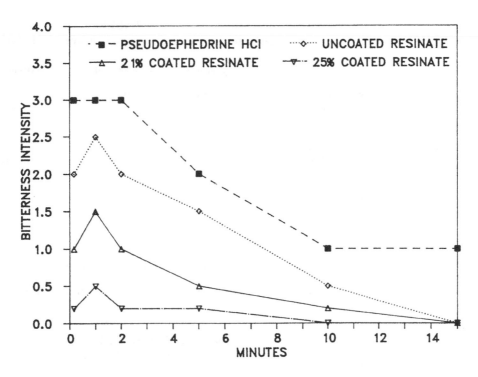

FIGURE 4. Pseudoephedrine bitterness intensity after holding in mouth for 10 sec. (From Borodkin, S. and Sundberg, D. P., *J. Pharm. Sci.*, 60, 1524, 1971. With permission.)

Biphetamine®, a capsule containing equal quantities of amphetamine and dextroamphetamine complexed to a sulfonic acid cation exchange resin,[13] has been used for several decades as an anti-obesity agent and for behavior control in children. The recommended dosing is one or two times per day. Although still considered an option, the dependence of release on gastrointestinal transit and fluid volumes would suggest that this method might be inferior to other controlled release alternatives.

B. TASTE COVERAGE IN CHEWABLE TABLETS

Many therapeutically useful drugs are quite bitter, limiting their utility in chewable tablets designed for pediatric or geriatric use. The ion exchange resin complex offers a method of overcoming this problem. This application is exemplified in taste masking of pseudoephedrine in the chewable Rondec® decongestant tablet.[14] This system involved absorbing pseudoephedrine into Amberlite®CG-50, a polymethacrylic acid ion-exchange resin (particle size range of 72 to 147 μm) to a level of 50 to 60% drug, using a column procedure. Additional taste protection was achieved by applying a 25% coating with an air suspension coater using a polymer mixture of 4:1 ethylcellulose:hydroxypropylmethyl-cellulose. Figure 4 illustrates the characteristics determined by a trained taste panel for the various forms of pseudoephedrine. A bioavailability study based on urinary excretion indicated complete drug absorption, although somewhat delayed compared to a capsule of pseudoephedrine HCl. The successful taste protection using this coated resinate technique was further demonstrated with dextromethorphan, ephedrine, and methapyriline. Table 3 lists some key characteristics of the compositions prepared.

C. BUCCAL ABSORPTION FROM GUM

Nicorette® is a widely used, patented product marketed as an adjunct to smoking cessation programs. It contains nicotine absorbed to a carboxylic acid ion exchange resin

TABLE 3
Drug Resinates for Taste Coverage Prepared with Amberlite® CG-

	Ephedrine	Pseudoephedrine	Dextromethorphan	M
Salt Used	Base	HCl	HBr	
Resin Cycle	H	Na	Na	
Resinate Potency, mg/g	645	552	522	
Dissolution:				
% after 1 min pH 6.7	26.7	32.1	4.9	
t(1/2) 0.08*N* HCl, min	0.2	0.1	0.1	
t(90%) 0.08*N* HCl, min	1.0	1.1	0.8	
% 24 h int fluid	98.1	92.5	30.4	
Bitterness Levels:[a]				
Salt	3	3	3	
Uncoated resinate	2	2	2	
Coated resinate	1/2	1/2	1/2	

[a]   Bitterness by Taste Panel: 3 = strong, 2 = moderate, 1 = slight.

From Borodkin, S. and Sundberg, D. P., *J. Pharm. Sci.*, 60, 1524, 1971. With permission.

TABLE 4
Dissolution Studies of Nicotine-Amberlite®
IRP-64 *M* Resinate

	Wt% released in			
Test conditions	2 min	5 min	10 min	20 min
Saline Solution	64%	66%	66%	66%
Artificial Saliva	54%	70%	70%	70%
Chewing — Study 2	18%	36%	61%	91%
Chewing — Study 1	18%	39%	65%	92%

(nicotine polacrilex) in a flavored chewing gum base, providing gradual drug r
absorption through the buccal mucosa as the gum is chewed.[15] The dosage is in
provide nicotine over a 30-min period, with the slow release being governed by
mechanical chewing activity and slow elution from the resin particles. Resin w
fine particle-size range was used to avoid grittiness that is inherent in most ion
resins. Some reported *in vitro* testing results are shown in Table 4. They show r
libration and incomplete release in fixed volume solutions, but continuous elu
chewing with fresh solvent (saliva) made available.

D. CONTROLLED RELEASE LIQUIDS

Probably the most advantageous application of ion exchange resins as drug
their use in controlled release liquids. Whereas a variety of alterntive methods are
in preparing controlled release solid products, the resin appraoch offers one of
usable in liquids. In the bottle, the ion exchange resins can keep the drug bound
suspension by keeping the liquid free of counterions. When ingested, the ions in
will initiate release from the resin at a gradual rate. If the properties of the drug-resin
do not give the desired controlled release rate, coating the particles with a rate-c
membrane can often achieve the target bioavailability. The Pennkinetic® system
by the Pennwalt Corporation is the most notable application of the ion exchan
controlled release liquid technique. The following paragraphs discuss several
release suspension products as examples:

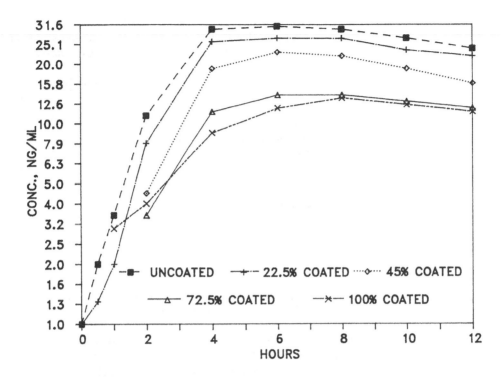

FIGURE 5.   Dextromethorphan blood levels — resinates with varying coating levels.

Delsym® (Dextromethorphan Polystirex) — Delsym® is a liquid suspension product designed to provide 12-h relief of coughs due to minor throat and bronchial irritation.[2] The active agent is dextromethorphan bound to a sulfonic acid ion exchange resin which is partially coated with ethylcellulose.[16] In a comparative bioavailability study, a single dose of the product was demonstrated to give blood levels of dextromethorphan comparable to two 6-h doses of dextromethorphan HBr solution over a 12-h period. Comparative steady state levels after 7 and 14 d were also demonstrated. The efficacy of this controlled release suspension has also been demonstrated in clinical studies.[17]

The report on the development of this product[16] describes a unique method for reproducibly controlling drug release rates. Both *in vitro* dissolution rates and *in vivo* bioavailability curves were obtained from suspensions containing varying levels of coated particles. The bioavailability curves are shown in Figure 5. They were thus able to establish an acceptable bioavailability profile and correlate the range to dissolution values. This could then be of considerable value in the manufacture of the product, where coating reproducibility is difficult. By establishing the bioavailability-dissolution correlation, different coating lots could be blended to achieve the right particle mix.

Penntuss® (Codeine and Chlorpheniramine Polistirex) — This is a combination product derived from the Pennkinetic® system intended for 12-h cough/cold relief. Both drugs are in the form of resinates bound to a sulfonic acid cation exchange resin, although the codeine-resinate particles are coated with ethylcellulose while the chlorpheniramine-resinate particles are uncoated.[18] Apparently, the chlorpheniramine has a much greater affinity for the resin, and the equilibrium-driven elution rate is sufficiently slow to provide adequate prolonged release. Conversely, the codeine-resin bonding is much weaker, and a rate-controlling membrane must be added.

The reported studies indicated that five formulations were evaluated, each employing codeine-resinate with different coating levels. Uncoated carbinoxamine was used in all five

TABLE 5

**Comparative Results from Five Formulations of Codeine and
Chlorpheniramine Resin Complexes**

	Formulation				
	A	B	C	D	E
Codeine:					
Dissolution 30 min %	34	37	30	52	57
Dissolution 3 h %	55	58	48	70	72
T_{max}, h	3.2	3.8	3.6	2.5	2.0
C_{max}, ng/ml	18.8	18.6	17.1	26.7	33.8
AUC(0—12 h), ng/hr/ml	140	142	128	161	195
Chlorpheniramine:					
Dissolution 30 min %	32	37	37	46	52
Dissolution 3 h %	58	66	64	73	77
Tmax, h	7.6	8.0	7.2	7.0	6.5
Cmax, ng/ml	7.0	7.0	7.0	8.1	9.5
AUC(0—12 h), ng/h/ml	164	161	153	176	181

From Amsel, L. P., Hinsvark, O. N., Rotenberg, K., and Sheumaker, J. L., Proc. Phar
Technol. Conf., Springfield, OR, 1984, 251.

formulations. Three formulations gave acceptable controlled release in bioavailabili
while the other two with insufficient coating, showed inadequate sustained relea
vivo results correlated well with dissolution testing allowing establishment of an
range based on *in vitro* dissolution studies. Chlorpheniramine bioavailability was
in all five formulations. Table 5 summarizes characteristics of the five suspensi
parisons of the selected resinate formula administered every 12 h to a control g
6 h showed equivalent blood level results. The control contained codeine sulfat
binoxamine maleate in the same suspension vehicle used in the suspension of
Figure 6 shows the plasma level curves over a 12-h period for both the resinate and
release formulation.

Liquifer® (Controlled Release Iron) — Liquifer® is a controlled release s
containing iron in the ferrous state bound to a sulfonic acid ion exchange resin.[6] It i
to provide supplemental iron as a once-a-day dosage in a pleasant-tasting liquid
opposed to sustained release dosages, where constant blood levels are desired, th
purpose for controlled release of iron is to prevent high concentrations of iron in th
which might cause gastrointestinal distress. The ion exchange resins are suited to th
because of their equilibrium-driven release. *In vitro* equilibration studies indicat
more than 25% of the iron would be solubilized in the stomach with normal repor
fluid levels.

$$(Re\text{-}SO_3^-)_2 Fe^{++} + 2H^+ \rightleftharpoons 2(Re\text{-}SO_3^- H^+) + Fe^{++}$$

In addition to reduced gastrointestinal irritation, the resinate form of iron allows
palatability, reduces tooth staining, and reduces the risk of toxic overdoses as co
conventional liquid products. These advantages can all be attributed to the eq
between soluble and bound iron. To assure maintenance of the iron in the fe
throughout storage, ascorbic acid is included in the suspension. Bioavailability stu
paring the resinate with marketed ferrous sulfate products established equivalenc
this controlled release dosage form and standard dosages. A series of clinical stu
both pediatric and adult patients established efficacy of the iron resinate by dem
restoration of normal hemoglobin, hematocrit, and serum iron levels.

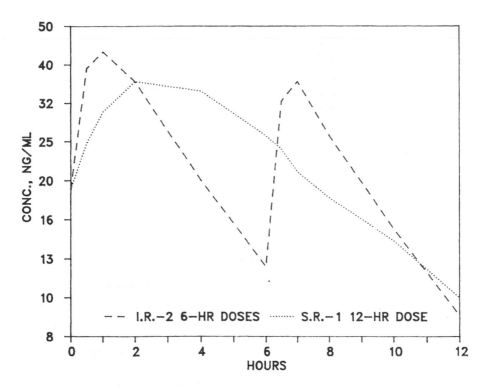

FIGURE 6. Comparative codeine plasma levels — immediate release vs. sustained resinate. (From Proc. Pharm. Technol. Conf., Washington, 1984, 257. With permission.)

Theophylline Controlled Release Liquid — Theophylline is a widely used asthma drug, used clinically in controlled release solid-dosage formulations. The desire to prepare a controlled release liquid product for pediatric use prompted considerable research activity. The ion exchange approach appears viable, although the extremely weak acidity of theophylline (pKa = 8.77) makes the task much more difficult. Although the drug may be absorbed on the resin, the binding is too weak to allow equilibrium-driven controlled release. This must be achieved by barrier coatings.

$$Re\text{-}N(CH_3)_3^+ \; THEOPH^- + Cl^- \rightleftharpoons Re\text{-}N(CH_3)_3^+ \; Cl^- + THEOPH^- \qquad (8)$$

Motycka et al[19] first reported on a theophylline resinate system for controlled release using anion exchange resins. *In vitro* release rates were controlled with ethylcellulose, hard paraffin, or both. Patel et al.[20] prepared a series of similar anion exchange resinates with 40% drug, using polymer coatings applied by the air suspension method to control drug release. Bioavailability studies in rats and dogs showed no significant differences between theophylline resinate and drug in solution. Crosslinkage percent and particle-size range had no effect. Microencapsulating the particles with ethylcellulose alone gave extended theophylline plasma levels over 10 to 14 h, but often with incomplete bioavailability. Incorporating 10 to 20% hydroxypropylmethylcellulose into the rate-controlling membrane led to complete bioavailability with acceptable release rates. Figure 7 shows some representative blood level curves in dogs.

E. PALATABLE LIQUIDS
Some drugs may be so bitter that conventional flavors and sweetness enhancers are insufficient to make them acceptable. A recent patent describes the use of a carbomer complex

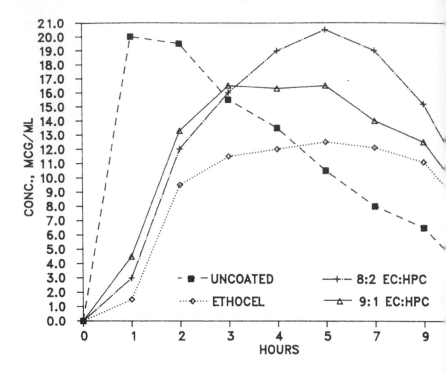

FIGURE 7.   Theophylline serum levels in dogs — resinates with varying coatings. (From Patel, ...
Ion exchange resin carriers for controlled release theophylline particles, Proc. 16th Annu. Symp. C...
Release Biomater., Pearlman, R. and Miller, J. A., Eds., Chicago, 1989, 63.)

to overcome the bitter taste of erythromycin and 6-*O*-methylerythromycin.[10] Altho...
bomer, a high molecular weight polyacrylic acid with very low crosslinking, ma...
classified as an ion exchange resin, it functions as one for this application. Stan...
boxylic acid resins are not porous enough to absorb these high-molecular weight an...

Although less bitter complexes could be achieved with potencies as high as 8(...
better taste protection was obtained with lower percentages of drug. Further imp...
in bitterness protection was obtained by coating with polymers to delay release in th...
Hydroxypropylmethylcellulose phthalate, an acid-insoluble polymer, proved best...
viding long-term taste stability in suspension products. A major problem to ove...
such taste protection applications is the aftertaste due to resinate particles remaini...
mouth. Table 6 lists some comparative taste evaluation results obtained by a train...

A crossover bioavailability study run using nine dogs showed that both unco...
particle coated 6-*O*-methylerythromycin-carbomer complex gave slightly higher ser...
than capsules of the unbound drug. The complex may provide faster dissolution than...
There was no difference between the coated and uncoated complex. The favora...
vailability results were later obtained in a human study using a palatable suspen...
mulation of 6-*O*-methylerythromycin-carbomer complex with approximat...
hydroxypropylmethylcellulose phthalate coating. Figure 8 shows the results of ...
using 21 subjects in a crossover study.

F. MISCELLANEOUS APPLICATIONS

Ion exchange resins have been advocated for use in a variety of topical app...
both to provide slow availability of active agents and for absorption of toxic mater...
have been tested as carriers for immobilized enzymes to provide extended activity at...
sites. Their use in providing faster dissolution of insoluble drugs compared to cry...

TABLE 6
Bitterness Evaluation of 6-*O*-Methylerythromycin Carbomer Complex in Suspensions — Particles Uncoated and Coated

Drug potency of complex %	Coated or uncoated	Final potency %	Bitterness[a] at 10 sec	Bitterness at 60 sec
58%	Uncoated	58%	0	1
58%	Coated	52%	0	0
62%	Uncoated	62%	0	2
62%	Coated	57%	0	0
70%	Uncoated	70%	1.5	2
80%	Uncoated	80%	2	3
80%	Coated	72%	0	2

[a] By taste panel: 3 = strong, 2 = moderate, 1 = slight.

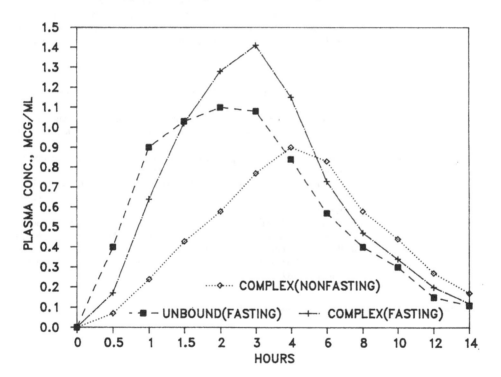

FIGURE 8. 6-*O*-Methylerythromycin bioavailability — coated carbomer complex vs. drug tablet.

been demonstrated. The use of ion exchange resins as controlled release drug carriers in injectable products can be visualized, but practical applications will probably require a biodegradable form.

Many other unidentified applications have undoubtedly been considered and evaluated. Ion exchange resins have unique and potentially valuable properties that should be exploited. Coupled with their established safety, the use of these polymers should always be an option in formulation design.

230 *Polymers for Controlled Drug Delivery*

REFERENCES

1. **Martin, G. L.,** *Ion Exchange and Adsorption Agents in Medicine,* Little, Brown, Boston, 1
2. **Barnhart, E. R.,** *Physicians' Desk Reference,* Medical Economics Company, Oradell, N.J.
3. **Calmon, C. and Kressman, T. R. E.,** *Ion Exchangers in Organic and Biochemistry,* Inters York, 1957.
4. **Borodkin, S. and Yunker, M. H.,** Interaction of amine drugs with a polycarboxylic acid resin, *J. Pharm. Sci.,* 59, 481, 1970.
5. **Van Abbe, N. J. and Rees, J. T.,** *J. Amer. Pharm. Ass. Sci. Ed.,* 49, 487, 1960.
6. **Borodkin, S.,** Iron-Resin Adsorbate, U.S. Patent 3,947,572, 1976.
7. **Deasy, P. B.,** *Microencapsulation and Related Drug Processes,* Marcel Dekker, New York,
8. **Borodkin, S. and Sundberg, D. P.,** Polycarboxylic acid ion-exchange resin adsorbates for t in chewable tablets, *J. Pharm. Sci.,* 60, 1523, 1971.
9. **Raghunathan, Y., Amsel, L., Hinsvark, O., and Bryant, W. J.,** Sustained release drug del I. Coated ion-exchange resin system for phenylpropanolamine and other drugs, *J. Pharm. S* 1981.
10. **Fu Lu, M. Y. and Borodkin, S.,** Antibiotic-Polymer Compositions, U.S. Patent 4,808,41 I
11. **Irwin, W. J., Belaid, K. A., and Alpar, H. O.,** Drug delivery by ion-exchange, Part IV. C complexes of ester pro-drugs of propranolol, *Drug Dev. Ind. Pharm.,* 14, 1307, 1988.
12. **Raghunathan, Y.,** Prolonged Release Pharmaceutical Preparations, U.S. Patent 4,221,778,
13. **Deeb, G. and Becker, B.,** Absorption of sustained-release amphetamine preparations in the *Appl. Pharmacol.,* 2, 410, 1960.
14. **Borodkin, S. and Sundberg, D. P.,** Chewable tablets including coated particles of pseudoep cation exchange resin, U.S. Patent 3,594,470, 1971.
15. **Lichtneckert, S., Lundgren, C., and Ferno, O.,** Chewable Smoking Substitute Composition 3,901,248, 1975.
16. **Amsel, L. P., Hinsvark, O. N., and Raghunathan, Y.,** Dissolution and blood level studie sustained release system, Proc. Res. Sci. Dev. Conf., Washington, D.C. Proprietary Assoc 94.
17. **Lilienfield, L. S. and Zapolski, E. J.,** Controlled releae dextromethorphan using advanced technology, *Curr. Ther. Res.,* 33, 692, 1983.
18. **Amsel, L. P., Hinsvark, O. N., Rotenberg, K. and Sheumaker, J. L.,** Recent advance release technology utilizing ion exchange polymers, Pro. Pharm. Tech. Conf., Sturges, M. B Springfield, OR, 1984, 251.
19. **Motycka, S., Newth, J. L., and Nairn, J. G.,** Preparation and evaluation of microencapsulat ion-exchange resin beads containing theophylline, *J. Pharm. Sci.,* 74, 643, 1985.
20. **Patel, J., Borodkin, S., and Hernandez, L.,** Ion exchange resin carriers for controlled release particles, Proc. 16th Ann. Symp. Controlled Release Biomater., Pearlman, R. and Miller, Chicago, 1989, 62.

Chapter 12

ANIMAL TESTING OF POLYMER BASED SYSTEMS

Kenneth R. Majors and Mitchell B. Friedman

TABLE OF CONTENTS

I. INTRODUCTION

More and more pharmaceutical products are being developed into controlle
delivery systems such as skin patches, or polymeric carriers such as microsph
liposomes. The goals of these alternative dosing forms are usually to provide a co
method for administering the active ingredient at a uniform and controlled rate.
such delivery systems, drugs which have a short half-life usually require frequent
be effective. The new delivery systems also provide alternatives to parenteral admir
of drugs that are too easily degraded to be taken orally. Putting drugs into micros
liposomal preparations may be used to provide selective distribution of a drug to
organs as well.

A major concern in the development of advanced dosage forms is the effect
alternative delivery systems might have on the safety of the active components(
the toxicological profile of the active ingredient will have been well established by
the novel delivery system is developed, and even the "inactive components" or e
may have been evaluated and found suitable for medical use. However, becaus
potential for adverse interactions or alterations in the way the drug is delivered to or di
in the body, the toxicologic profile of the new dosage form could be quite differ
that of the active ingredient alone. Thus, the controlled release formulations may
sidered a new entity for toxicity evaluation.

This chapter will describe animal tests which are used to evaluate the toxicit
active and inactive ingredients, as well as the combinations found in the new dosag

II. TOXICOLOGY TESTS

A. ACUTE TOXICITY
1. General Description

An acute toxicity test is conducted to determine the adverse effects of single,
large doses of a test material in animals. Generally, several groups of animals, usu
or rats, are treated one time with a range of dose levels, and overt toxic manifestat
as abnormal behavior, changes in body weight gains, and deaths are monitored a
intervals for the next few days or weeks. If deaths occur at more than one dose l
of several statistical methods,[1,2] may be used to estimate a median lethal dose (L
LD_{50} value may be defined as the dose of a compound which theoretically would
to 50% of a given population of animals. Although lethality is often a principal en
acute toxicity tests, other adverse effects are also undesirable, and must be includ
toxicological assessment. In addition, valuable information can be gained in the un
ing of overdose situations.

2. Route of Administration

The route of administration can greatly affect the toxicity of test materials. In
the greatest effects and the most rapid responses occur following intravenous admir
Orally administered compounds must pass first through the liver, and a large perc
the dose may be metabolized or detoxified before entering the systemic circulation. I
routes of administration, e.g., intravenous, intramuscular, etc. avoid this so-cal
pass effect." Depending on the site of application, topically applied agents must pas
a generally effective diffusion barrier to reach the systemic circulation, and, althoug
some metabolism can take place here as well.

The routes of administration used in acute toxicity studies usually are the sar
intended clinical routes. However, a comparison of the effects that occur when
routes of administration are used may provide information about the absorption of t

Likewise, comparison of the acute toxicity of different formulations can be a useful screening technique. In some countries, more than one route of administration is required by their regulatory agencies, with a more "bioavailable" parenteral route requested even though the intended route is oral.

3. Vehicle

Water or aqueous suspensions such as 0.2% hydroxypropylmethylcellulose (HPMC) are typically used in acute toxicity tests to dissolve or suspend solid test agents. Alternate vehicles such as corn oil may be used in some instances, but other solvents which may have their own inherent toxicity are avoided. Such factors as pH and osmolarity are important considerations. Intravenous administration of a hypotonic solution, can lead to hemolysis. For example, extremes in pH can lead to tissue damage at the site of administration.

4. Uses of Acute Toxicity Data

Acute toxicity data are often the toxicologist's first available indication of the potential hazard of a given compound or formulation. The results of acute toxicity tests might reveal effects not seen in longer-term studies where lower dosages are used and tolerance may develop. An LD_{50} value may be used to categorize the material according to its acute toxicity. The following classification system was adapted from the one described by Gleason et al.[3]

LD_{50} value	Toxicity rating
Less than 5 mg or 0.5 mcl/kg	Super toxic
5—50 mg or ml/kg	Extremely toxic
50—500 mg or ml/kg	Very Toxic
0.5—5 gm or ml/kg	Slightly toxic
above 15 gm or ml/kg	Practically nontoxic

Acute toxicity data are often useful in making comparisons of similarly-tested materials. For example, the data may indicate that a polymeric controlled-release formulation is more or less toxic than the active ingredient by itself. Thus, these data may provide preliminary indication of whether the active ingredient is being made "bioavailable," and the rate at which an active ingredient is reaching the systemic circulation. If a formulation produces an LD_{50} value that is higher than expected based on its concentration, it may be supposed that either not all of the active ingredient is being made bioavailable or that the ingredient is being delivered or absorbed at a reduced rate. An LD_{50} value that is lower than expected would indicate that the bioavailability of the active ingredient has been increased, that another component of the formulation is toxic in itself, or that an interaction with another component is enhancing the toxicity of the active ingredient. Such circumstances show why testing of the formulation without the active ingredient can also be important.

Often, a formulation does not cause deaths at the maximum feasible dosage, and an LD_{50} cannot be determined. In these cases, overt signs of toxicity or exaggerated pharmacologic activity instead of lethality may be used to compare the relative toxicities and bioavailability of formulations.

If one is comparing the acute toxicity of more than one active ingredient, it is important that the dose-response curves be similar. Dose-response curves which deviate significantly from parallelism may be an indication of dissimilar mechanisms of toxicity.

A number of factors such as species, strain, length of fasting prior to oral dosing, rate of intravenous administration, ambient temperature, and even the number of animals per cage are known to affect the results of acute toxicity tests. Thus, caution must be taken in comparing acute toxicity data (e.g., LD_{50} values) generated at different laboratories, or even data from the same laboratory produced at different times. Although qualitatively useful, quantitative comparisons of LD_{50} values can be misleading. Due to the relatively high degree

of biological variation, comparison of values is most descriptive when there is v
gence.

The usefulness of acute toxicity data are quite limited for predicting the effe
might occur in humans after a long exposure to a clinical dosage. The biologica
to a single massive dose may differ greatly from the response to repeated therapeu
and, therefore, acute toxicity results are not intended to be used to predict effects
except in relation to an accidental overexposure or intentional misuse. Likewis
sorption, distribution, and metabolism profile of a drug may also be distorted b
doses employed in this type of study.

Currently, there is considerable concern about the use of large numbers of a
acute toxicity studies.[4] While it is true that using large numbers of animals simply t
the precision of LD_{50} values is unwarranted, properly conducted acute toxicity t
a reasonable number of animals can provide a rapid source of valuable informati

B. SUBCHRONIC AND CHRONIC TOXICITY
1. General Description

Subchronic and chronic toxicity studies are designed to detect adverse effects c
treatments on growth and behavior of animals as well as functional or morpholo
on major organs. A well-designed study will determine the maximum dose level t
species will tolerate without any adverse effect (no-effect dosage), as well as det
adverse effects that occur at higher dosages. The results of these studies may t
decide whether or not a drug is safe for testing in man, and at what dose, and
the clinician about the side effect most likely to be seen in clinical trials.

Subchronic toxicology studies may last from 2 weeks up to 3 months, where
studies are usually defined as those lasting 6 months or longer. The duration of s
and chronic studies are usually multiples of the anticipated length of clinical studi
lines have been published by the U.S.[5] and foreign regulatory agencies[6] which pro
duration of the preclinical toxicology studies that are necessary before a new comp
be administered in clinical studies. These regulatory requirements are discusse
detail in the following chapter.

Usually, a new compound will be tested for 2 weeks to 1 month in two spec
rodent and one a non-rodent. Two-week studies in two species are the minimum re
before a single dose of a new compound may be given in a clinic in the U.S. Long
studies may then be conducted concurrently with the initial clinical trials so that the
toxicology data are available at the time that longer and more comprehensive cli
are begun. One-month studies will support clinical trials lasting up to 2 weeks, anc
6-month and 1-year studies support proportionately longer clinical trials. Generally
all countries require a similar scheme to support the safety of clinical trials. Th
of studies is determined by the duration of intended treatment once efficacy
established. For example, an antibiotic may require studies of a 6-month durat
their relatively short dosing period. An antihypertensive will require 6-month,
2-year studies due to the chronic nature of the drug therapy involved. Such testing
by an appropriate route of administration.

2. Species

Worldwide requirements are for use of both a rodent and a non-rodent speci
adult rats and dogs are used most often in subchronic and chronic toxicity studies
species, particularly monkeys, may be used when there is data to suggest that the
response to the drug in that species will be more like that of man. Subchronic
the antiviral agent zidovudine (azidothymidine) were conducted in rats and cy
monkeys when metabolism studies determined that dogs didn't glucuronidate near

of an administered dose as did monkeys, rats, and humans.[7] In addition to metabolic differences, bioavailability due to differing absorption may determine the choice of species to be used. Young animals are used in subchronic and chronic studies primarily for the reason that effects on growth are more easily discernible in rapidly growing animals. Other considerations as to species may relate to the pharmacologic activity of a drug. Dogs, for example, are notorious for their heightened emetic response. Drugs that may produce emesis are therefore best tested in an alternate non-rodent species. Rabbits are unusually sensitive to certain antibiotics, and therefore may "overpredict" the toxicity of a given antibiotic agent.

3. Routes of Administration

The routes of administration chosen for subchronic and chronic studies usually are the same as the intended clinical route. If more than one clinical route is likely, toxicity studies may be conducted by each potential route. Complete repetition of all testing is not required if it can be clearly demonstrated that the alternate routes are not leading to a toxic response unique to that route. Topical application of a drug can lead to sensitization, for example. Intravenous administration can lead to much higher peak blood levels than other routes, thus possibly producing toxicity at a fraction of the oral dose. Alternatively, some drugs can be more toxic when administered orally as opposed to intravenously. This is due to the presence of an "absorption phase" in which systemic exposure may be increased. Systemic exposure is generally quantified by measuring the area under the graph of the plasma drug concentration vs. time, commonly referred to as the "area under the curve" or "AUC."

4. Dose Levels

The dosages used in subchronic and chronic studies generally are more clinically relevant than the enormous doses employed in acute toxicity studies. Data from preliminary dosage-range-finding assays or preceding subchronic studies are used to select three or four dosage levels. The lowest dosage level that is selected is usually at, or several multiples of, the intended clincial dosage, but is projected not to be toxic, based on the preliminary data. The highest dose level is selected to produce toxicity without excessive mortality. It is important that definite adverse effects be elicited at the higher dosages so that clinicians may be forewarned of which organ systems might be affected by the agent as well as its potential side effects. Intermediate dosage levels are intended to produce milder effects so that dose-response relationships might be established.

Even the lowest dosages used in subchronic and chronic studies are often many multiples of the intended clinical or therapeutic dosages. The reason for administering exaggerated dosages is that the number of animals in a typical toxicology study is minute compared to the potential number of patients who may eventually receive the drug. Because of normal variability, not all animals or humans will respond equally to the same dosage. Giving animals larger dosages than the intended clinical dosage decreases the likelihood that an effect would not be detected simply because a large enough population was not used.

5. Observations

During subchronic studies, the animals are carefully observed for changes in physical appearance or behavior, periodic eye exams are conducted, and body weights and food consumption are monitored on a regular basis. Cardiovascular and other physiologic parameters may also be measured when warranted. Blood samples are collected from all animals during and after the treatment period for comprehensive clinical, chemical, and hematologic analyses. Similarly, urine samples are collected for urinalysis.

6. Anatomic Pathology

At the end of the dosing period the animals are euthanized and necropsied to look for any gross changes in internal structures, and samples of all major organs and ti⸮ collected for histopathology. The tissues are usually fixed in formalin, embedded in sections, and placed on glass slides, and then stained with hematoxylin and eosin⸮ aration for examination under the light microscope. A smaller list of tissues may be and specially prepared for electron microscopic evaluation; such examinations m⸮ particular importance in evaluating disposition or fate of polymeric microcapsules

7. Recovery Groups

Often, a portion of the animals in two or more test groups, usually the contro⸮ highest dosage group, will be retained without treatment for an additional lengt⸮ (usually 2 weeks or 1 month) after the end of treatment to determine whether adver⸮ of the treatment regimen are readily reversible. Most adverse effects will dimini⸮ compound is eliminated from the body, but irreversible changes may also occur. to organs which are able to regenerate rapidly, such as the gastrointestinal tract or⸮ are more likely to be reversible than damage to the nervous system, for exampl⸮ doesn't regenerate.

8. Blood Level Data

Plasma concentrations of the test article are periodically monitored during su⸮ and chronic toxicity tests to provide evidence of absorption (except when the dr⸮ ministered intravenously), and to test for accumulation or increased metabolic ca⸮ is particularly important to know how plasma drug levels from polymeric controlle⸮ systems compare with those from standard modes of drug delivery.

C. CARCINOGENICITY

Studies designed to assess the carcinogenic capability of a test article are ⸮ conducted in mice and rats. The procedures used in these tests are similar to othe⸮ tests except that dosing in these studies are carried out over the majority of the⸮ lifespan of the species, i.e., 18 months in mice, and 2 years in rats. Special att⸮ paid to the detection of masses, i.e., suspected tumors, during the life of the a⸮ well as during the subsequent post-mortem histopathologic examinations. Untreat⸮ hicle-treated control animals will spontaneously develop a number of tumors du⸮ lifetime, and significant increases in the tumor burden or reductions in the time th⸮ appear are considered indicative that the test agent is carcinogenic in that specie⸮ numbers of animals (often 50 or 60/sex/dosage level) are used in these studie⸮ meaningful statistical analyses may be carried out on tumor incidences, and so tha⸮ may be useful for assessing carcinogenic risk in humans.

Proper dosage selection for carcinogenicity tests can be difficult. Dosages th⸮ high may produce premature deaths, overshadowing toxicity or overwhelming the ⸮ capability of the animals, predisposing them to tumor development. Dosages tha⸮ low may underpredict the carcinogenic potential of the compound. The highest d⸮ carcinogenicity studies are set at the maximum tolerated dosage for that species as de⸮ in a preceding 90-day study for that purpose. The maximum tolerated dosage (⸮ been defined as the ''highest dose of the test agent given during the chronic study⸮ be predicted not to alter the animals' normal longevity from effects other than⸮ genicity,''[8] and is usually set at a dosage that causes no more than a 10% decrease⸮ gain below normal. The definition of an MTD does vary somewhat from country t⸮ and even agency to agency. There are those who believe that overt signs of toxi⸮ than body weight changes should be used as an acceptable endpoint.

D. LOCAL IRRITATION

In addition to evaluations for untoward systemic effects, controlled release syst⸮

as dermal patches and injectable formulations should be evaluated for the potential to produce tissue irritation at the site of administration. These tests are relatively easy to perform and take very little time.

1. Skin Irritation

Materials intended for dermal application are usually tested for the potential to cause adverse local irritation on the skin of albino rabbits. The rabbit skin is generally considered at least as sensitive as human skin, and has become the standard animal model for these type of tests. For this reason, a great deal of data exist which can allow for meaningful comparison between compounds as well as for extrapolating effects to man. The material is applied to the shaved skin on the backs of rabbits, and left in place or reapplied for periods proportional to the intended clinical duration. The reaction of the skin to the test material is evaluated by periodic gross examination of the treatment site during the testing period, and then by histologic examination of the treated skin at the end of the exposure period.

2. Vein Irritation

Intravenous irritation potential of parenterally administered products is commonly evaluated by injecting the formulation into the marginal ear vein of rabbits. The veins are observed grossly during treatment and frequently thereafter for signs of local effects such as local swelling and redness. On the day after the treatment, the rabbits are euthanized, and samples of the treated ear veins are collected for histological examination. Care is taken that the portions of the vein collected are located immediately proximal to the end of the intravenous needle or catheter so that chemically-induced effects are not confounded by iatrogenically-induced vein damage. Some test materials may require repeated infusions over several days to determine their irritant potential.

3. Muscle Irritation

The local muscle irritation potential of parenteral formulations is commonly evaluated in rabbits as well. A dose of the formulation is injected into a sacrospinalis muscle, a large muscle mass located on both sides of the spinal column of rabbits. The hair over the injection site is shaved before treatment so that the site may be examined frequently for evidence of local irritative effects. Samples of blood are collected from the rabbits before treatment and at intervals thereafter for measurement of serum creatine phosphokinase (CPK) activities. CPK is an enzyme found in muscle tissue, and muscle damage will produce marked elevations in CPK. Some of the rabbits are euthanized on the day after treatment for collection of muscle samples for histopathology. The remaining rabbits may be retained and examined later to evaluate the reversibility of the muscle damage.

D. SENSITIZATION

Sensitization studies are conducted to determine whether a material will produce allergic reactions. These are adverse reactions where pre-exposure to the agent is required before the toxic effect will occur. Initial contacts with an allergy-producing agent will induce the body to produce antibodies, and subsequent exposure to the same agent will result in an antigen-antibody reaction, i.e., an allergic response.

There are a number of animal test designs which may be used to test for sensitization. Howver, the Hartley guinea pig is common to most of these tests. The Buehler test,[9] the Magnusson-Kligman maximization test,[10] and the Freund's Complete Adjuvant test[11] are three tests for testing compounds for contact or dermal sensitization. The initial phase of these tests, called the induction phase, consists of repeatedly applying the test material to the skin of the animals or, in the case of the Freund's Complete Adjuvant test, injecting the agent intradermally. Typically a 2-week period follows in which the animals are monitored but not treated. This intermediate phase allows the animals to develop antibodies to the test

material. Finally, a challenge dose of material is applied to the animals, and signs
response are looked for that can range from swelling and inflammation to an an
response and lead to the death of the animal.

E. REPRODUCTIVE FUNCTION

Since polymers may be utilized with a wide variety of drugs from different t
categories, it is important to assess reproductive function when these new delivei
are utilized. Not only is it important to evaluate the consituents of a delivery sy
also the changes that can occur in the bioavailability of the drug being delivered. It
for example, that some drugs such as caffeine are teratogenic when high peak
achieved, whereas drugs such as trimethadione are more dependent upon the area
plasma concentration curve (AUC).[12] In the former case, we know that caffeine
commonly consumed, is not associated with teratogenesis due to the fact that
orally, and therefore high peak plasma levels are not achieved due to the relat
absorption of the drug from the gastrointestinal tract. This absorption phase leads
AUC, and therefore considerable systemic exposure, but peak values are limite
thadione, on the other hand, although also administered orally, is associated w
genesis. Experimental findings indicate that peak blood levels are not as importar
drug as AUC, or the duration of systemic exposure.

In testing for effects on reproductive potential, three phases of testing are i
stituted. The first phase or Segment I study is a general fertility and reproduc
which involves the treatment of both male and female rats with the test materia
by mating. The females are treated throughout gestation and parturition. The i
offspring, their general condition, and viability are assessed, as well as various
parameters, depending upon the regulatory requirements being considered. Repi
pups from the various dosage groups are allowed to produce a subsequent genera
is also similarly evaluated.

The second phase of testing or Segment II involves two species, usually rats a
This phase of testing is designed to evaluate the teratogenic potential of the tes
In these tests, pregnant animals are treated with the test material throughout the
gestation when major organogenesis is taking place. Prior to parturition, anime
thanized, and the pups are examined for evidence of skeletal and visceral deforr

The third and final phase of testing is Segment III which involves the study c
and postnatal effects in rats. The pregnant animals are treated both during ges
throughout parturition and lactation until the offspring are weaned. During this i
uation of litter size, viability, behavioral and overall functional performance o
takes place.

As mentioned earlier, there are cetain regulatory requirements for behavioi
which may come into play that can effect the design of these various studies. It is
to recognize that novel delivery systems which themselves may be biologicall)
have profound effects on the toxicity of the drugs being delivered. Only throu
testing can it be determined that all regulatory and scientific issues have been a(

III. METABOLISM AND ELIMINATION

Although metabolism is somewhat outside the range of this particular chi
improtant for the scientist developing a new drug delivery system to have some aj
of the generation and application of these data. The importance of pharmacok
been brought up as it relates to toxicology and encompasses many of the quantitat
of metabolism. Delivery systems can markedly influence the absorption, distrib
tabolism, and elimination of a drug, thus affecting both the pharmacology and
of the compound.

Tissue distribution studies using radiolabelled drug can yield important information as to target organ effects. Mass balances can be determined by collecting urine, feces, and somtimes even bile. These studies can also determine the preferential routes of elimination and determine if changes have occurred as a result of the new delivery system. Such data can be effective in protecting that segment of the patient population that may be suffering from altered kidney function, for example, when it is determined that the major route of elimination is through the urine.

IV. CONCLUSIONS

Not all of the studies described above may be required for a new polymer-based product. Evaluation of existing toxicity data for individual ingredients and similar preparations may reduce the toxicology requirements considerably. Comparisons of the absorption, distribution, metabolism, and elimination of the active ingredients between existing and alternate formulations may assist in deciding what tests are necessary.

As can be seen from the preceding discussion, the toxicology of a previously untested substance can be involved, i.e., expensive and time consuming. Thus, the selection of nonactive components of polymer-based alternative dosing forms must be made carefully. Selecting previously tested materials may eliminate the necessity of reproducing extensive toxicology studies. On the other hand, development of unique and potentially useful adjuncts must not be diminished because of inadequate existing toxicology data.

REFERENCES

1. **Finny, D. J.**, *Probit Analysis*, Cambridge University Press, Cambridge, 1971.
2. **Litchfield, J. T. and Wilcoxon, F. C.**, A simplified method of evaluating dose-effect experiments. *J Pharmacol. Exp. Ther.* 96, 99, 1949.
3. **Gleason, M., Groselin, R., Hodges, H., and Smith R.**, *Clinical Toxicology of Commercial Products*, 3rd ed., Williams and Wilkins, Baltimore, 1976.
4. **Goldberg, A. M. and Frazier, J. M.**, Alternatives to animals in toxicity testing. *Sci. Amer.*, 261, 24, 1989.
5. **Goldenthal, E.**, Current views on safety evaluation of drugs, *FDA Pap.*, 13, 1968.
6. **Alder, S. and Zbinden, G.** *National and International Drug Safety Guidelines*, MTC, Verlag G. Zbinden, Zollikon, Switzerland, 1988.
7. **Ayers, K. M.**, Preclinical toxicology of zidovudine, *Am. J. Med.*, 85 (Suppl. 2A), 186, 1988.
8. **Sontag, J., Page, N., and Saffiotti, U.**, Guidelines for Carcionogen Bioassay in Small Rodents, in DHEW Publication No. (NIH) 76-801, National Institute of Health, Bethesda, MD, 1976.
9. **Buehler, E. V.**, Experimental skin sensitization in the guinea pig and man, *Arch. Dermatol.* 91, 171, 1965.
10. **Magnusson, B., and Kligman, A. M.**, The identification of contact allergens by animal assay, *J. Invest. Dermatol.*, 52, 268, 1969.
11. **Kleack, G.**, Identification of contact allergens: predictive test in animals, in *Dermatology and Pharmacology, Advances in Toxicology*, Marzulli, F. N. and Maibach, H. I., Eds., Hemisphere Publishing Co., Washington, D.C., 1977, chap. 9.
12. **Heine, Nau and Scott, J. J., Eds.**, Interspecies comparison and maternal/embryonic-fetal drug transfer, *Pharmacokinetics in Teratogensis*, CRC Monograph 1, CRC Press, Boca Raton, FL, 1987, 82.

Chapter 13

REGULATORY REQUIREMENTS FOR NEW DRUG SUBMISSIONS

Frederick A. Gustafson and Richard D. Kiernan

TABLE OF CONTENTS

I. INTRODUCTION

The approval of new drugs, biological products, and devices in the United St
responsibility of the commissioner of the Food and Drug Administration (FDA)
position appointed by the President. The regulatory process by which such new
are approved by the FDA is delineated in great detail in the Code of Federal Re
Title 21—Food and Drugs. The Code of Federal Regulations (CFR) contains
general and permanent rules issued by the federal government and published in t
Register, which is a government publication allowing for the dissemination of r
and legal notices to the public.

Title 21 CFR consists of nine volumes covering 1300 "parts" or sections
general, cover the requirements for drugs (parts 300 through 460), biologics
through 680) and devices (parts 800 through 899). The authority for the federal g
to issue regulations which are binding on the public rests with two laws passed by
(1) the Federal Food, Drug and Cosmetic Act, which assures the safety and e
drugs and devices, and (2) the Public Health Service Act, which assures the
efficacy of biological products.

The regulatory process for securing FDA approval of a new drug, biologic,
is complex and time-consuming, and it requires careful management of time and
(Figure 1). The FDA is faced with the same time/resource constraints as the phar
industry in fulfilling its obligation to allow only safe, effective products to be mad
to the medical profession to treat the many diseases plaguing mankind today. It i
in the best interests of all namely, the FDA, industry, academia, the medical p
and, most important, consumers who may eventually become patients, to fulfill the
approval requirements efficiently, thoroughly, and expeditiously.

This chapter takes a close look at the specific regulatory requirements whic
met before a new product will be approved by the FDA. The discussion will c
on new drugs and drug delivery systems rather than devices or biological produc
basic principles of data development and interaction with the FDA hold true fo

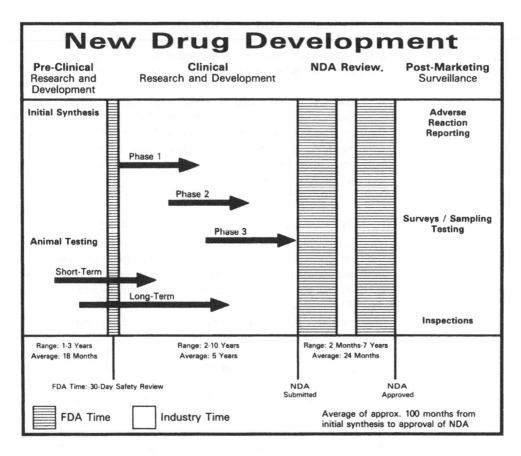

New Drug Development

Pre-Clinical Research and Development	Clinical Research and Development	NDA Review.	Post-Marketing Surveillance

Initial Synthesis

Phase 1

Phase 2

Phase 3

Animal Testing

Short-Term

Long-Term

Adverse Reaction Reporting

Surveys / Sampling Testing

Inspections

| Range: 1-3 Years Average: 18 Months | Range: 2-10 Years Average: 5 Years | Range: 2 Months-7 Years Average: 24 Months | |

FDA Time: 30-Day Safety Review

NDA Submitted

NDA Approved

FDA Time Industry Time Average of approx. 100 months from initial synthesis to approval of NDA

FIGURE 1.   The regulatory process for obtaining FDA approval for a new drug.

classes of products. A brief review of the legislative history of food and drug law will serve as a backdrop for understanding the basis for the regulations and the importance of fulfilling the regulatory requirements for new drug approval. The two specific applications required for approval of a new drug or drug delivery system will be discussed: (1) the *Investigational New Drug Exemption*, or IND, which allows the new drug sponsor to investigate the new drug in human subjects and patients to establish its safety and efficacy in treating a specific disease state; and (2) the *New Drug Application*, or NDA, which is a specific request by the sponsor for approval to market a new drug based on preclinical animal toxicity data; clinical data; adequate manufacturing controls information, to assure conformance to current good manufacturing practice; and adequate product labeling, to assure the safe and effective use of the product based on the clinical data generated under the new drug IND. Finally, we will present a brief discussion of the benefits of interaction between the new drug sponsor and the FDA reviewing scientists at appropriate points during the IND and NDA review process.

II. A BRIEF REVIEW OF LEGISLATIVE HISTORY

The cornerstone of the authority of the FDA to regulate new drugs in the U.S. is the Food, Drug and Cosmetic Act (F, D & C Act) of 1938. Together with several key amendments, the 1938 F, D & C Act forms the basis for requiring a new drug sponsor to demonstrate the safety and efficacy of the drug based on data from adequate and well-controlled animal toxicity studies and human clinical studies.

A. FOOD AND DRUG ACT OF 1906

The Food and Drug Act of 1906 represents the first real federal drug law to co
quality of drugs. However, it only required that drugs meet official standards of
and purity, but did not require the seller to substantiate the labeling claim.

B. FEDERAL FOOD, DRUG AND COSMETIC ACT OF 1938

This represents a complete revamping of the 1906 law, which Congress recog
inadequate and obsolete. Introduced in the Senate in 1933, it was passed in 1938 c
a tragedy in the U.S.; an elixir of sulfanilamide dissolved in diethylene glycol (ar
killed more than 100 people, mostly children. The 1938 Act, for the first time,
evidence of safety before a drug could be marketed; however, there was still no req
in the Act for demonstration of efficacy.

C. KEFAUVER-HARRIS AMENDMENTS OF 1962

Again, another tragedy preceded the passage of the 1962 amendments to the Fo
and Cosmetic Act. A drug being marketed in Europe, thalidomide, was linked to birt
in thousands of babies. Thalidomide was, at that time, under review in the U.S
FDA, but not yet approved. As a result of the publicity surrounding the thalidomide
the 1962 amendments were passed, requiring substantial evidence of *effectiveness* (in
to *safety* in the 1938 Act) prior to marketing. The FDA applied the effectiveness req
retroactively to all new drugs approved since 1938, and those without adequate effe
data were ordered off the market. It made the remaining drugs, i.e., those drugs v
FDA determined were safe and effective, eligible for Abbreviated New Drug App
or ANDAs, which, in essence, allows any company to file an ANDA for those n
approved between 1938 and 1962 *without* submitting safety and efficacy data. Th
provision allows for generic equivalents of marketed drugs to be made available, i
competition and thereby lowering drug prices for the consumer. Any drugs marke
to 1938, with some exceptions, were allowed to remain on the market, i.e., th
considered by the FDA to be "grandfathered" because they were generally recog
the medical profession as safe and effective.

D. DRUG PRICE COMPETITION AND PATENT TERM RESTORATION OF 1984

Also known as the Waxman-Hatch Act, this legislation provides ANDA eligi
those new drugs approved between 1962 and September 1, 1984. It also allows c
to recoup a portion of the 17-year patent life (up to a total of 5 years) for new dru
on the length of time the new drug was being reviewed by the FDA prior to appr

E. KEY DEFINITIONS

Throughout this chapter, a number of regulatory terms will be referred to on
basis. In order to facilitate an understanding of the discussions of INDs and ND
regulatory terms will be defined.

- IND — Intvestigational New Drug application (also known as "Notice of Investigational Exemption for a New Drug").
- NDA — New Drug Application.
- ANDA — Abbreviated New Drug Application — for a generic equivale established drug, which requires no safety or efficacy data.
- Sponsor — A person who takes responsibility for, and initiates, a clinical inv of a new drug under an IND.
- Investigator — A person who conducts a clinical investigation under an IN

- New Drug — A drug not generally recognized by qualified experts as safe and effective for a particular disease.
- Drug Substance — The active ingredient intended to diagnose, treat, cure, or prevent disease or affect a body structure or function of the body, excluding intermediates used in the synthesis of such ingredient.
- Drug Product — The finished dosage form (tablet, capsule, solution) that contains the drug substance, generally, but not necessarily, in association with other ingredient(s).
- Institutional Review Board (IRB) — Any board, committee, or other group formally designated by an institution to review, to approve the initiation of, and to conduct periodic review of biomedical research involving human subjects.

III. CONTENT OF AN INVESTIGATIONAL NEW DRUG APPLICATION (IND)

A full discussion of the procedures and requirements for investigating new drugs, as well as the content of an IND, is clearly delineated in 21 CFR 312 Investigational New Drug Application. The reader is referred to this document for a more detailed discussion of the IND procedure than is presented in this section. Generally speaking, there are three major categories of information included in an IND, namely:

1. Animal toxicity study results, confirming that the drug dose proposed in the clinical studies is safe.
2. Drug formulation information, including specifications and testing methods for the active ingredient(s) and finished dosage form; proposed manufacturing procedure for the new drug substance and new drug product; and stability data on the new drug substance and new drug product.
3. Proposed clinical protocols for the clinical study plan, and all existing human experience with the new drug.

A. ANIMAL TOXICITY DATA

The requirements for animal toxicity testing to support clinical studies of a new drug under an IND have been thoroughly discussed in Chapter 11. The completed studies conducted under Good Laboratory Practice (GLP) regulations, 21 CFR 58, are submitted in the IND and should address the following:

1. The pharmacological effects and mechanisms of action of the drug, and any information known on the drug's absorption, distribution, metabolism and excretion;
2. The effects of the drug on reproduction and the developing fetus;
3. Any special studies related to a particular route of drug delivery, e.g., topical, inhalation, as well as any *in vitro* studies intended to evaluate drug toxicity. These data should demonstrate the safety of the new drug product at the proposed clinical dosage requirements.

B. CHEMISTRY, MANUFACTURING, AND CONTROLS INFORMATION

All available information on the composition, manufacturing procedure, specifications, and test methods for both the new drug substance and the new drug product should be submitted. Adequate stability data on the new drug substance and new drug product, to assure that they are within acceptable chemical and physical specifications for the duration of the planned clinical studies, should also be included. Any major scale-up from pilot scale production to larger scale production to support expanded clinical studies will usually require submitting an IND amendment describing any changes to the initial chemistry, manufacturing, and controls processes.

C. PROPOSED CLINICAL PLAN

The major item in an IND submission is the proposed clinical study plan to de the efficacy of the new drug product to treat the intended disease-state or cond safety of the new drug product at the dosage levels proposed in the clinical s previously been confirmed by animal toxicity studies. Generally speaking, clini tigation of a new drug product consists of three sequential phases, although they m during the course of the clinical investigation. The number of subjects generall in each of these phases is stated here, but it varies depending on the drug proc investigated.

1. Three Phases of Clinical Studies

Phase 1 represents the initial introduction of the new drug product into huma 1 studies are closely monitored, and usually involve normal volunteers, but ca patients as well. The studies are designed to determine (1) metabolism and phar actions, and (2) possible early evidence of effectiveness. (There are typically from subjects and/or patients.)

Phase 2 represents controlled clinical studies in patients with the disease or the new drug product is intended to treat. These studies are closely controlled and r and are intended to develop efficacy data and evaluate side effects and risks assoc the use of the new drug product. (Number of patients: typically no more than several

Phase 3 represents expanded controlled and uncontrolled studies. These s generally conducted when there is preliminary evidence that the drug has efficacy of patients: from several hundred to several thousand).

2. Clinical Investigator Brochure

Prior to the initiation of clinical studies, the sponsor of the IND is required each clinical investigator with an investigator's brochure containing the following in about the new drug:*

(a)   A brief description of the drug substance and the formulation, including the formula, if known.
(b)   A summary of the pharmacological and toxicological effects of the drug and, to the extent known, in humans.
(c)   A summary of the pharmacokinetics and biological disposition of the drug and, if known, in humans.
(d)   A summary of information relating to safety and effectiveness in humans from prior clinical studies. (Reprints of published articles on such studie appended when useful.)
(e)   A description of possible risks and side effects to be anticipated on the bas experience with the drug under investigation or with related drugs, and of p or special monitoring to be done as part of the investigational use of the d

3. Content of Clinical Protocols

Clinical protocols are required for each planned study in sufficient detail to FDA reviewing medical officer to assess that the safety and rights of all subjects are In addition, especially in Phase 2 and 3 studies, the FDA medical officer will k that the study design will result in adequate data to permit an evaluation of the dr and effectiveness. The protocols should be written with sufficient flexibility to anticipated modifications of a minor nature in study design. A major modific

---

*   21 CFR 312.23(a)5.

protocol, however, will require a protocol amendment, which will be discussed in the next section. Protocols are required to contain the following:**

(a) A statement of the objectives and purpose of the study.
(b) The name and address, and a statement of the qualifications (curriculum vitae or other statement of qualifications) of each investigator, and the name of each sub-investigator (e.g., research fellow, resident) working under the supervision of the investigator; the name and address of the research facilities to be used; and the name and address of each reviewing Institutional Review Board.
(c) The criteria for patient selection and for exclusion of patients, and an estimate of the number of patients to be studied.
(d) A description of the design of the study, including the kind of control group to be used, if any, and a description of methods to be used to minimize bias on the part of subjects, investigators, and analysts.
(e) The method for determining the dose(s) to be administered, the planned maximum dosage, and the duration of individual patient exposure to the drug.
(f) A description of the observations and measurements to be made to fulfill the objectives of the study.
(g) A description of clinical procedures, laboratory tests, or other measures to be taken to monitor the effects of the drug in human subjects and to minimize risk.

In listing (b) above, reference is made to "a statement of the qualifications of each investigator." This statement is obtained from each investigator on a Form FDA 1572 (see Figure 2). The Institutional Review Board (IRB) referred to in the same listing is a group of individuals designated by the institution where the clinical study is to be conducted, whose responsibility it is to review and approve the proposed clinical protocol with the express purpose of assuring the protection of the rights and welfare of the participating human subjects. The responsibilities of the IRB are clearly delineated in 21 CFR 56.

D. SUBMITTING THE IND

Once the animal toxicity studies have been completed, the manufacturing procedures, related specifications and test methods prepared, and the documents for the proposed clinical plan finalized, the IND may now be assembled and submitted to the FDA. The format to be followed is presented in an FDA cover sheet, Form FDA 1571 (see Figure 3).

1. Formatting the IND

Form FDA 1571 spells out the specific information required in the IND necessary for the FDA to adequately review of the proposed clinical studies. In conjunction with Form FDA 1571, the sponsor should refer to 21 CFR 312.23 for a detailed discussion of each section provided for in Form FDA 1571. The IND submission must include the original application and two copies. There is a specific numbering system required for the original submission and all subsequent submissions. The initial IND is to be numbered "000." Each subsequent submission of an amendment, additional data, etc., must be numbered chronologically in sequence, e.g., "001, 002." The initial submission should be sent to the following address:

> Central Document Room
> Center for Drugs and Biologics
> U.S. Food and Drug Administration

** 21 CFR 312.23(a)6 iii.

DEPARTMENT OF HEALTH AND HUMAN SERVICES
PUBLIC HEALTH SERVICE
FOOD AND DRUG ADMINISTRATION
STATEMENT OF INVESTIGATOR
(TITLE 21, CODE OF FEDERAL REGULATIONS (CFR) Part 312)
(See instructions on reverse side)

Form Approved OMB No 0910-0014
Expiration Date November 30, 1987

NOTE: No investigator may participate in an investigation until he/she provides the sponsor with a completed, signed Statement of Investigator Form FDA 1572 (21 CFR 312 53(c))

1 NAME AND ADDRESS OF INVESTIGATOR

2 EDUCATION, TRAINING, AND EXPERIENCE THAT QUALIFIES THE INVESTIGATOR AS AN EXPERT IN THE CLINICAL INVESTIGATION OF THE DRUG FOR THE USE UNDER INVESTIGATION ONE OF THE FOLLOWING IS ATTACHED

☐ CURRICULUM VITAE ☐ OTHER STATEMENT OF QUALIFICATIONS

3 NAME AND ADDRESS OF ANY MEDICAL SCHOOL, HOSPITAL OR OTHER RESEARCH FACILITY WHERE THE CLINICAL INVESTIGATION(S) WILL BE CONDUCTED

4 NAME AND ADDRESS OF ANY CLINICAL LABORATORY FACILITIES TO BE USED IN THE STUDY

5 NAME AND ADDRESS OF THE INSTITUTIONAL REVIEW BOARD (IRB) THAT IS RESPONSIBLE FOR REVIEW AND APPROVAL OF THE STUDY(IES)

6 NAMES OF THE SUBINVESTIGATORS (e g, research fellows, residents, associates) WHO WILL BE ASSISTING THE INVESTIGATOR IN THE CONDUCT OF THE INVESTIGATION(S)

7 NAME AND CODE NUMBER, IF ANY, OF THE PROTOCOL(S) IN THE IND IDENTIFYING THE STUDY(IES) TO BE CONDUCTED BY THE INVESTIGATOR

8 ATTACH THE FOLLOWING CLINICAL PROTOCOL INFORMATION

☐ FOR PHASE 1 INVESTIGATIONS, A GENERAL OUTLINE OF THE PLANNED INVESTIGATION INCLUDING THE ESTIMATED DURATION OF THE STUDY AND THE MAXIMUM NUMBER OF SUBJECTS THAT WILL BE INVOLVED

☐ FOR PHASE 2 OR 3 INVESTIGATIONS, AN OUTLINE OF THE STUDY PROTOCOL INCLUDING AN APPROXIMATION OF THE NUMBER OF SUBJECTS TO BE TREATED WITH THE DRUG AND THE NUMBER TO BE EMPLOYED AS CONTROLS, IF ANY, THE CLINICAL USES TO BE INVESTIGATED, CHARACTERISTICS OF SUBJECTS BY AGE, SEX, AND CONDITION, THE KIND OF CLINICAL OBSERVATIONS AND LABORATORY TESTS TO BE CONDUCTED, THE ESTIMATED DURATION OF THE STUDY, AND COPIES OR A DESCRIPTION OF CASE REPORT FORMS TO BE USED

9 COMMITMENTS

I AGREE TO CONDUCT THE STUDY(IES) IN ACCORDANCE WITH THE RELEVANT, CURRENT PROTOCOL(S) AND WILL ONLY MAKE CHANGES IN A PROTOCOL AFTER NOTIFYING THE SPONSOR EXCEPT WHEN NECESSARY TO PROTECT THE SAFETY, THE RIGHTS, OR WELFARE OF SUBJECTS

I AGREE TO PERSONALLY CONDUCT OR SUPERVISE THE DESCRIBED INVESTIGATION(S)

I AGREE TO INFORM ANY PATIENTS, OR ANY PERSONS USED AS CONTROLS, THAT THE DRUGS ARE BEING USED FOR INVESTIGATIONAL PURPOSES AND I WILL ENSURE THAT THE REQUIREMENTS RELATING TO OBTAINING INFORMED CONSENT IN 21 CFR PART 50 AND INSTITUTIONAL REVIEW BOARD (IRB) REVIEW AND APPROVAL IN 21 CFR PART 56 ARE MET

I AGREE TO REPORT TO THE SPONSOR ADVERSE EXPERIENCES THAT OCCUR IN THE COURSE OF THE INVESTIGATION(S) IN ACCORDANCE WITH 21 CFR 312 64

I HAVE READ AND UNDERSTAND THE INFORMATION IN THE INVESTIGATOR'S BROCHURE, INCLUDING THE POTENTIAL RISKS AND SIDE EFFECTS OF THE DRUG

I AGREE TO ENSURE THAT ALL ASSOCIATES, COLLEAGUES, AND EMPLOYEES ASSISTING IN THE CONDUCT OF THE STUDY(IES) ARE INFORMED ABOUT THEIR OBLIGATIONS IN MEETING THE ABOVE COMMITMENTS

I AGREE TO MAINTAIN ADEQUATE AND ACCURATE RECORDS IN ACCORDANCE WITH 21 CFR PART 312 62 AND TO MAKE THOSE RECORDS AVAILABLE FOR INSPECTION IN ACCORDANCE WITH 21 CFR 312 68

I WILL ENSURE THAT AN IRB THAT COMPLIES WITH THE REQUIREMENTS OF 21 CFR PART 56 WILL BE RESPONSIBLE FOR THE INITIAL AND CONTINUING REVIEW AND APPROVAL OF THE CLINICAL INVESTIGATION I ALSO AGREE TO PROMPTLY REPORT TO THE IRB ALL CHANGES IN THE RESEARCH ACTIVITY AND ALL UNANTICIPATED PROBLEMS INVOLVING RISKS TO HUMAN SUBJECTS OR OTHERS ADDITIONALLY I WILL NOT MAKE ANY CHANGES IN THE RESEARCH WITHOUT IRB APPROVAL, EXCEPT WHERE NECESSARY TO ELIMINATE APPARENT IMMEDIATE HAZARDS TO HUMAN SUBJECTS

I AGREE TO COMPLY WITH ALL OTHER REQUIREMENTS REGARDING THE OBLIGATIONS OF CLINICAL INVESTIGATORS AND ALL OTHER PERTINENT REQUIREMENTS IN 21 CFR PART 312

INSTRUCTIONS FOR COMPLETING FORM FDA 1572
STATEMENT OF INVESTIGATOR:

1 Complete all sections Attach a separate page if additional space is needed

2 Attach curriculum vitae or other statement of qualifications as described in Section 2

3 Attach protocol outline as described in Section 8

4 Sign and date below

5 FORWARD THE COMPLETED FORM AND ATTACHMENTS TO THE SPONSOR
The sponsor will incorporate this information along with other technical data into an Investigational New Drug Application (IND) INVESTIGATORS SHOULD NOT SEND THIS FORM DIRECTLY TO THE FOOD AND DRUG

DEPARTMENT OF HEALTH AND HUMAN SERVICES
PUBLIC HEALTH SERVICE
FOOD AND DRUG ADMINISTRATION
INVESTIGATIONAL NEW DRUG APPLICATION (IND)
(TITLE 21, CODE OF FEDERAL REGULATIONS (CFR) Part 312)

Form Approved OMB No. 0910-0014
Expiration Date: November 30, 1987

NOTE: No drug may be shipped or clinical investigation begun until an IND for that investigation is in effect (21 CFR 312.40)

1 NAME OF SPONSOR

2 DATE OF SUBMISSION

3 ADDRESS (Number, Street, City, State and Zip Code)

4 TELEPHONE NUMBER (Include Area Code)

5 NAME(S) OF DRUG (Include all available names Trade, Generic, Chemical, Code)

6 IND NUMBER (If previously assigned)

7 INDICATION(S) (Covered by this submission)

8 PHASE(S) OF CLINICAL INVESTIGATION TO BE CONDUCTED ☐ PHASE 1 ☐ PHASE 2 ☐ PHASE 3 ☐ OTHER _____ (Specify)

9 LIST NUMBERS OF ALL INVESTIGATIONAL NEW DRUG APPLICATIONS (21 CFR Part 312), NEW DRUG OR ANTIBIOTIC APPLICATIONS (21 CFR Part 314), DRUG MASTER FILES (21 CFR 314.420), AND PRODUCT LICENSE APPLICATIONS (21 CFR Part 601) REFERRED TO IN THIS APPLICATION

10 SERIAL NUMBER
_ _ _

IND submissions should be consecutively numbered. The initial IND should be numbered "Serial Number: 000." The next submission (i.e., amendment, report, or correspondence) should be numbered "Serial Number: 001." Subsequent submissions should be numbered consecutively in the order in which they are submitted

11 THIS SUBMISSION CONTAINS THE FOLLOWING (Check all that apply) ☐ INITIAL INVESTIGATIONAL NEW DRUG APPLICATION (IND)

PROTOCOL AMENDMENT(S)
☐ NEW PROTOCOL
☐ CHANGE IN PROTOCOL
☐ NEW INVESTIGATOR

INFORMATION AMENDMENT(S)
☐ CHEMISTRY/MICROBIOLOGY
☐ PHARMACOLOGY TOXICOLOGY
☐ CLINICAL

IND SAFETY REPORT(S)
☐ INITIAL WRITTEN REPORT
☐ FOLLOW-UP TO A WRITTEN REPORT

☐ RESPONSE TO FDA REQUEST FOR INFORMATION ☐ ANNUAL REPORT ☐ RESPONSE TO CLINICAL HOLD

☐ GENERAL CORRESPONDENCE ☐ REQUEST FOR REINSTATEMENT OF IND THAT IS WITHDRAWN, INACTIVATED, TERMINATED OR DISCONTINUED ☐ OTHER _____ (Specify)

Refer to the designated CFR citations before checking any of the following

☐ TREATMENT IND 21 CFR 312.35(b) ☐ TREATMENT PROTOCOL 21 CFR 312.35(a) ☐ CHARGE REQUEST NOTIFICATION 21 CFR 312.7(d)

FOR FDA USE ONLY

CDR/DIND/DGD RECEIPT STAMP	DDR RECEIPT STAMP	IND NUMBER ASSIGNED
		DIVISION ASSIGNMENT

FORM FDA 1571 (8/87)   PREVIOUS EDITION IS OBSOLETE

CONTENTS OF APPLICATION

12 This application contains the following items: (check all that apply)

☐ 1 Form FDA 1571 [21 CFR 312.23(a)(1)]
☐ 2 Table of contents [21 CFR 312.23(a)(2)]
☐ 3 Introductory statement [21 CFR 312.23(a)(3)]
☐ 4 General investigational plan [21 CFR 312.23(a)(3)]
☐ 5 Investigator's brochure [21 CFR 312.23(a)(5)]
☐ 6 Protocol(s) [21 CFR 312.23(a)(6)]
   ☐ a Study protocol(s) [21 CFR 312.23(a)(6)]
   ☐ b Investigator data [21 CFR 312.23(a)(6)(iii)(b)] or completed Form(s) FDA 1572
   ☐ c Facilities data [21 CFR 312.23(a)(6)(iii)(b)] or completed Form(s) FDA 1572
   ☐ d Institutional Review Board data [21 CFR 312.23(a)(6)(iii)(b)] or completed Form(s) FDA 1572
☐ 7 Chemistry, manufacturing, and control data [21 CFR 312.23(a)(7)]
   ☐ a Environmental assessment or claim for exclusion [21 CFR 312.23(a)(7)(iv)(e)]
☐ 8 Pharmacology and toxicology data [21 CFR 312.23(a)(8)]
☐ 9 Previous human experience [21 CFR 312.23(a)(9)]
☐ 10 Additional information [21 CFR 312.23(a)(10)]

13 IS ANY PART OF THE CLINICAL STUDY TO BE CONDUCTED BY A CONTRACT RESEARCH ORGANIZATION? ☐ YES ☐ NO

IF YES, WILL ANY SPONSOR OBLIGATIONS BE TRANSFERRED TO THE CONTRACT RESEARCH ORGANIZATION? ☐ YES ☐ NO

IF YES, ATTACH A STATEMENT CONTAINING THE NAME AND ADDRESS OF THE CONTRACT RESEARCH ORGANIZATION, IDENTIFICATION OF THE CLINICAL STUDY, AND A LISTING OF THE OBLIGATIONS TRANSFERRED

14 NAME AND TITLE OF THE PERSON RESPONSIBLE FOR MONITORING THE CONDUCT AND PROGRESS OF THE CLINICAL INVESTIGATIONS

15 NAME(S) AND TITLE(S) OF THE PERSON(S) RESPONSIBLE FOR REVIEW AND EVALUATION OF INFORMATION RELEVANT TO THE SAFETY OF THE DRUG

I agree not to begin clinical investigations until 30 days after FDA's receipt of the IND or on earlier notification by FDA. I also agree not to begin or continue clinical investigations covered by the IND if those studies are placed on clinical hold. I agree that an Institutional Review Board (IRB) that complies with the requirements set forth in 21 CFR Part 56 will be responsible for the initial and continuing review and approval of each of the studies in the proposed clinical investigation. I agree to conduct the investigation in accordance with all other applicable regulatory requirements

16 NAME OF SPONSOR OR SPONSOR'S AUTHORIZED REPRESENTATIVE	17 SIGNATURE OF SPONSOR OR SPONSOR'S AUTHORIZED REPRESENTATIVE	
18 ADDRESS (Number, Street, City, State and Zip Code)	19 TELEPHONE NUMBER (Include Area Code)	20 DATE

(WARNING: A willfully false statement is a criminal offense U.S.C. Title 18, Sec. 1001.)

*U.S. GPO 1987-0-181-338/64852

FIGURE 3.   Form FDA 1571, the format and content of an Investigational New Drug Application (IND).

Park Building, Room 214
12420 Parklawn Drive
Rockville, MD 20852

The FDA Central Document Room will assign the IND to the appropriate
drug division, and the sponsor will be notified that all subsequent submissions to
should be sent to the reviewing drug division address.

The clinical studies may not commence until the IND goes into effect, which
after the FDA receives the IND. The FDA notifies the sponsor in writing of th
IND was received, or the FDA notifies the sponsor that the IND has been put on
hold." A clinical hold will be imposed if the FDA determines, during its initial
the IND, any of the following:

(a)   Human subjects may be exposed to unreasonable and significant risk.
(b)   The clinical investigators named in the IND are not qualified to conduct th
(c)   The investigator brochure is misleading, erroneous, or incomplete.
(d)   The IND is inadequate to assess the risks to the human subjects to be stud
        clinical plan will not result in meaningful clinical data.

The new drug product must not be shipped to an investigator named in the
30 days after the FDA receives the IND, and the investigator must not administ
drug product to a human subject until the IND goes into effect. That is, if the
on clinical hold by the FDA, the investigator must not administer the drug pr
human subject until the FDA removes the clinical hold on the study. The FDA
the sponsor when the clinical hold is removed, and the sponsor must then notify
tigators that the clinical study may begin.

The sponsor may request a waiver of the 30-day waiting period following i
mission of the original IND. The FDA will notify the sponsor if the clinical stud
initiated prior to the end of the 30-day waiting period. Once the IND has been
and the clinical studies have begun, it is important that the sponsor keep the IN
by reporting to the FDA changes to what was submitted in the original IND
information that is of significance to the continued clinical evaluation of the new d
changes or amendments to the IND follow.

2. Protocol Amendments

Included in this type of IND amendment are (a) the addition of a new pr
changes to an existing protocol; and (c) the addition of a new clinical investigat

(a) New Protocol

— Any clinical study plan not already included in the IND requires the submis
new protocol as a protocol amendment. The amendment should be clearly marked
Amendment: New Protocol," and contain a copy of the new protocol and a brief
of the most clinically significant differences between it and previous protocols. '
conducted under a new protocol may be implemented immediately provided the ne
has been submitted to the FDA and it has been approved by the appropriate IR

(b) Changes to an Existing Protocol

— Any change to a protocol already in an IND that *significantly* affects the sa
human subjects, the scope of the investigation, or the scientific quality of the
be submitted to the FDA as a protocol amendment.

The sponsor must decide if the change meets the criteria in the above parag significant protocol changes may be included in the Annual Report discussed later in this chapter. The amendment should be clearly marked "Protocol Amendment: Change in Protocol", and contain a brief description of the change and reference to the IND submission (by date and three-digit submission number) that contained the original protocol. The studies conducted under the revised protocol may be implemented immediately, provided the protocol amendment has been submitted to the FDA and approved by the appropriate IRB.

(c) Addition of a New Investigator
— The addition of a new investigator requires the submission of a protocol amendment clearly marked "Protocol Amendment: New Investigator" and containing the investigator's name, qualifications to conduct the investigation, reference to the previously submitted protocol, and a signed Form FDA 1572. Once the investigator has been added to the study, the new drug may be shipped to the investigator. The FDA must be notified of the new investigator by the sponsor within 30 days of the addition.

3. Information Amendments
Any essential information not covered by either a Protocol Amendment, an IND Safety Report, or the Annual Report must be reported to the IND in the form of an information amendment. The amendment should be clearly marked "Information Amendment: Chemistry, Manufacturing, and Control" or "Information Amendment: Pharmacology-Toxicology," or other descriptive terminology to identify the nature of the information being submitted. The kinds of information to be submitted in an information amendment include new toxicology, chemistry, or other technical information; or the discontinuance of a clinical investigation. The information amendment should state the nature and purpose of the submission in an organized presentation of the data supporting the amendment. The sponsor may request the FDA to comment on the submission. Information amendments should be sumitted as necessary, but preferably not more than every 30 days.

4. IND Safety Reports
The sponsor is required to notify the FDA and all participating clinical investigators, in writing, of any adverse experience *associated with the use of the investigational drug* that is both *serious* and *unexpected*. The underlined portions of the previous sentence are critical to the need for submitting IND Safety Reports. Unless the adverse experience meets the definitions of these italicized portions, it should be submitted in the Annual Report, which is discussed later on in the chapter. The following terms and definitions are key to determining the need to submit an IND Safety Report:

Associated with the use of the drug — A reasonable possibility that the experience may have been caused by the drug.

Serious — Any experience suggesting a significant hazard, contraindication, side effect, or precaution, including any human experience that is fatal or life-threatening, permanently disabling, requires inpatient hospitalization, or is a congenital anomaly, cancer, or overdose.

Unexpected — Any experienec not identified in nature, severity, or frequency in the current investigator brochure.

If the adverse experience meets all three of the above definitions, the sponsor must notify the FDA and all clinical investigators *in writing, within 10 working days* of becoming aware of the experience. The sponsor shall also notify FDA *by telephone within 3 working days* of any unexpected, fatal, or life-threatening experience associated with the use of the investigational drug. All written and telephone communication must be made to the FDA drug division at the Center for Drug Evaluation and Review responsible for the IND. The sponsor is required to investigate all safety reports and submit any relevant follow-up information to the FDA when available.

5. Annual Reports

The sponsor is required to submit an annual IND progress report on the clinic
tigation of the drug in a specific format (21 CFR 312.23), including both individu
information and a general summary of information pertinent to the drug:

(a) Individual Study Information

— A summary of which studies were completed and of those in progress, i.e., n
patients entered, completed, or dropped out, and a brief description of the study r

(b) Summary Information

— A summary of (1) the most frequent and serious adverse experience by the bod
(2) all IND safety reports; (3) all subjects who died or dropped out because o
experience, whether or not drug related; (4) any information relative to the acti
drug (dose response, bioavailability, etc.) (5) preclinical animal studies; and (6)
ufacturing changes.

The Annual Report should also discuss the clinical plan. Any revisions to th
brochure should be summarized and a new brochure submitted, as well as any si
revisions to Phase I protocols not previously submitted in a protocol amendment. Th
Report should also summarize any significant foreign marketing developments for
i.e., approval, withdrawal, or suspension from marketing for whatever reason.

6. Treatment INDs

In order to facilitate the availability of promising investigational drugs to desp
patients with serious or life-threatening diseases, the FDA has established what
as the Treatment IND. It allows the use of the investigational drug by patients not
in the clinical trials. The FDA has established the following criteria for allowing T
IND status to investigational drugs:

(a)   The drug is intended to treat a serious or immediately life-threatening disea
(b)   There is no other comparable drug or therapy to treat the disease.
(c)   The drug is covered by an IND, and is being investigated in controlled clinica
(d)   The IND sponsor is actively seeking marketing approval of the drug.

The FDA may deny the treatment use of an investigational drug if there is in
evidence of its safety and efficacy for the targeted patient population. All the
requirements for the sponsor and the clinical investigator, i.e., informed consent, IR
and approval, safety reports, etc., remain in effect for treatment use.

E. RESPONSIBILITIES OF THE SPONSOR

The sponsor of an IND has overall responsibility to assure that the clinical inv
is conducted according to the information submitted to the FDA. The sponsor m
qualified investigators; provide them with necessary information to conduct th
effectively; select qualified clinical monitors to review the progress of the studies a
conformance to the protocols and the clinical study plan; and provide required comm
to the FDA and all participating investigators relative to significant new adverse ex
or risks associated with the investigational drug. The sponsor must control the d
of the drug only to qualified investigators included in the IND, and must maintair
records showing this disposition. The sponsor is required to permit the FDA to re
copy records relative to any clinical investigation conducted under an IND. Th
must submit all required IND reports, as outlined in Section III D of this chapter

F. RESPONSIBILITIES OF THE INVESTIGATOR

The investigator has the primary responsibility to assure that the clinical study is conducted according to the approved protocol; to protect the rights, safety, and welfare of the subjects; and to control the disposition and proper use of the assigned investigational drugs assigned to the investigator. In the event the investigation is terminated or completed, the investigator is responsible for returning the unused supply of drug to the sponsor. The investigator must maintain accurate records of the disposition of the drug. The investigator is required to maintain accurate and complete case histories on all subjects in the clinical investigation and furnish all required reports to the sponsor, i.e., progress reports, safety reports, and a final close-out report of the completed study. The investigator must comply with all requirements of 21 CFR PART 50 — *Protection of Human Subjects*, and 21 CFR PART 56 — *Institutional Review Boards*, with respect to patient informed consent and IRB approval of the clinical plan. The investigator must report any proposed changes to the clinical plan or any significant problems associated with the investigational plan to the IRB. The investigator is required to permit the FDA to review and copy records relative to any clinical investigation conducted under an IND.

IV. CONTENT OF A NEW DRUG APPLICATION (NDA)

A. FDA AUTHORITY FOR NDA

The Food, Drug and Cosmetic Act requires that FDA preapprove all "new drugs" prior to their entry into the marketplace. Title 21 of the CFR, in Section 314, sets forth the procedures to gain market approval from the FDA through the NDA process. An NDA approval is granted only after an exhaustive study of the drug by regulators at the FDA. These individuals review the information gathered and submitted by the sponsor in order to reach a conclusion that the proposed drug is efficacious and may be used safely within the constraints provided in the labeling.

B. MARKETING EXCLUSIVITY

In certain cases, the sponsor may obtain marketing exclusivity upon approval of an NDA, i.e., no other firm may obtain FDA approval for the same drug or indication unless the firm also conducts clinical studies under an IND and files an original NDA for approval. If the NDA is for the initial marketing of the drug, exclusivity may be obtained for the remainder of the patent life, provided no challenges to the patent are encountered. Even if the NDA is not for the initial marketing of the drug, exclusivity still may be obtained if, for example, the sponsor of the application performed clinical studies to determine a new use for the drug product.

C. FDA DRUG REVIEW CLASSIFICATION SYSTEM

In order to assure that the limited resources of the FDA are devoted to the most important tasks involved, the Agency has developed a rating system to provide guidance for their review staff. When the application is received by the FDA, it is analyzed to determine its category assignment. The advantages of drug classification are many, and assures that an NDA for a new chemical entity (NCE) determined to be useful in fighting a serious disease is deemed more important than an NDA for an already marketed drug being used for a new purpose. The classification assigned by the FDA tells the public and the scientific world at large the importance the Agency places on the application.

When received in a review division, the application is assigned a spot in the review queue, depending on the classification provided. The FDA classifies a drug submission using a combination of numbers and letters. The numbers represent the type of drug substance (DS) contained in the drug product (DP), and the letter represents the therapeutic potential.

TABLE 1
FDA Drug Classification System

Class 1 — a new molecular entity/new chemical entity (NME/NCE) consisting of a drug substance the subject of an application at FDA

Class 2 — a new salt, ester, or derivative of a previously approved drug substance

Class 3 — a new formulation of a previously approved drug substance

Class 4 — a new combination of two (or more) previously approved drug substances

Class 5 — a drug already approved and marketed by another sponsor

Class 6 — a drug already approved and marketed by the same sponsor

Index 1AA — a rating reserved for new therapies for life-threatening conditions, such as drugs to tre related conditions

Index A — a drug that offers important therapeutic gains over those therapies already approved

Index B — a drug that offers modest therapeutic gains over those therapies already approved

Index C — a drug that offers no therapeutic gain over those therapies already approved

Index D — a special drug, with known risks, but providing the only effective treatment for a specif

Index E — a drug proposed to satisfy a DESI (Drug Efficacy Study Implementation) notice, or for a the Counter use)

Index F — a drug reserved for pediatric use

Index H — an orphan drug

Index M — a drug currently marketed in a foreign country, but not in the U.S.

Index P — a drug made important by packaging rather than by the drug substance

Index S — a "sensitive" drug, due to wide publicity or interest from Congress

Index T — a drug with known toxicity problems

TABLE 2
Structure of Offices of Drug Review I and II

The Office of Drug Review I is currently reponsible for the:
> Pilot Drug Evaluation Unit (HFN-007)
> Division of Cardio-Renal Drug Products (HFN-110)
> Division of Neuropharmacologic Drug Products (HFN-120)
> Division of Oncologic and Pulmonary Drug Products (HFN-150)
> Division of Medical Imaging, Surgical and Dental Drug Products (HFN-160))
> Division of Gastrointestinal and Coagulation Drug Products (HFN-180)

The Office of Drug Review II is currently responsible for the:
> Division of Metabolism and Endocrine Drug Products (HFN-810)
> Division of Anti-Infective Drug Products (HFN-815)
> Division of Anti-Viral Drug Products (HFN-530)

The listings are shown in Table 1. The FDA's drug review effort is divided i review divisions. The divisions report through the Office of Drug Review I, and of Drug Review II. The Office structures are provided in Table 2.

1. Filing Considerations

Within 60 days after receiving an application, the FDA will determine v application may be "filed." When the FDA agrees that an application may be f made a preliminary determination that the application is sufficiently complete comprehensive review to proceed.

The FDA may refuse to file an NDA if it

- Does not contain a completed application form.
- Is not submitted in the form required by the regulations.
- Is deemed incomplete because it does not contain sufficient information in the regulations.
- Does not contain an environmental impact analysis report.
- Does not contain an English translation of included foreign language stud

For each nonclinical laboratory study, the application must contain a statement that the study was conducted in compliance with Good Laboratory Practice Regulations, 21 CFR 58, or explain why it was not subject to those regulations. If it does not, the FDA will refuse to file the application. The FDA will also refuse to file the application if the drug product is already marketed in accord with an approved application, or it the drug product is subject to licensing by the FDA under the Public Health Service Act.

Within 180 days after the FDA-accepted date of filing, plus any agreed upon extensions to the review period, the FDA will either approve the application or afford the opportunity for a hearing to resolve remaining issues, including a non-approvable letter.

2. Classifications

The mechanisms for speed review of an NDA depend on the classification provided by the FDA, and the completeness and accuracy of the application. The only way to effectively deal with the enormous workload at the FDA is for the sponsor to follow the NDA through the review process. The sponsor should determine exactly who is performing the review, and the current stage of the review process.

D. APPLICATION FORMAT

The format for submitting applications to the FDA is set by regulations; 21 CFR Section 314.50, states: ''Applications... are required to be submitted in the form and contain the information, as appropriate for the particular submission.'' The application must contain all sections applicable to the drug under review. For an NCE, the application will usually contain an index, a detailed summary, tabulations of patient data, case report forms, and five different technical sections (six if the drug is a microbiological entity). These technical sections are discussed in detail later in this chapter.

The entire application must be well organized, since one of the criteria for refusal to file an application is a lack of organization. The FDA maintains guidelines on the format and content of an application to assist in its preparation. They are available from The Hearing Clerk's Office, Food and Drug Administration, 5600 Fishers Lane, Rockville, MD 20857. Figure 4 is a copy of form FDA 356-H showing, in outline form, the content of the application.

Two copies of an original application are required: an *archival* copy and a *review* copy. Both should be identical in content, with the exception that the archival copy is required to contain three copies of analytical methods to be used by the FDA to validate the testing methods for the new drug substance and the new drug product. Additionally, copies of the labeling for the drug product are included in the archival copy as are the case report forms and tabulations.

The application is required to contain:

- The name of the sponsor
- The date
- The application number, if previously assigned
- The name of the drug in the application
- The dosage form and strength
- The route of administration
- The indentification number of all INDs and Drug Master Files (DMF) referenced in the application
- The intended use of the drug product.

The application should also state whether it is an original, a resubmission, a supplement, or an amendment to an application under review. It should contain a checklist of all enclosures, and the legal signature of the sponsor or the agent.

CONTENTS OF APPLICATION

This application contains the following items: (Check all that apply)

1. Index

2. Summary (21 CFR 314.50 (c))

3. Chemistry, manufacturing, and control section (21 CFR 314.50 (d) (1))

4. a. Samples (21 CFR 314.50 (e) (1)) (Submit only upon FDA's request)

    b. Methods Validation Package (21 CFR 314.50 (e) (2) (ii)

    c. Labeling (21 CFR 314.50 (e) (2) (ii))

        i. draft labeling (4 copies)

        ii. final printed labeling (12 copies)

5. Nonclinical pharmacology and toxicology section (21 CFR 314.50 (d) (2))

6. Human pharmacokinetics and bioavailability section (21 CFR 314.50 (d) (3)).

7. Microbiology section (21 CFR 314.50 (d) (4))

8. Clinical data section (21 CFR 314.50 (d) (5))

9. Safety update report (21 CFR 314.50 (d) (5) (vi) (b))

10. Statistical section (21 CFR 314.50 (d) (6))

11. Case report tabulations (21 CFR 314.50 (f) (1))

12. Case reports forms (21 CFR 314.50 (f) (1))

13. Patent information on any patent which claims the drug (21 U.S.C. 355 (b) or (c))

14. A patent certification with respect to any patent which claims the drug (21 U.S.C. 355 (b) (2) or (j) (2) (A))

15. OTHER (Specify)

I agree to update this application with new safety information about the drug that may reasonably affect the statement of contraindications, warnings, precautions, or adverse reactions in the draft labeling. I agree to submit these safety update reports as follows: (1) 4 months after the initial submission, (2) following receipt of an approvable letter and (3) at other times as requested by FDA. If this application is approved, I agree to comply with all laws and regulations that apply to approved applications, including the following:

1. Good manufacturing practice regulations in 21 CFR 210 and 211
2. Labeling regulations in 21 CFR 201
3. In the case of a prescription drug product, prescription drug advertising regulations in 21 CFR 202
4. Regulations on making changes in application in 21 CFR 314.70, 314.71, and 314.72
5. Regulations on reports in 21 CFR 314.80 and 314.81
6. Local, state and Federal environmental impact laws

If this application applies to a drug product that FDA has proposed for scheduling under the controlled substances Act, I agree not to market the product until the Drug Enforcement Administration makes a final scheduling decision

NAME OF RESPONSIBLE OFFICIAL OR AGENT	SIGNATURE OF RESPONSIBLE OFFICIAL OR AGENT	DATE

ADDRESS (Street, City, State, Zip Code)		TELEPHONE NO. (Include Area Code)

DEPARTMENT OF HEALTH AND HUMAN SERVICES	Form Approved: OMB No. 0910-0001
PUBLIC HEALTH SERVICE	Expiration Date: August 31, 1989

FOOD AND DRUG ADMINISTRATION

APPLICATION TO MARKET A NEW DRUG FOR HUMAN USE OR AN ANTIBIOTIC DRUG FOR HUMAN USE

(Title 21, Code of Federal Regulations, 314)

FOR FDA USE ONLY		
DATE RECEIVED		DATE FILED
DIVISION ASSIGNED	NDA/ANDA NO. ASS

NOTE: No application may be filed unless a completed application form has been received (21 C.F.R. Part 314)

NAME OF APPLICANT

DATE OF SUBMISSION

TELEPHONE NO. (Include Area Code)

ADDRESS (Number, Street, City, State and Zip Code)

NEW DRUG OR ANTIBIOTIC APPLICATION NUMBER (If previously issued)

DRUG PRODUCT

ESTABLISHED NAME (e.g., USPUSAN)	PROPRIETARY NAME (If any)

CODE NAME (If any)	CHEMICAL NAME

DOSAGE FORM	ROUTE OF ADMINISTRATION	STRENGTH(S)

PROPOSED INDICATIONS FOR USE

LIST NUMBERS OF ALL INVESTIGATIONAL NEW DRUG APPLICATIONS (21 CFR Part 312), NEW DRUG OR ANTIBIOTIC APPLICATIONS (21 CFR Part 314), AND DRUG MASTER FILES (21 CFR 314.420) REFERRED TO IN THIS APPLICATION:

INFORMATION ON APPLICATION

TYPE OF APPLICATION (Check one)

☐ THIS SUBMISSION IS A FULL APPLICATION (21 CFR 314.50) ☐ THIS SUBMISSION IS AN ABBREVIATED APPLICATION (ANDA) (21 CFR 314.55)

IF AN ANDA, IDENTIFY THE APPROVED DRUG PRODUCT THAT IS THE BASIS FOR THE SUBMISSION

HOLDER OF APPROVED APPLICATION

NAME OF DRUG		

STATUS OF APPLICATION (Check one)

☐ PRESUBMISSION   ☐ AN AMENDMENT TO A PENDING APPLICATION   ☐ SUPPLEMENTAL APPLICATION

The application must contain a comprehensive index showing the location by volume and page of the information discussed in the summary (see next paragraph), as well as the technical sections and any supporting information contained in the application. This comprehensive index is located in the archival section.

1. Overall Summary of the NDA

The overall summary should contain:

- The proposed text of the labeling for the drug, with footnotes directing the reviewer to the summary and technical section of the NDA supporting the inclusion of each statement in the labeling.
- A statement identifying the pharmacologic class of the drug, and a discussion of the scientific rationale for the drug and its intended use.
- A brief discussion of the foreign marketing history of the drug.
- A list of the foreign countries where approval has been granted, as well as a list of those countries, if any, where approval has been withdrawn.
- A brief summary of each technical section.
- A discussion of the benefits and risks associated with the drug, including any planned postmarketing studies to be conducted.

2. Chemistry, Manufacturing, and Controls Section

The Chemistry, Manufacturing, and Controls section (CMC) must contain sufficient information to allow the reviewer to conclude that the drug product will have the characteristics of identity, strength, quality, and purity it purports to possess.

The preparation and/or synthesis of the drug substance must be described, including the name and address of the manufacturer, the actual manufacturing procedure and purification processes, and the process controls utilized during manufacturing and packaging. Any alternate synthetic procedures, in-process controls, or specifications must be fully described.

Information on the drug product must include a list of all components (ingredients) used in its manufacture, and a statement about its composition. It should also contain a statement about the specifications and test methods for each component of the drug product. The name and address of each component manufacturer must be included, along with a description of the manufacturing and packaging procedures and in-process controls necessary to assure the quality and purity of the final drug product.

For both the drug substance and the drug product, reference may be made to the current issues of the U.S. Pharmacopeia (USP)/National Formulary (NF). It should be noted, however, that the FDA may refuse to accept reference to these compendia, requiring methods of analysis to be included in the individual application. The application must also include either a claim for exclusion or an environmental assessment of the effect of manufacture of the drug substance and the drug product on the environment.

Once the actual date on which the application is to be filed has been determined by the sponsor, the sponsor may elect to make an "early" pre-submission of the information in the CMC section. The FDA will accept such an "early" submission between 90 and 120 days *before* filing of the remainder of the NDA. It is suggested that the sponsor take advantage of this "early" submission provision of the regulations, since early resolution of CMC questions may avoid delays in approving the NDA.

3. Nonclinical Pharmacology and Toxicology Section

The nonclinical pharmacology and toxicology section must describe, with the aid of tables and graphs, information on nonclinical studies of the drug. All tables should be clearly identified and captioned, and summary tables should permit comparison of selected results from all dosage groups and relevant controls, on the same page.

A discussion should be included on the studies of the pharmacological acti
drug in relation to the therapeutic indication, as well as studies that define its pha
properties or are otherwise pertinent to possible adverse effects. This section o
must include study results of the toxicological effects of the drug as they relate to tl
clinical uses of the drug, including studies assessing its acute, subacute, and chron
carcinogenicity; and studies relating to the particular mode of administration o
Studies demonstrating the effect of the drug on reproduction and on the develo
as well as studies of the absorption, distribution, metabolism, and excretion o
must be included and described. For each nonclinical laboratory study that is su
Good Laboratory Practice (GLP) regulations, the application must contain a stat
the study was conducted in accord with these regulations.

4. Human Pharmacokinetics and Bioavailability Section

This section of the NDA describes the human pharmacokinetic and bioavaila
A description of each of the bioavailability and pharmacokinetic studies performed
including a description of the analytical and statistical methods used in each stu
included. It should also contain a statement with respect to the performance of tl
compliance with the IRB regulations. If human bioavailability studies were not
the application contains information supporting a waiver of this requirement.

If the CMC section contains specifications to assure bioavailability, this se
contain a rationale for establishing the specification or analytical method, includ
support the rationale. Data on the pharmacokinetics and metabolism of the drug
and the bioavailability and/or bioequivalence of the drug product must be demo

The NDA, if it is for an antiinfective drug product, must contain informat
microbiology of the drug product in a sixth technical section, as mentioned e
scriptions of the biochemical basis of the action of the drug on microbial phys
antimicrobial spectra of the drug, any known mechanisms of resistance to the
clinical microbiology laboratory methods needed for effective use of the dru
included.

5. Clinical Data Section

The clinical data section must contain a description of each clinical pharmacc
performed, as well as an analysis of each such study. It must compare the human
studies, and must contain a description and analysis of each controlled study a
description of each uncontrolled study. It must contain a description and analy
other data from any source, foreign or domestic, including clinical investigations
elsewhere.

The clinical data section must also contain an integrated summary of the da
strating substantial evidence of efficacy, dosage and administration, and provide
dosage and frequency of dosing. It must address modifications made for su
patients. This section is required to contain summaries and updates of safety i
on the drug product, pertinent animal data, demonstrated and potential adver
clinically significant interactions, and other safety considerations such as epide
studies of related drugs.

This section must contain a description of statistical analyses, and the filed
must be periodically updated with new safety data. These updates must be provide
after the inital NDA submission; following receipt of any approvable letter; and a
by the FDA. If the drug product has abuse potential, the application must describe
related to abuse, provide an analysis of studies related to abuse, and include a
of overdosage studies.

The clinical data section must also contain an integrated summary of risks an a statement on each study regarding IRB approval (or the reasons for lack of such approval); a statement for each study on informed consent; a statement on outside research contractors used in conducting any clinical study; and, if original patient records were audited by the sponsor, a list identifying each such study so audited.

6. Statistical Section

The statistical section must describe the statistical evaluation of each controlled clinical study, including the documentation and supporting statistical analyses used in evaluating the safety of the drug product.

7. Samples and Labeling

The FDA performs laboratory validation of selected tests for the drug substance and drug product included in the CMC section. Upon FDA request, the NDA sponsor is required to submit samples of the drug substance, the drug product, and any reference standards for laboratory validation. These samples should be sufficient to allow the FDA to perform each test described in the application three times. The FDA review chemist will inform the sponsor of the location(s) of the FDA laboratory taking part in the validation effort. If the CMC section has been updated since initial NDA submission, the validation package provided to the laboratories should include any updated information relevant to laboratory validation.

The archival copy of the NDA must include, as stated earlier, three copies of analytical methods for the drug substance and drug product, including a description of each sample, specifications, and a detailed description of testing methods. This description must include supporting data for accuracy, specificity, precision, and ruggedness. It must include complete certificates of analysis (the sponsor's test results), and copies of the label and all labeling. The archival copy is also expected to include patient case report tabulations, case report forms, and any additional data deemed pertinent by the sponsor or specifically requested by the FDA.

E. PREPARING AND FILING AN NDA

In order to properly prepare and submit an NDA, many departments in a drug firm must become involved. These include, but are not limited to, the medical, statistical, and toxicology departments, as well as development (including pharmaceutical, chemical, and analytical), quality assurance, and production and engineering. It should be remembered that the CMC section may be submitted early and, therefore, would probably undergo a separate review.

The sponsor must also designate the specific internal department responsible for coordinating the submission. This is usually the Regulatory Affairs Department, working in conjunction with a project planning function. These areas determine the timetable for submission, and the estimated time for review and approval of the application once it has been filed.

Sufficient time must be allocated for a proper assembly and in-house review of the submission. It should be remembered that one criterion for the refusal of the FDA to file an application is its finding of a lack of completeness. After assembly, the completed application should be routed for review and approval by the senior staff involved with the drug development process. For timely reviews, the application may be divided, as will be done at the FDA, to allow specific departments to review their portions of the applicaiton.

The development areas should devote their review efforts to their specific areas of expertise. Toxicologists should review the toxicology technical section, the biostatisticians the bioavailability section, etc. It is critical that knowledgeable members of the medical staff review the clinical technical section. All reviewing disciplines should carefully review the overall summary.

During the in-house review, revisions and changes to the data in the applica
sometimes necessary. An in-house procedure should be developed to determine wh
of revisions would be cause for a complete re-review of the application, and whic
be allowed with a less critical review. Certainly, any error should be highlighted
partment review, but is should be unnecessary for a complete re-review of such
When the application is deemed complete, the form should be signed by the ap
official.

When the reviews are complete, the application should be photocopied for fi
submission purposes. It is very important that the completed application filed with
be identical to the copy kept in the sponsor's files, for when the questions arrive
FDA reviewer, they are usually identified by volume and page number.

There are many articles and publications devoted to filing a computer-assist
(CANDA), and the reader may refer to these publications for information on that
submission. FDA provides guidance on submitting the archival copy of an applic
microfiche, and the reader may refer to that guideline, entitled "Submission in M
of the Archival Copy of an Application," available from the FDA Hearing Clerk'

There are many ways to submit an application to FDA. It can be sent by U.
Service regular mail, delivered by courier, or presented in person by personnel rep
the firm. No matter how delivery is made, a receipt showing the date and location
should be obtained. This can usually be effected by providing a second copy of
letter to be stamped and signed by the receiving FDA official. This receipted copy
important if the application is misfiled or lost at the FDA. The proof of receipt
expedite treatment, but will enable the FDA to insert the application into the revie
in approximately the position it should have been.

F. DEFICIENCY LETTERS/NON-APPROVABLE LETTERS

As the review progresses at the FDA, the FDA reviewers may have questions co
the information provided in the application. The reviewer can communicate with the
by telephone, mail, or by meetings in person at the FDA. It is very beneficial to the
to be able to respond to questions before they become part of a deficiency lett
communication saves both time and scarce resources.

Deficiencies in applications can consist of several matters, including a lack o
information, or misleading, unclear, or erroneous data or information. Such deficie
lead to a delay in approval of the application, or a refusal to approve the applicati
In the situation of misleading or erroneous data, the deficiency can lead to an FDA ir
of the sponsor, clinical investigator, and/or contract organizations involved with
of the drug product.

FDA reviewers usually make every effort to alert the sponsor to deficencies wl
be corrected while the review is ongoing. This is particularly the case in the CMC
FDA reviewers will usually inform the sponsor of additional information needed
the review to be completed.

The regulations provide for a "90-day meeting," if one is desired by the spor
purpose of this meeting is to inform the sponsor of the progress being made in the
and to provide a listing of deficiencies already found in the application. Generally,
day meeting" is restricted to drugs classified as 1AA, 1A, 1B, or 1C.

G. APPROVABLE VS. APPROVAL LETTERS

As various FDA disciplines complete their review of the NDA, their conclu
written and sent to the supervisor of their discipline for review and approval.
pharmacology, medical, clinical, and CMC reviews are complete, the Consum
Officer (CSO) takes the various drafts of the reviews and prepares a letter for the

Director to sign, as well as an approval package with additional information supporting the conclusions reached by the individual disciplines. The Division Director is already familiar with the specific drug, for as the review has progressed, the Division "Rounds" have covered the drug and its review in detail.

If the FDA believes that the application is basically "approvable" but certain conditions still have to be met, certain additional information is still required to be submitted, or some labeling changes remain to be made, the application cannot be approved. In those situations, FDA will prepare and issue an "approvable letter." The approvable letter will be sent if FDA believes that it can approve the application when the requested information is provided, or when specific conditions are met. The approvable letter will set forth the conditions of approval, listing the information required or the conditions to be met.

The approvable letter requires the sponsor to respond within 10 days after receipt of the letter. The sponsor may either file a request for a hearing, withdraw the application, or notify the FDA of its intent to satisfy the requirements of the approvable letter.

When all conditions are met for approval, the FDA will issue the formal *approval* letter. This is done after the FDA determines that the drug meets the statutory standards for approval including safety and effectiveness, adequate manufacturing and controls, and appropriate labeling.

If the only deficiencies in the application pertain to editorial or other minor problems in the labeling, an approval letter can also issue. In this case, the approval is conditional until the sponsor provides corrections as required.

The approval letter will also set forth certain conditions of approval, such as a commitment to conduct post-approval Phase 4 studies, or to provide for submission of additional data after approval.

H. FINAL MARKETING APPROVAL

As time for the approval draws near, production should begin to scale up to full-size batches of drug product, if this has not already been done. Production of the drug product should commence in order to build up sufficient inventories to fill the shipping pipe line once permission to market has been received. Production, quality assurance, marketing, and regulatory affairs departments must work closely together to assure that production takes place within the contraints set forth in the application.

At times, the FDA will require the submission of market packages of the drug product. If this is a requirement for approval, the submission should be coordinated with regulatory affairs and quality assurance departments. It should be determined where and how the market samples will be delivered.

I. COMMITMENTS TO GAIN APPROVAL

It may be necessary to commit to provide additional manufacturing information, stability updates, or clinical data in order to satisfy the conditions of the approval letter. The approval letter will set forth the time frame for submission of the additional information, although it will usually be on a quarterly basis.

J. PERIODIC REPORTS

The regulations set forth the content and frequency of post-approval reports to the application. Generally, barring conditions in the approval letter, these reports are due to be filed on an annual basis within 60 days of the anniversary date of approval of the application.

K. CHANGES TO APPROVED APPLICATIONS

Once the application is approved, changes made to it may require the approval of the FDA. The regulations set forth the types of supplements and the approval scheme necessary

for each. In general, prior FDA approval is required for clinical submissions, inclu
for additional indications, etc. The only exception appears to be those supplements
use of the drug by providing tighter controls on labeling, safety, reduction in i
etc.

The supplemental application, no matter what type of approval scheme is
required to contain full information for each change. For those submissions no
prior FDA approval, the application shall state the date on which the changes
into effect. In the case of notification by submission in the annual report, the
shall not only contain full information of the type required in a normal supple
plication, but shall also inform the FDA of the date when the change was effect

Generally, supplements that provide increased assurance of compliance witl
ifications do not require prior approval. These include new or tighter specifica
new, revised, or changed nonregulatory test methods. Changes made to the labe
or strengthen a statement about warnings, contraindications, precautions, adverse
drug abuse potential, dependence, overdosage, dosage and administration (includi
tions for the safe use of the product) do not require prior approval. Similarly, cha
to the labeling to delete false, misleading, or unsupported indications or claims
tiveness may be effected without prior approval.

A supplement to use a different facility to manufacture the *drug substance*
into effect without prior approval, provided that the process in the new facilit
differ from that in the current facility, and that the new site has been inspected
last 2 years for that or a similar process.

Supplements providing for changes to the *drug substance* to relax or delete a sp
or regulatory method, or to change the synthesis of the drug substance, includir
or route of synthesis, require prior approval. Supplements providing for a differ
to manufacture the drug substance, when the process differs from that currently
or where the site has not been inspected in the last 2 years, also require prior a

Supplements involving the *drug product* that require prior approval include tl
or delete an ingredient (with the exception of an ingredient added solely for co
may be removed without prior approval); to change the formulation; to relax
specification; or to establish or delete a regulatory method. Changes in the man
the drug product, including changing or relaxing an in-process control, or use of
facility or establishment to manufacture, process or pack the drug product, req
approval.

The following changes to the approved container and closure system requir
proval: to change the specification for the container or closure; to change a
analytical method for the container or closure; to change the size of the containe
exception of a change for a solid oral dosage form which does not require prior
the same container and closure system is used); and to extend the expiration per
drug product based on a nonapproved, revised, or modified stability protocol. Ii
cation does not provide for reprocessing/reworking the drug product, it is necessar
prior approval to do so.

In the regulations, any change not specified as requiring prior approval,
without prior approval, are reported in the annual report. The regulations classify
report category as the residual location for all changes not specified elsewhere.
include changes to comply with an official compendium; changes in labeling no
a change in dosage strength/form; and changes to provide a new description in tl
of the drug product and how it is supplied, along with any editorial or similar
labeling. Deletion of an ingredient intended solely for color, and extension of the
date using an approved protocol with full term data, may be included in the ann
A change within the container and closure system from one HDPE material (Hi

Polyethylene) to another for solid dosage forms, using a USP protocol or a protocol in the application, may be reported in the annual report, as may the addition or deletion of alternate analytical methods.

V. INTERACTION WITH THE FDA

Communication between the sponsor and the reviewing FDA drug division is very important during both the IND phase of clinical investigation and the NDA review phase. The majority of that communication takes place in written form through the submission of the original IND and NDA applications, and subsequent IND and NDA amendments. Some communication occurs by telephone between the sponsor and the FDA Division Consumer Safety Officer (CSO). However, there are times when the most effective communication between FDA and the sponsor is a meeting where issues can be discussed openly and completely. These meetings are almost always conducted at the FDA headquarters and arranged through the CSO. A request for a meeting is generally communicated by the sponsor in writing, stating clearly the reason for the meeting, along with a proposed agenda and list of sponsor attendees. The sections which follow describe the most effective meetings in communicating with FDA to assure timely review and approval of a new drug for marketing.

A. PRE-IND MEETING

A sponsor may request a meeting with the FDA prior to filing an IND in order to review the proposed clinical plan for the new drug. This interchange of information can be very helpful to both parties to assure an orderly review of the IND when submitted, as well as a timely initiation of the clinical program after the FDA 30-day review period. A discussion at this point will avoid any misconceptions by the sponsor about the scope of its clinical plan in order to determine the safety and efficacy of the new drug. This can be particularly helpful in minimizing expenditures of time and money, and will help expedite the drug development and evaluation process.

B. END OF PHASE 2 MEETING

The purpose of a meeting at this point is to determine whether it is safe to proceed to Phase 3 based on clinical data gathered in Phase 1 and Phase 2 studies. The sponsor should request the meeting and provide sufficient background information of the proposed Phase 3 clinical plan. Adequate summaries of the Phase 1 and 2 studies, specific Phase 3 protocols, and proposed labeling claims for the drug should also be included.

C. PRE-NDA MEETING

The purpose of this meeting is to reduce any potential delays in the initial NDA review by uncovering any unresolved problems; to identify those studies the sponsor has determined to be the pivotal studies, i.e., the adequate and well-controlled studies on which the drug will be determined to be safe and effective; and to acquaint the FDA reviewers with the drug and its intended use. A pre-NDA meeting allows the FDA reviewers to discuss with the sponsor the most informative and efficient way to present and format the data, and the best methods to use in the statistical evaluation of the data. Again, sufficient time should be allowed by the sponsor (approximately 1 month) to allow the FDA to review the sponsor's summary of the clinical studies to be included in the NDA, its proposed format for organizing the NDA, and any other information requested by the FDA or considered germane to the meeting by the sponsor.

D. MEETINGS DURING THE NDA REVIEW PERIOD

The sponsor has the right and the obligation to check on the progress of the review of the application filed with the FDA. These rights and obligations may be satisfied in several

ways. In attempting to satisfy the sponsor's right to know, a balance must be est
between that right and the actual need for the progress check to take place. The mo
calls and visits the FDA reviewer has, the less opportunity he or she has to review th
application.

The NDA sponsor must select an individual or a specific functionary within t
nization who will have the responsibility to interact with FDA reviewers on a regul
These individuals must have a great deal of tact and common sense. They must kn
to interact effectively with people, and must be familiar with the application in que
is best to limit direct access to FDA reviewers so that the sponsor can keep trac
negotiations regarding the application.

Although an occasional unscheduled "drop in" visit may be tolerated by the
respond to a quick question, constant interruptions lead to lower productivity in t
review process. In most cases, it is better to contact the FDA Consumer Safety
(CSO) in charge of the application to schedule a meeting. In many cases, question
asked of the CSO, and answers relayed back to the sponsor. For major interacti
FDA rightfully insists on a presubmitted agenda and a formal meeting. At this
meeting, additional information may be provided, and questions may be asked and re
to.

To telephone the reviewer, the call should be placed to the CSO. The CSO, in con
with the reviewer and the reviewer's supervisor, can decide on the merit of a t
conference and aid in setting up such a conference. It should be noted that the
required to maintain records of all telephone conversations. Decisions and agreements
during a telephone conversation can be binding.

At the conclusion of any formal meeting or telephone conference, the sponsc
provide written notification to the FDA concerning the subject matter discussed. T
munication will allow the FDA to correct any inconsistencies between the sponse
clusions and those of the FDA.

Chapter 14

BEYOND TODAY'S TECHNOLOGY

Peter J. Tarcha and R. Saul Levinson

TABLE OF CONTENTS

I. INTRODUCTION

In recent years, new pharmaceutical technologies and scientific advances discovered and developed at an astounding rate. In fact, it is difficult for th practitioner or pharmaceutical scientist to stay current and well versed in more areas of specialized interest. The profusion of technology in the pharmaceutica especially those related to drug delivery systems, has caused a good deal of conf in some instances confrontation, between pharmaceutical scientists, pharmaceu keting experts, those who pay medical costs, and the consumer.

Specifically, the medical need and cost/benefit advantages of controlled delive have been the subject of heated debate. The basis of the controversy deals with the between convenience and therapeutic advantages of controlled delivery system ample, with the transdermal controlled delivery of nitrates in the prophylaxis of is difficult to demonstrate therapeutic advantage over oral and/or sublingual nitra Here, the use of transdermal or oral controlled release delivery systems offer cor and one could argue that convenience leads to increased patient compliance to the drug regimen. However, third party payers, especially federal and state governm to encourage the use of the lowest cost conventional drug delivery system where cut therapeutic advantage of a more sophisticated delivery system cannot be e onstrated. Clearly, it is in the best interest of both the patient and industry to ce development of controlled delivery systems based on the therapeutic benefits th had over the secondary benefit of convenience.

Do rational therapeutic benefits from controlled drug delivery exist? The foll while not complete, enumerates several examples:

1.   Antihistamines. Controlled delivery, for example, timed release (micro)cap to smooth out peaks and valleys in plasma drug levels, allowing consistent an activity and minimizing the intensity of side effects such as drowsiness, c some of these agents.
2.   Broncholdilators. Controlled delivery tends to minimize subthreshold druჳ that a constancy in bronchodilation can be achieved, usually with lower dosage. Tedral® SA, a slow-dissolving, layered matrix, is one example bronchodilator delivery system.
3.   LH-RH Agonists. It has been shown that leuprolide acetate, encapsulated pheres of polylactic/polyglycolic acid copolymer (Lupron®), can be deli sustained manner for 1 month, and therapeutic levels are maintained at one total amount required by daily injection of the analog solution.

Of course, drug delivery system design can achieve more than controlled active moieties. A scan of journals, recent scientific meetings, and the current paten certainly indicates that major advances in understanding and improving the gastro transdermal, and transmucosal absorption profile of many troublesome drug ent curring with novel drug delivery systems. This short chapter gives a subjective ᴎ suggestions for further research in selected areas, where polymers can play a role in drug delivery.

II. POLYMERS FOR PARENTERAL DELIVERY

A. DISGUISING DRUG CARRIERS FROM THE RETICULOENDOTHE SYSTEM (RES)

Poly(ethylene oxide)-based polymers have been found to have a mediating et reticuloendotheial system. Abuchowski[1] found that catalyse and bovine serum al

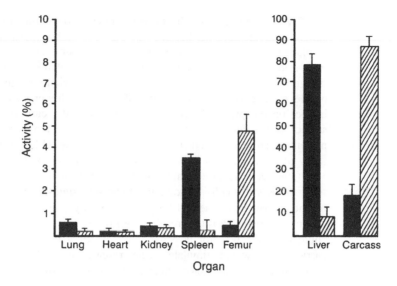

FIGURE 1.   Distribution of ^{131}I-labeled polystyrene microspheres in various organs following intravenous administration.[12] (■): uncoated microspheres; (▨): poloxamer 407 coated microspheres. (From Illum, L. and Davis, S.S., Targeting of colloidal particles to bone marrow, *Life Sci.*, 40, 1553, 1987. With permission.)

their immunogenicity after conjugation with poly(ethylene glycol) (PEG). In more recent studies it was shown by Sehon and Lee[2] that a variety of antigens could be rendered nonantigenic and tolerogenic by conjugation to monomethoxy poly(ethylene glycols). PEG's of higher molecular weight were more effective in reducing antigenicity, and the tolerogenicity increased with the level of conjugation. In addition, the PEG conjugates studied were capable of surpressing the IgE response to their native counterparts in both nonimmunized and sensitized mice and rats.

The mechanism of this apparent immunosuppression remains to be elucidated; however, it has been suggested that the conjugates are not effectively processed by macrophages.[3] The potential applications of these findings are significant and far-ranging. It may be possible to design allergens for use in tolerizing regimens, where the entity would not only be nonantigenic, but elicit immunosuppression of future IgE responses to the native analog as well. Such conjugation methods may also find applications in the blood substitute field where a variety of crosslinked and polymerized hemoglobins are being developed, and the potential for anaphylactic reactions is a concern.

A related phenomenon is the ability of poly(ethylene oxide)-based materials to divert uptake by the liver. Illum and Davis found almost a 50% reduction of liver uptake of polystyrene latex particles coated with poloxamer 407, a polyethylene oxide/polypropylene oxide block copolymer surfactant, compared to uncoated particles.[4] This was consistent with the subsequent finding that this same surfactant was particularly effective in reducing the uptake of the coated particles by macrophages *in vitro*.[5] As a result, a larger proportion of particles are available for possible therapeutic advantage in other areas of the body. Further studies by Illum and Davis[6] showed selective uptake by the bone marrow in rabbits, as shown in Figure 1. Kreuter and Troster[7] recently screened nine surfactants for their effects on the body distribution of ^{14}C-labeled poly(methyl methacrylate) latex particles. They hoped to correlate these results to a physical property of the amphiphile, namely, contact angle. A good correlation was not made; however, the study did show that poloxamers 908 and 337 were the most effective at reducing liver uptake of the particles. Chapter 10 extensively reviews the pharmaceutical applications of poloxamers.

The studies to date on the surface property effects on particle distribution have
simple adsorption to modify the surface. It can be questioned whether the surf.
displaced with time by serum proteins. It is possible that these encouraging effects
increased if the poly(oxyethylene) chains are covalently bound to the particle surf.
design of colloidal hydrogels for drug delivery, where a significant percentage of t
of the particle is composed of crosslinked oxyethylene chains, could have a si₂
impact on the practicability of injectable colloidal carriers. Once the mechanisr
surface interactions of particles with Kupffer cells and macrophages is better und
polymers can be designed specifically to evade the RES. Another avenue of resear
study of the cell membranes of bacteria already possessing this ability.

It has been suggested that the body distribution of polymer colloids may be shift
from the Kupffer cells by lowering their size significantly.[8] To this end, Lenaer
recently developed a method for producing polycyanoacrylate polymer colloids in t
20 nm size range. Positive results from future *in vivo* studies on such ultra-small
could open the way for possible treatment of a broader array of diseases with
carriers. This would stimulate further research not only into optimization of the b
tribution of synthetic nanoparticles, but optimal designs for improved safety as we

B. DRUG TARGETING

The targeting of therapeutic agents will take on a greater urgency motivate
growing epidemic of fatal HIV infection in the Western world. Rapidly growing
efforts into drugs which suppress the replication of the HIV virus are discoverin
which could be effective; however, acute toxicity may limit their use. Approach.
at targeting drugs against hepatitis, localized in the hepatic cells, may be a spring.
strategies for selective delivery of anti-HIV drugs, since hepatic cells can harbor
virus.

Galactosylated proteins such as lactosaminated serum albumin (L-SA) specific.
hepatocytes after binding to receptors for galactosyl-terminated glycoproteins.[10,11]
al.[12] showed that conjugates of L-SA with 9β-*d*-arabinofuranosyl-adenine 5'-monop.
(ara-AMP) exhibited selectivity for uptake by hepatocytes in mice infected with E.
virus hepatitis. The drug, ara-AMP, was released in active form, and inhibited DNA
in the liver. The conjugated drug showed four to five times longer duration of action c
to free drug, and toxicity was not observed when administered at 1 to 2 mg/g body

Targeting anti-HIV drugs to the monocyte/macrophage lineage can potentiall
complished by the administration of a drug contained in polymer colloids. The re
foreign particles by phagocytic mechanisms is very efficient in that intravenousl
istered colloids can be totally removed within a few minutes.[13] It is known that HI
the macrophage and monocytes by either phagocytic mechanisms or through th
antigen expressed on this cell population; however, the exact mechanism is not y.
(see Krowka et al.[14]). It has been reported that after infection with subsequent dev.
of opportunistic infections, there is a marked decrease in chemotatic response of
ocyte,[15] though no significant difference exists in the ability of these cells from AIDS
to phagocytize or kill fungi.[16] Hence, the administration of antiviral agents via a
carrier may be a means of interdicting or retarding the HIV disease.

C. DESIGNING BIODEGRADABLE SYNTHETIC CARRIERS

The pioneering work in human patients, of the Johns Hopkins/MIT groups shou.
the safety issues relating to the use of certain biodegradable polymers *in vivo*. T
involved the use of polyanhydride implants containing anticancer drugs, after su.
section of brain tumors. Through the efforts of other groups, certain poly(lactid.
colide) microspheres are approved for human use and are already being used in drug

If these systems continue to be successful from a safety standpoint, one might expect that futher efforts will result in reformulation of these and other biodegradable polymers, such as polyphosphazines, polyphosphates, polyiminocarbonates, and polyorthoesters, all of which have degradable backbones, into more easily administered dosage forms. Nonaqueous dispersion technology could be used to form nano- or microparticles that contain drug, and these carriers could be reconstituted into suspension with normal saline immediately before use. Appropriate nontoxic steric stabilizers could be used (e.g., poloxamers), and the dosage form could be administered as a subcutaneous or possibly intramuscular injection.

Most studies on polymer colloids as injectable drug delivery systems have used model particles which are not easily biodegraded. If such systems are to become safe, and hence commercially viable, quantitative breakdown and elimination of the carrier must be achieved in a reasonable time. Promising candidates will be polymers which not only become soluble via breakdown of crosslinks or hydrolysis of substituents, but have degradable backbone linkages as well.

Except for the polycyanoacrylates, research activity on acrylic polymer colloids having hydrolizable chain backbones has been scarce. As mentioned in Chapter 9, the incorporation of carbon dioxide into the backbone of polyolefins is possible.[17] Monomeric acrylate pro-drugs could potentially be polymerized with carbon dioxide via a nonaqueous latex process. Alternatively, pseudo-latexes might be formed from many of these materials if the linear polymer can be dissolved in a suitable solvent (see Chapter 9).

D. HEMOGLOBIN-BASED RESUSCITATIVE FLUIDS

More than 30 years have passed since the first attempts to microencapsulate hemoglobin as artificial red cells by T.M.S. Chang at McGill University. Since that time many advances have taken place in the field of synthetic hemoglobin-based blood substitutes, and there was at least one type undergoing human trials, until recently. Studies of this nature, especially those involving the administration to human subjects, seemed to indicate initially that it is possible to prepare sterile and fairly nontoxic oxygen carriers from purified and chemically modified hemoglobins. Some unexplained adverse reactions in human subjects have caused the FDA to halt clinical trials in September 1989, raising fundamental questions about the safety of these products.[28] With further research, preparations which can demonstrate safety in humans will provide countless opportunities as drug carriers for I.V. administration.

The most common approaches for producing hemoglobin-based resuscitative fluids are encapsulation of hemoglobin into liposomes or chemical modification of soluble hemoglobin. The chemical alterations can include crosslinking of the tetramer to improve stability; pyridoxylation to shift the oxygen saturation curve towards that of whole blood and polymerization to increase the circulating half-life in the body. Polypeptide and other drug conjugates of these modified myoglobins could serve as pro-drugs or active therapeutic entities. Naturally, the toxicity of the conjugate would have to be determined, but much of the basic groundwork on the base reagent will already be in place. An added advantage of a hemoglobin-based carrier is that these proteins seem to be only weakly immunogenic, if at all.

III. POLYMERS FOR ORAL DELIVERY

A. ABSORPTION OF POLYPEPTIDE DRUGS FROM THE GI TRACT

It has been recognized that some important new therapeutic drug entities will be difficult to successfully administer via the oral route because of molecular size or chemical/physical instabilities that occur within the gastrointestinal tract. Specifically, the peptide drugs are a prime example of these new and rather important entities. In recent years, significant research attention has been turned to the development of pharmaceutical techniques that could facilitate successful oral absorption of peptide drugs. In general, most of these techniques either utilize

mechanical protection to shield the peptide molecule from the hostile gastroint
vironment, or combine protection with a variety of techniques to increase the
potential of these difficult-to-absorb drug molecules. Unfortunately, the publish
regarding these techniques indicate that difficulty in achieving significant levels o
drug after oral administration still remains. A careful analysis of the problems i
the oral delivery of peptides will yield a number of rather troublesome facts:

1. Peptides do not diffuse well across biological membranes.
2. Peptides are easily destroyed by hostile gastrointestinal juice and enzymes
3. Peptides, as a class, exhibit poor water solubility, or tend to "associate" i
   limiting the extent of an absorption pool that would be necessary for suffic
   brane transport.

It should be clear from an analysis of these facts that the successful oral c
peptides will require more than molecular shielding by embedding the drug in a
core, or the use of simple absorption enhancers that are coadministered with
Innovative experimentation and thought needs to be applied to successfully s
problems. For example, a rational approach may be to piggyback a peptide moi
physiologically occurring compound that is known to be absorbed by a natural
mechanism, e.g., a nutrient or vitamin.

Another approach may be to utilize the absorption mechanisms used physiol
the absorption of fats through the lymphatic system. In this approach, the fo
polymer/peptide complexes that exhibit good fat solubility may allow the desir
of enhancing the absorption of the peptide complex through the lymph if the com
be uncoupled after absorption. Several studies in the literature indicate that w
decapeptides, the dissolution of the peptide in fat, followed by emulsification p
administration, can dramatically affect the extent of oral absorption.[18,19,20,21] C
experimental observations be further enhanced by the selection of polymer/peptide
that increase fat solubility? The concept of modifying the partition coefficient of a p
drug has been studied by Hashimoto et al., who showed that palmitic acid can be
to insulin, increasing its hydrophobicity, without significant loss of biological a

Further consideration along these lines leads to consideration of incorporating
into a physical unit containing polymeric compounds that have the ability to ass
dispersible units ("association colloids"). In this case, a polymeric surfactant with
to micellize at low concentration may provide both the spatial protection and the
or dispersibility in fat, allowing the absorption of the micellar unit containing
via its association with a fat molecule or a fat emulsion globule (chylomicron). I
vein, an emulsion globule, wherein the peptide is incorporated in the interior of t
may be explored. If this fat globule was constructed to be similar to chylomicra i
and other physical/chemical characteristics, one may observe absorption enhance
peptide as the globule approaches the intestinal membrane and disassembles p
sorption, as is the case in the absorption of dietary fat. If this disassembly occu
to the membrane, the required diffusion path for the peptide may be exceedir
resulting in enhanced absorption. The "synthetic chylomicron," by its very ar
could provide the protection needed to keep enzyme, acid, and other reactants
the peptide molecule. In fact, a very recent article by Cho and Flynn demonstra
insulin formulation, which gives serum levels of active insulin in humans, con
subcutaneous doses, using only one to three times the injected dosage level.[23]
mulation was comprised of water-in-oil microemulsion, where the insulin an
inhibitor was contained in the water phase, and the oil phase contained lecithin, no
fatty acids, and cholesterol.

IV. STABILIZATION OF POLYPEPTIDE DRUGS

Specific protein-based ligands having an affinity for the polypeptide drug might be an avenue for providing increased circulating stability. The binding of whole antibodies or subunits to the drug before administration could increase the half-life. Recombinant DNA techniques allow us to potentially synthesize only the active binding regions, or parts thereof. The moiety could be modified during synthesis or afterwards to have the appropriate drug affinity so as to maintain reasonable therapeutic availability of the drug.

Neocarzinostatin, a proteinaceous antitumor agent, has been conjugated to a synthetic copolymer of styrene-maleic anhydride.[24,25] Studies to date with this and other macromolecular anticancer agents have been recently reviewed by Maeda and Matsumura.[26] The studies indicate increased stability, lower clinical toxicity, more than tenfold increase in circulating half-life and high accumulation in tumor tissue and lymph nodes, compared to the unconjugated drug. Further design and development, perhaps to incorporate biodegradability, seem interesting.

One of the principal strategies in the oral delivery of peptide drugs is their protection from the proteolytic enzymes in the lumen of the gastrointestinal tract. It may be possible that polymer/peptide complexes could be constructed to spatially interfere with the cleavage of peptide bonds.

The introduction of easily biodegradable chain linkages into polymers which normally form hydrogels should make such materials more viable as delivery systems for polypeptide drugs. The immobilization of such drugs should increase their stability towards enzyme catalyzed degradation as outlined by Berezin et al.[27] for autolysis of immobilitzed proteases. This effect is attributed to a reduction of translational diffusion of the immobilized molecules.

V. CONCLUSION

It is interesting and somewhat constructive to observe and listen to the "experts" in drug delivery at symposia and meetings. In recent years the scientific spokespersons from leading pharmaceutical companies and academic centers have apparently come to the conclusion that the oral delivery of peptide drugs is impossible, and that the very administration of such agents by any other route of administration is precluded due to the antigenic nature of these drug agents. Meanwhile, in the research laboratories around the world, some rather exciting discoveries regarding the nature of peptide drugs and their activity *in situ* are being made and reported. Additionally, information on new delivery systems, such as pulmonary delivery devices, intranasal delivery devices, and transdermal electrical devices are being reported. It appears to the knowledgeable observer that the doomsayers have not considered what may be possible with technologies and discoveries just being made, or with such science that has yet to be investigated.

History indicates that the drug delivery scientist needs to continue to probe, observe, discover, and develop relevant technologies despite negative philosophies being articulated regarding the absorption of peptides.

It is instructive to reflect on the short history of biotechnology. Just a few decades ago the scientific literature was filled with negative opinion regarding the feasibility of preparing human insulin via biosynthetic techniques. Needless to say, the technologies developed, and the product is a current marketplace reality. There are countless other examples in recent decades regarding the successful commercialization of concepts and technologies where, early in the development of these products, negative opinion abounded.

Finally, it can be generally agreed that the adoption of new and technologically advanced drug delivery systems will not occur unless significant cost advantages over existing technologies are evident. But cost should be thought of in a broader sense then the sum of research, development, manufacturing, and marketing expense. Improved therapy and patient compliance ultimately reduce the cost of health care; and in these cost cont times, these advantages can be translated into significant savings in the cost of p health care.

REFERENCES

1. **Abuchowki, A.**, Effect of covalently attached polyethylene glycol on the immunogenicity and enzymes, Ph.D. thesis, Rutgers University, New Brunswick, 1976.
2. **Sehon A. H. and Lee W. Y.**, Suppression of IgE antibodies with PEG-modified allergens, Meet. Am. Acad. Allergy, Phoenix, AZ, Abstract No. 167, 1978.
3. **Lee, W. Y. and Sehon A. H.**, Surpression of reaginic antibodies, *Immunol. Rev.*, 41, 201, 1
4. **Illum. L. and Davis, S. S.**, The organ uptake of intravenously administered colloidal partic altered using a non-ionic surfactant (Poloxamer 338), *FEBS Lett.*, 167, 79, 1984.
5. **Illum, L., Jacobsen, L. O., Muller, R. H., Mak, E., and Davis, S. S.**, Surface characteris interaction of colloidal particles with mouse peritoneal macrophages, *Biomaterials*, 8, 113, 19
6. **Illum, L. and Davis, S. S.**, Targeting of colloidal particles to bone marrow, *Life Sci.*, 40, 15
7. **Kreuter, J. and Troster, S.**, Influence of the surface properties of ^{14}C-poly(methyl methacry particles, Proc. 16th Intl. Symp. Controlled Release Bioactive Mater., Chicago, 1989, No. 60
8. **Douglas, S. J., Illum, L. and Davis, S. S.**, *J. Colloid Interface Sci.*, 103, 154, 1985.
9. **Lenaerts, V., Raymond, P., Juhasz, J., Simard, M. A., and Jolicoeur, C.**, New meth preparation of cyanoacrylic nanoparticles with improved colloidal properties, *J. Pharm. Sci.*, 1989.
10. **Wilson, G.**, Effect of reductive lactosamination on the hepatic uptake of bovine pancreatic ribc dimer, *J. Biol. Chem.*, 253, 2070, 1978.
11. **Krantz, M. J., Holtzman, N. A., Stowell, C. P., and Lee, Y. C.**, Attachment of thiogl proteins: enhancement of liver membrane binding, *Biochemistry*, 15, 3963, 1976.
12. **Fiume, I., Bassi, B., Budi, C., Mattioli, A., and Spinosa, G.**, Drug targeting in antiviral che A chemically stable conjugate of 9-β-*d*-arabinofuranosyl-adenine 5'-monophosphate with lact albumin accomplished a selective delivery of the drug to liver cells, *Biochem. Pharmacol.*, 35,
13. **Illum, L. and Davis, S. S.**, The targeting of drugs parenterally by use of microspheres, *J. Pa Technol.*, 36, 242, 1982.
14. **Krowka, J. F., Moody, D. J., and Stites, D. P.**, Immunological Effects of HIV Infectio *Pathogenesis and Treatment*, Chap. 10, Levy, J. A., Ed., Marcel Dekker, 1989.
15. **Smith, P. D., Ohura, K., Masur, H., Lane, H. C., Fauci, R. S., and Wahl, S. M.** Monocy in acquired immune deficiency syndrome: defective hemotaxis, *J. Clin. Invest.* 74, 2121, 198
16. **Washburn, R. G., Tuazon, C. U., and Bennet, J. E.**, Phagocytic and fungicidal activity of from patients with acquired immunodeficiency syndrome, *J. Infect. Dis.*, 151, 565, 1985.
17. **Soga, K., Hosoda, S., and Ikeda, S.**, Copolymerization of carbon dioxide and some diene c *Makromol. Chem.*, 176, 1907, 1975.
18. **Tarr, B. D., and Yalkowsky, S. H.**, Enhanced intestinal absorption of cyclosporin in rats throug of emulsion droplet size, *Pharm. Res.*, 6, 40, 1989.
19. **Jensen, B. K.**, The effect of different fatty acids on the intestinal lymphatic absorption of cyc after oral administration in the rat, *Diss. Abst. Int.*, 49 (12), 1, 1988.
20. **Reymond, J. P., and Sucker, H.**, *In vitro* model for cyclosporin intestinal absorption in lip *Pharm. Res.*, 5, 673, 1988.
21. **Veda, C. T., Lemaire, M., Gsell, G., and Nussbaumer, K.**, Intestinal lymphatic absorptio porin-A following oral administration in an olive oil solution in rats, *Biopharm. Drug Dispo* 1983.
22. **Hahimota, M., Takada, K., and Muranishi, S.**, Sythesis of palmitoyl derivatives of insul biological activities, *Pharm. Res.*, 6, 171, 1989.
23. **Cho, Y. W. and Flynn, M.**, Oral delivery of insulin, *Lancet*, Dec. 23/30, 1518, 1989.
24. **Maeda, H., Takeshita, J., and Kanamaru, R.**, A lipophilic derivative of neocarzinostatin conjugation of an antitumor protein antibiotic, *Int. J. Pept. Protein Res.*, 14, 81, 1979.
25. **Meade, H., Ueda, M., Morinaga, T., and Matsumoto, T.**, Conjugation of poly(styrene-co-I derivative to the antitumor neocarzionstatin: pronounced improvements in pharmacological pr *Med. Chem.*, 29, 455, 1985,

26. **Maeda, H. and Matsumura, Y.,** Tumoritropic and lymphotropic principles of macromolecular drugs, *CRC Critical Reviews in Therapeutic Drug Carrier Systems,* 6, 193, 1989.
27. **Berezin, I. V., Klibanov, A. M., Goldmacher, V. S., and Martinek, K.,** in *Methods of Enzymology,* Vol. 44, Mozbach, K., Ed., Academic Press, New York, 1976, 571.
28. *Business Week,* May 21, 1990, .

INDEX

A

Printed and bound by CPI Group (UK) Ltd, Croydon, CR0 4YY

23/10/2024

01778245-0009